Progress in Epileptic Disorders
Volume 12

**Outcome
of Childhood Epilepsies**

Progress in Epileptic Disorders
International Advisory Board

Aicardi Jean, *France*
Arzimanoglou Alexis, *France*
Baumgartner Christoph, *Austria*
Brodie Martin, *UK*
Cross Helen, *UK*
Duchowny Michael, *USA*
Elger Christian, *Germany*
French Jacqueline, *USA*
Glauser Tracy, *USA*
Gobbi Giuseppe, *Italy*
Guerrini Renzo, *Italy*
Hirsch Edouard, *France*
Kahane Philippe, *France*
Luders Hans, *USA*
Meador Kimford, *USA*
Moshé Solomon L., *USA*
Noachtar Soheyl, *Germany*
Noebels Jeffrey, *USA*
Palmini André, *Brazil*
Perucca Emilio, *Italy*
Pitkanen Asla, *Finland*
Ryvlin Philippe, *France*
Scheffer Ingrid, *Australia*
Schmitz Bettina, *Germany*
Schmidt Dieter, *Germany*
Serratosa José, *Spain*
Shorvon Simon, *UK*
Tinuper Paolo, *Italy*
Thomas Pierre, *France*
Tuxhorn Ingrid, *USA*
Wolf Peter, *Denmark*

Progress in Epileptic Disorders
Volume 12

Outcome
of Childhood Epilepsies

Willem F. Arts
Alexis Arzimanoglou
Oebele F. Brouwer
Carol Camfield
Peter Camfield

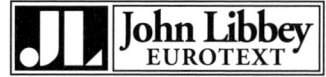

ISBN: 978-2-7420-1102-5
ISSN: 1777-4284
Vol. 12

Published by
Éditions John Libbey Eurotext
127, avenue de la République, 92120 Montrouge, France
Tel.: +33 (0)1 46 73 06 60
Website: www.jle.com

John Libbey Eurotext
42-46 High Street, Esther, Surrey, KT10 9KY
United Kingdom

© 2013, John Libbey Eurotext. All rights reserved.

Unauthorized duplication contravenes applicable laws.
It is prohibited to reproduce this work or any part of it without authorisation of the publisher or of the Centre Français d'Exploitation du Droit de Copie (CFC), 20, rue des Grands-Augustins, 75006 Paris.

Contents

Foreword IX

List of participants XII

Entrance criteria and outcome measures in pediatric epilepsy clinical trials
    Deborah Hirtz 1

Is it possible to predict the outcome of childhood epilepsy?
    Peter Camfield, Carol Camfield 17

Prognostic factors for recurrence after a first unprovoked seizure in childhood
    Shlomo Shinnar 25

Newly diagnosed epilepsies:
clinically relevant conclusions from global studies on outcome
    Willem F. Arts 33

Does treatment with antiepileptic drugs influence the long-term outcome of newly diagnosed epilepsies?
    Alexis Arzimanoglou 45

The influence of convulsive status epilepticus on outcomes of childhood epilepsy
    Richard Chin 53

Mortality in children with epilepsy
    Oebele F. Brouwer 61

Immune-related mechanisms of seizures: insights from experimental models
    Teresa Ravizza, Silvia Balosso, Valentina Iori, Federica Frigerio,
    Annamaria Vezzani 71

Febrile infection-related epilepsy syndrome (FIRES):
pathogenesis, treatment, and outcome
A large cohort and update
    Uri Kramer 83

Are idiopathic epilepsy syndromes in neonates always "benign?"
    Federico Vigevano, Maria Roberta Cilio, Domenico Serino, Lucia Fusco 91

Neonatal epilepsy and underlying aetiology (other than idiopathic): to what
extent do the seizures and the EEG abnormalities influence outcome?
    Georgia Ramantani 99

Infantile spasms: what matters more?
Seizures, EEG, underlying aetiology, or treatment?
    Andrew L. Lux 109

Lennox-Gastaut syndrome: nosographic limits and long term outcome
    Giuseppe Capovilla, Alberto Verrotti 121

Dravet syndrome
What matters more: seizures or the underlying aetiology?
    Ingrid E. Scheffer 133

Epileptic encephalopathy with continuous spike-waves during slow-wave
sleep including Landau-Kleffner syndrome: what determines the outcome?
    Patrick Van Bogaert 141

Outcome of idiopathic generalized epilepsy and the role of EEG discharges
    Elaine C. Wirrell 149

Refractory childhood epilepsy: comparing the outcome of medical *versus*
surgical treatment
    Michael Duchowny 163

Adult outcome of childhood-onset, cause unknown (cryptogenic),
MRI-negative, focal epilepsy
    Carol Camfield, Peter Camfield 173

Focal non-idiopathic epilepsies: does outcome after epilepsy surgery depend
on the localization of the epileptogenic zone in frontal and temporal lobe
epilepsy?
    Ingrid Tuxhorn 179

Outcome after epilepsy surgery of MRI-negative non-idiopathic focal
epilepsies
    Thomas Bast 191

Outcome when malformations of cortical development (MCD) are the cause
   Hans Holthausen, Tom Pieper, Manfred Kudernatsch, Ingmar Blümcke 203

Timing of antiepileptic drug withdrawal after pediatric epilepsy surgery
   Kees P.J. Braun, Kim Boshuisen 217

Anxiety and depression in children with epilepsy
   Julianne Giust, David W. Dunn 225

Health perception and socio-economic status of childhood onset epilepsy
   Ada T. Geerts 237

What if quality of life better expressed outcomes for epilepsy?
   Kathy Nixon Speechley 253

Foreword

From 15 to 18 November, 2012, 49 experts in the field of childhood epilepsy convened in The Hague, The Netherlands, for a workshop entitled: *Outcome of Childhood Epilepsies*. The workshop was held within the framework of the "Progress in Epileptic Disorders" workshops, organized by the journal *Epileptic Disorders*. The 2012 workshop was held in The Hague on the occasion of the 25th anniversary of the Dutch Study of Epilepsy in Childhood, and the members of the Dutch study group felt indeed very honoured to host so many distinguished guests.

The Dutch Study of Epilepsy in Childhood (DSEC) started in 1987 as a prospective cohort study of children with newly diagnosed epilepsy. The children were recruited from four hospitals in three adjacent cities in The Netherlands and the almost 500 children recruited over a period of four years were considered to contain roughly 70–80% of all incident cases in the referral area of the participating hospitals.

The original study group consisted–in alphabetical order–of Willem Arts, Oebele Brouwer, Ada Geerts, Boudewijn Peters, Hans Stroink and Cees Van Donselaar, and, sticking together as a group despite changes in the respective careers, we were able to continue the follow-up of the cohort until quite recently. Altogether, the DSEC produced about 50 papers in peer-reviewed journals, six theses, and countless contributions to international congresses and meetings. Most of this output concerned research on the outcome of the epilepsy of these children. Without aiming for completeness, we can mention the outcome after a single unprovoked seizure (Stroink), the outcome of newly diagnosed epilepsy (Arts, Geerts), the outcome after withdrawal of AEDs (Brouwer, Peters, Geerts), mortality (Brouwer, Callenbach), quality of life and psychosocial outcome (Carpay, Geerts), cognitive outcome (Geerts, Oostrom, Peters, Schouten), outcome predictability (Arts, Boerrigter, Geelhoed, Geerts), and intractability (Arts, Geerts).

Many of the contributions were realized only after intensive collaboration by and discussions with experts in the field like Carol and Peter Camfield, Anne Berg, Shlomo Shinnar, Matti Sillanpää, David Chadwick, Richard Appleton and many, many others. The 25th anniversary of the DSEC for us marked an excellent occasion to acknowledge their contributions and express our gratitude for it.

The background of the workshop was on the one hand the availability of many outcome data from cohort studies, trials and other studies on (treatment of) childhood-onset epilepsy. We felt that a state-of-the-art survey of the available data was now timely. On the other hand, it had already become clear that our knowledge on outcome of childhood epilepsy in general and of specific types of epilepsy and of treatment modalities in particular is as yet by far insufficient to base sound, evidence-based treatment strategies on. The workshop therefore also aimed to identify the lacuna's in our knowledge and define research topics in this area for the years to come.

We really enjoyed three days of exciting discussions, and we hope that the readers of this book will agree with us that altogether, this is a state-of-the-art review as good and as up-to-date as one can get.

We are very grateful for having had the opportunity to organize this workshop. Our thanks go especially to Alexis Arzimanoglou, editor-in-chief of *Epileptic Disorders*, who opened up the possibility to embed the workshop within the "Progress in Epileptic Disorders" series, and was of great help with the content and organization, and to the other two members of the scientific committee, Carol and Peter Camfield. And of course, this also gives us the opportunity to gratefully acknowledge the enduring friendship, trust and hospitality we experienced from "The Camfields" during many years!

We thank all speakers and discussants who did such a great job, especially those who wrote a chapter and later revised it, incorporating the remarks and suggestions made during the sometimes heavy discussions. Special thanks go to Mrs. Florence Marsy from ANT Congress who did all the practical organizational work and to UCB Pharma for their continuing support for the "Progress in Epileptic Disorders" workshops. We gratefully acknowledge their unrestricted educational grant.

Finally, we also wish to thank John Libbey Eurotext Editions and their editor, Mrs Anne Chevalier, for their help in publishing this book soon after the workshop, eliminating our textual and linguistic mistakes.

Willem F. Arts, Oebele F. Brouwer

Outcome of Childhood Epilepsies
Progress in Epileptic Disorders Workshop
The Hague, The Netherlands
November 2012

Scientific Committee
Willem F. Arts (The Netherlands), Alexis Arzimanoglou (France), Oebele F. Brouwer (The Netherlands), Carol Camfield (Canada), Peter Camfield (Canada)

List of participants

Willem F. Arts, Erasmus MC, Sophia Kinderziekenhuis, Rotterdam, The Netherlands, w.f.m.arts@erasmusmc.nl

Alexis Arzimanoglou, Epilepsy Sleep & Pediatric Neurophysiology Department, University Hospitals of Lyon (HCL), Lyon, France, aarzimanoglou@orange.fr

Stéphane Auvin, Neurologie Pédiatrique, Hôpital Robert-Debré, Paris, France, stephane.auvin@rdb.aphp.fr

Nadia Bahi-Buisson, Hôpital Necker-Enfants Malades, Université Paris-Descartes, Service de Neuropédiatrie et Maladies Métaboliques, Paris, France, nadia.bahi-buisson@inserm.fr

Thomas Bast, Klinik für Kinder und Jugendliche Epilepsiezentrum Kork, Kehl-Kork, Germany, TBast@epilepsiezentrum.de

Thomas Blauwblomme, Service de Neurochirurgie Pédiatrique, Hôpital Necker Enfants-Malades, Paris, France, tblauwblomme@hotmail.com

Kees Braun, Rudolf Magnus Institute of Neuroscience, University Medical Center, Utrecht, The Netherlands, k.braun@umcutrecht.nl

Oebele F. Brouwer, Department of Neurology, University Medical Center Groningen, University of Groningen, Groningen, The Netherlands, o.f.brouwer@umcg.nl

Peter Camfield, Department of Pediatrics, Dalhousie University and the IWK Health Centre, Halifax, Canada, camfield@dal.ca

Carol Camfield, Department of Pediatrics, Dalhousie University and the IWK Health Centre, Halifax, Canada, camfield@dal.ca

Giuseppe Capovilla, Child Neuropsychiatry Department, Epilepsy Center "C. Poma Hospital", Mantova, Italy, pippo.capovilla@aopoma.it

Richard Chin, Neurosciences Unit, Child Life and Health, University of Edinburgh, Edinburgh, United Kingdom, R.Chin@ed.ac.uk

Helen Cross, Neurosciences Unit UCL, Institute of Child Health, London, United Kingdom, h.cross@ucl.ac.uk

Thierry Deonna, Unité de Neurologie et de Neuroréhabilitation Pédiatrique, Département Médico-Chirurgical de Pédiatrie CHUV, Lausanne, Switzerland, th.deonna@bluewin.ch

Mike Duchowny, University of Miami, Miller School of Medicine, Florida International University College of Medicine, Miami, USA, michael.duchowny@mch.com

David Dunn, Riley Child and Adolescent Psychiatry Clinic, Indiana University School of Medicine, Indianapolis, USA, ddunn@iupui.edu

Melissa Filippini, Child Neurology Unit, IRCCS, Neurological Science Institut of Bologna, Ospedale Maggiore "C.A. Pizzardi", Bologna, Italy, melissa.filippini@libero.it

Annick Fonteyne, Revalidatiecentrum voor kinderen en jongeren Pulderbos, Zandhoven, Belgium, Annick.Fonteyne@revapulderbos.be

Stefano Francione, Centro per la chirurgia dell'epilessia "Claudio Munari", Ospedale Niguarda Ca' Granda, Milano, Italy, stefano.francione@gmail.com

Ada Geerts, Department of Neurology, Erasmus MC, Rotterdam, The Netherlands, mail@adageerts.nl

Giuseppe Gobbi, Child Neurology Unit IRCCS Neurological Science Institute of Bologna Ospedale Maggiore "C.A. Pizzardi", Bologna, Italy, giuseppe.gobbi@ausl.bologna.it

Renzo Guerrini, Pediatric Neurology Unit and Laboratories Children's Hospital A. Meyer-University of Florence, Florence, Italy, r.guerrini@meyer.it

Bruce Hermann, Department of Neurology, University of Wisconsin, Madison, USA, hermann@neurology.wisc.edu

Deborah Hirtz, National Institute of Neurological Disorders and Stroke, NIH, Bethesda, Maryland, USA, dh83f@nih.gov

Hans Holthausen, Neuropediatric Clinic and Clinic for Neurorehabilitation-Epilepsy-Center for Children and Adolescents, Vogtareuth, Germany, hansholthausen@gmx.de

Philippe Kahane, Epilepsy Unit Neurology & Psychiatry Department Grenoble University Hospital, Grenoble, France, philippe.kahane@ujf-grenoble.fr

Uri Kramer, Pediatric Neurology Unit, Tel Aviv Sourasky Medical Center, Tel Aviv University, Tel Aviv, Israel, umkramer@netvision.net.il

Lieven Lagae, KU Leuven, Neuro-musculo-skeletal Research Unit, Leuven, Belgium, lieven.lagae@uzleuven.be

Andrew Lux, Bristol Royal Hospital for Children, Bristol, United Kingdom, andrew.lux@bristol.ac.uk

Wendy Mitchell, Childrens Neurology Hospital Los Angeles, Los Angeles, USA, WMitchell@chla.usc.edu

Brian Neville, Neurosciences Unit UCL, Institute of Child Health, London, United Kingdom, B.Neville@ich.ucl.ac.uk

John Pellock, Division of child Neurology, Virginia Commonwealth University, Richmond, USA, jpellock@mcvh-vcu.edu

Georgia Ramantani, Universitätsklinikum Freiburg; Epilepsiezentrum im Neurozentrum, Freiburg, Germany, georgia.ramantani@uniklinik-freiburg.de

Victoria San Antonio, Universitätsklinikum Freiburg; Epilepsiezentrum im Neurozentrum, Freiburg, Germany, victoriasanantonio@gmail.com

Ingrid Scheffer, Florey Institute and Department of Medicine and Department of Paediatrics, University of Melbourne, Royal Children's Hospital, Melbourne, Australia, scheffer@unimelb.edu.au

Shlomo Shinnar, Comprehensive Epilepsy Management Center Montefiore Medical Center, Albert Einstein College of Medicine, New York, USA, sshinnar@aol.com

Matti Sillanpaa, Department of Public Health, University of Turku, Turku, Finland, matti.sillanpaa@utu.fi

Kathy Speechley, Schulich School of Medicine & Dentistry Western University, London, Ontario, Canada, kathy.speechley@lhsc.on.ca

Ulrich Stephani, Klinik für Neuropädiatrie Universitätsklinikum Schleswig Holstein Campus, Kiel, Germany, stephani@pedneuro.uni-kiel.de

Hans Stroink, Department of Neurology, St. Elisabeth Hospital, Nijmegen, The Netherlands, stroink.h@gmail.com

Petra Tijink-Callenbach, University Medical Centre Groningen, Department of Neurology, Groningen, The Netherlands, p.m.c.tijink@umcg.nl

Ingrid Tuxhorn, Pediatric Epilepsy Rainbow Babies and Children's Hospital Case Western Reserve University, Cleveland, USA, Ingrid.Tuxhorn@UHhospitals.org

Patrick Van Bogaert, Université Libre de Bruxelles (ULB), Department of Pediatric Neurology, Hôpital Erasme, Brussels, Belgium, pvanboga@ulb.ac.be

Cees Van Donselaar, Maasstad Ziekenhuis, Rotterdam, The Netherlands, cees@vandonselaar.net

Onno Van Nieuwenhuizen, Rudolf Magnus Institute of Neuroscience, University Medical Center, Utrecht, The Netherlands, OnnovanNieuwenhuizen@umcutrecht.nl

Annamaria Vezzani, IRCCS-Istituto di Ricerche Farmacologiche "Mario Negri", Milano, Italy, annamaria.vezzani@marionegri.it

Federico Vigevano, Neuroscience Department Bambino Gesù Children's Hospital, Rome, Italy, vigevano@opbg.net

Patty Vinning, Department of Neurology, Johns Hopkins Hospital, Baltimore, USA, evining@jhmi.edu

Elaine Wirrell, Child and Adolescent Neurology, Mayo Clinic, Rochester, USA, Wirrell.elaine@mayo.edu

Entrance criteria and outcome measures in pediatric epilepsy clinical trials

Deborah Hirtz

National Institute of Neurological Disorders and Stroke, NIH, Bethesda, Maryland, USA

In April 2011, a National Institute of Neurological Disorders and Stroke (NINDS) workshop was held to identify problems in recent epilepsy clinical trials and to propose new approaches, including recommendations for selection criteria that could be widely used and that would augment the efficient, appropriate and safe recruitment for new trials (Fertig et al., 2012). Clearly one single set of selection criteria would not fulfill the needs of all trials, but it would be easier to compare trial results if entry criteria and measured outcomes were similar. The workshop recommendations were intended as suggestions for a framework which could be modified as appropriate for any specific trial. The discussion focused on epilepsy trials involving primarily adults. However, lowering the age limit in general to 12 years was recommended, with the caveat that applicable preclinical and clinical safety and PK studies have been done in this age group.

One of the roadblocks to a common set of entrance criteria for epilepsy trials is the etiologic heterogeneity of the epilepsies and epilepsy syndromes. Many trials are for add-on therapies, and stability of the current AEDs can be a problem. Another issue is that patients with other stable but chronic conditions are excluded, making the results less applicable to real-world settings. To facilitate the conduct and comparability of trials, the NINDS has developed epilepsy common data elements (CDEs) (Loring et al., 2011). These generally apply to ages 12-75, unless a pediatric population is the specific target of the study. This chapter will present recommendations from the workshop and the CDEs specifically with regard to pediatric epilepsy trials, and will give examples of criteria used in several recent NINDS sponsored studies. These will include definitions of treatment-resistant epilepsy, seizure types, and other eligibility criteria. Recently recommended outcome measures will also be presented, mainly from the NINDS common data elements, as well as suggestions to approaches to measuring quality of life as an outcome in pediatric epilepsy trials.

Study entry criteria

Entrance criteria as recommended in the workshop

Seizure type: Focal seizures must have a focal onset according to current ILAE criteria. At least some of the seizures must be observable. If there is no impairment of consciousness, there must be ictal EEG correlation. Primary generalized seizures must: fulfill criteria for either a genetic epilepsy or unknown cause (idiopathic); have one of the following generalized seizure types: typical absence, myoclonic seizures, and generalized tonic-clonic, with absence of other seizure types, and have an EEG or report that demonstrates generalized spike-wave of ≥ 3 Hz.

Drug resistant epilepsy: For definition of drug resistance, the 2009 ILAE definition (Kwan et al., 2010) was used: "Failure of adequate trials of 2 tolerated and appropriately chosen and used AED schedules to achieve sustained seizure freedom". For those trials requiring study of refractory or drug resistant epilepsy, there should be at least 2 years from the onset of the patient's treatment with AEDs, as prior to this time the prognosis and course cannot be considered intractable.

Seizure rates: Although no minimum monthly rate was suggested, most trials exclude those with less than 3 seizures per month. This can vary depending on the study design. It is critical that the seizure rate can be counted, and that seizure diaries can be kept by the patient or a reliable observer.

EEG, imaging: The panel recommended that for focal epilepsy an EEG is not mandatory. However, if there is an EEG pattern not consistent with focal epilepsy, then the subject should be excluded. If focal seizures are without impaired consciousness, or if there are only subjective sensory symptoms, then there must be an ictal EEG correlation. An EEG is needed to screen for focal epilepsy with secondary generalization which may clinically present as primary generalized epilepsy. EEG confirmation should be required for generalized epilepsy of genetic origin with > 3 Hz generalized spike waves. The EEG itself should meet minimum standards and include activation procedures. In general, imaging studies should be available, with MRI strongly preferred.

AEDs: In general, patients enrolling in trials should be on a stable AED regimen for at least 28 days and be taking no more than 3 concomitant AEDs. The use of felbamate or vigabatrin, both associated with potential severe side effects, should not automatically cause exclusion. The aplastic anemia and hepatic failure that are associated with felbamate usually are seen within the first 6 months to one year, so it would be safe to include a patient who had been on the drug for at least a year (Pellock et al., 2006). For Vigabatrin, history of use for at least 2 years was recommended as most visual field changes occur between 6 months and 2 years (Kalviainen & Nousiainen, 2001) with documentation of visual field examinations would need to be available.

Psychopathology: If there is any psychiatric comorbidity which is unstable, and changes may be needed in medication, exclusion from a trial is probably warranted. However, a condition such as depression that is stable on medication should not be a cause for exclusion. The issue of suicidality is of critical relevance due to the potential for exacerbation by AEDs as per the current FDA warning. Therefore it was recommended that patients with a history of a suicide attempt within the past two years, a history of multiple attempts, or with any active suicide plans or ideation in the most recent 6 months should be excluded and referred for clinical psychiatric care if this is not already in place. In addition, psychiatric, neurological, or medical comorbidities that could impair the subject's ability to follow study procedures would be reason for exclusion.

Other abnormalities: The group recommended that there be no limitations on BMI or weight unless there is a pharmacokinetic reason (*e.g.*, lipid solubility). Exclusion for abnormal blood values should be only if they are clinically relevant, for example in the case of new onset elevation of LFT's. Abnormalities such as chronic anemia or mild hyperglycemia should not be cause for automatic exclusion.

Entrance criteria used in the Childhood Absence Epilepsy trial

A double-blind, randomized controlled trial of the efficacy and tolerability of initial monotherapy for children with newly diagnosed childhood absence epilepsy compared 3 medications: ethosuximide, valproic acid, and lamotrigine (Glauser *et al.*, 2010). The primary outcome was freedom from treatment failure at week 16 or week 20. The secondary outcome was evidence of attentional dysfunction on the Conners' continuous performance test at the 16 or 20-week visit or earlier if treatment was discontinued. Calculations of sample size were based on the ability to detect a 20% difference in freedom from failure rates at 16 weeks.

This study enrolled children ages 2.5 to 13 years who met the following entry criteria: 1) new onset childhood absence epilepsy diagnosed according to the ILAE classification; 2) bilaterally synchronous and symmetric spike waves of 2.7 to 5 Hz with a normal background, and at least one seizure lasting 3 seconds or greater on a one hour waking video EEG; 3) weight at least 10 kg, BMI < 99%; 4) normal CBC and serum levels of aspartate aminotransferase and alanine aminotransferase and serum bilirubin. The girls enrolled had to be premenarchal.

Additional exclusion criteria were: AEDs for ≥ 7 days before randomization, history of another nonfebrile seizure type, a history consistent with juvenile absence (later onset, less frequent absence seizures, more frequent generalized tonic-clonic seizures, and higher frequency (> 3Hz) generalized spike wave discharges) or myoclonic absence epilepsy (*e.g.*, generalized tonic-clonic or myoclonic seizures), a history of severe skin reaction to medication, a history of ASD or major psychiatric disorder, or a history of a clinically significant medical condition. Baseline neuropsychological measures were: Age-appropriate Conners Continuous Performance Test (CPT-II for children ≥ 6 years, and K-CPT for children 4-6 years (Conners, 2002); standardized tests of verbal and nonverbal (Wechler 2003, Brown *et al.*, 1997) intelligence, vocabulary (Dunn & Dunn, 1997), learning skills (Sheslow & Adams, 2003), visual-motor integration (Beery *et al.*, 1997), executive function (Heaton *et al.*, 1993), academic achievement (Wilkinson, 1993; Woodcock *et al.*, 2007), behavior (Achenbach & Rescorla, 2001), and quality of life (Sabaz *et al.*, 2009).

Entrance criteria used in the ERSET trial

The question of whether early epilepsy surgery is beneficial to patients with intractable seizures was addressed by the early randomized surgery epilepsy trial (ERSET) (Engel *et al.*, 2010). This was a multicenter randomized controlled parallel group clinical trial of patients with mesial temporal lobe epilepsy (MTLE) who were 12 years old or older with disabling seizures for no more than 2 consecutive years following adequate trials of at least 2 AEDs. In addition, for subjects to be eligible they had to be candidates for surgical resection based on a standardized presurgical evaluation protocol.

The intent of this study was to enroll teenagers and young adults, who had been considered to have intractable epilepsy for a relatively short period of time. Subjects were to have been within a 2-year window of a diagnosis of pharmacoresistance. This concept is difficult to apply as TLE often has a stuttering course. In this study, the definition of pharmacoresistant was "persistent disabling seizures despite prior trials of at least 2 AEDs, one of which had to have a monotherapy indication." Persistent was defined as: "a) on average at least one day every 2 months when at least one seizure occurred; and b) no more than 6 months between seizures during the 2 years prior to enrollment." In order to make sure that the cohort enrolled was early in the course of intractability, if patients had active epilepsy prior to this 2-year period, there had to be no period of pharmacoresistance for 2 consecutive years or more. Additional exclusionary criteria were more than 4 secondarily generalized seizures per year for more than 3 years, or more than 1 incident of nonfebrile status epilepticus.

The definition in this study of "disabling" seizures was: seizures that resulted in loss of awareness, *e.g.*, complex partial or generalized tonic-clonic, or a change in behavior that interfered with ability to carry out usual activities or were noticeable to others. Seizures that were simple partial that were noticeable only to the patient and during which patients could carry out usual activities did not qualify as disabling.

This was a study of patients with a specific seizure type, but additional types of seizures were allowed. Postictal confusion after complex partial seizures was a requirement. If auras were reported, they had to exclude primary sensory symptoms but could include autonomic, psychic, olfactory, gustatory or nonspecific somatosensory symptoms. Other exclusions were a history of serious cerebral insult after age 5, a progressive neurological disorder, nonepileptic psychogenic seizures, or any focal neurological deficits.

Seizures were diagnosed as mesial temporal lobe by history but confirmed using video EEG monitoring. EEG criteria for exclusion were contralateral or extratemporal ictal onsets, persistence of extratemporal or strongly contralateral focal interictal spikes or slowing, or generalized interictal spikes.

An additional feature of the study was the use of a baseline daily seizure log for one month which allowed confirmation of reported seizure frequencies. Also, baseline QOL and psychosocial measures were obtained.

There was adjudication by a central EEG committee. Ictal semiology was classified as: ipsilateral onset temporal lobe seizures, extratemporal onset of seizures, or contralateral onset. There were 4 types of seizures included:

- Simple partial seizures without impairment, that is with no alteration of consciousness, not noticeable by an observer, and not interfering with normal activities. This type of seizure could also be called an aura.
- Simple partial seizures with impairment of activities that may be noticeable by an observer, but without any alteration of consciousness.
- Complex partial seizures that do involve an alteration of consciousness, but do not progress to bilateral tonic and/or clonic motor involvement.

- Secondarily generalized seizures with alteration of consciousness and progression to bilateral tonic and/or clonic movements.

Baseline evaluations: EEG: Video EEG monitoring was done in inpatient units using standard 10-20 electrode placements.

Neuroimaging: MRI scans and PET scans were interpreted at each site but then were also reviewed by a central committee. Central adjudication was used for any conflicting interpretations.

Neuropsychological testing was done at baseline, 1 and 2 years. Because in the ERSET study the youngest subjects were age 12 years, the battery focused on adult testing. Tests of memory used were: the Rey auditory verbal learning test (Schmidt, 1996), Wechsler scale-revised, logical memory subtest (Wechsler, 1987) and BRIEF visuo-spatial memory subtest-revised (Benedict, 1997). Test of word finding used: Boston naming test (Kaplan et al., 2001). Attention: Digit span (Wechsler 1997), Trail making test and motor speed: grooved pegboard (Strauss et al., 2006).

Psychopathology: screening at baseline was done using the Achenbach child behavior checklist (CBCL) (Achenbach, 1991) and the mini international psychiatric interview (MINI) (Sheehan et al., 1994) for those ages 16 and over. For those under age 16, the Kiddie schedule of affective disorders and schizophrenia (K-SADS) was used. (Kaufmann et al., 1997). A summary diagnosis was made using both parent and subject responses to these questionnaires. If any psychiatric diagnosis was suspected, a psychiatric interview was performed with the MINI addendum.

Outcome variables

CAE trial

The primary outcome was the rate of freedom from failure; failure criteria were persistence of absence seizures, a generalized tonic-clonic seizure at any time, significant drug related systemic toxicity (*i.e.*, platelet count < 50,000/cmm, absolute neutrophil count < 500/cmm, liver enzymes > 10 times upper limit, moderately severe rash, pancreatitis, or increased BMI > 3x baseline), or withdrawal initiated by a parent or physician. The secondary outcome was attentional dysfunction as measured by the Connors Continuous Performance Scale.

ERSET

In most pediatric epilepsy trials, seizure reduction is the entire or a component of the primary outcome, often measured as median percent reduction in seizure frequency from baseline, or alternatively as the percentage of patients who have a specific reduction in seizure frequency from baseline, *i.e.*, a responder rate. In the ERSET trial, the primary outcome variable was freedom from disabling seizures. This was determined in the second year of follow up, using patient reported seizure logs and report forms. There was a seizure adjudication committee that reviewed all new seizure types that occurred during follow up and classified them. The secondary outcome was overall seizure frequency and frequency by seizure type. Other secondary outcomes were health related quality of life scales, which were done at baseline and again at 6 months. Other questionnaires and ancillary measures of cognitive function, with questions regarding medical issues, employment, education, use of community support, and driving were used.

■ Recommendations for neuropsychological outcome measures from the ninds common data elements

There are a large number of recommended neuropsychology instruments for ages 6-16 years as well as ages ≤ 5 years from the NINDS Common data elements: http://www.commondataelements.ninds.nih.gov/epilepsy.aspx#tab=Data_Standards.

Also see: http://www.commondataelements.ninds.nih.gov/epilepsy.aspx#tab=Overview

The following section on neuropsychological outcomes summarizes information found on these websites. Neuropsychological evaluation in children must take into consideration the developmental trajectory, so is more complex that the evaluation of adults. The NINDS CDEs cover relevant cognitive domains across a variety of pediatric epilepsy syndromes. The recommended tests are for use by appropriately trained psychologists or neuropsychology technicians under appropriate supervision. (Loring *et al.*, 2011; Loring & Hermann, 2011).

■ Testing for the 6-16-year old range

Intelligence Quotient (IQ)

It is important to formally assess IQ in children with pediatric epilepsy because there is a high rate of disability and because IQ is important in assigning school resources and accommodations. Formal IQ tests recommended: the Wechsler intelligence scale for children (WISC-IV, fourth edition) or Wechsler abbreviated scale of intelligence, or a WISC-R short form. There is also a Spanish version. This is the most common test of general cognitive ability. Included are measures of working memory and processing speed. The fourth version no longer includes VIQ or PIQ summary scores. Instead there are four factor based scales: verbal concept index, working memory index, perceptual reasoning index, and processing speed index. This test is sensitive to epilepsy-related cognitive problems in clinically referred children with a high seizure burden, and is sensitive to verbal expressiveness, working memory, and processing speed issues. The WASI uses 4 subtests to generate FSIQ, VIQ and OIQ scores. It can span all the way from 6 to 89 years and so has an advantage for studies of both adults and children. However, the scores do not include working memory or processing speed, and both of these are more sensitive to both disease and treatment effects. The CDE's recommend that the WASI VIQ and PIQ be considered as comparable to WISC-IV VCI and PRI, and that a general ability index be calculated.

Learning and memory

There is a children's memory scale such as the California Verbal Learning Test for Children (CVLT-C) is a learning task containing words that can be associated in categories. There are five learning trials of 15 words each, followed by a single trial. After that, recall of the initial word list is requested, so the measures obtained are a learning score, which is the sum across the five trials, and also a measure of delayed free recall. There is also the pediatric Rey Auditory Verbal Learning Test (AVLT), but there is no information about one being more sensitive than the other and the CVLT-C was recommended because it covers a larger age range. The alternative test for adolescents, particularly in the 15-17 age range, is the AVLT. A Spanish version of the CVLT is available.

Language

Language function in children requires grammatical as well as lexical knowledge, and requires specialized assessment. Epilepsy may have a broad impact on the child's ability to communicate, and this may negatively affect academic and social development. A recommended and commonly used specific test for language is the Boston Naming Test, which also has a Spanish version. This is sensitive to naming problems following surgical resection of the language dominant hemisphere. Some studies have suggested this test is sensitive to linguistic impairment associated with TLE. Other measures from this test include the number of semantic and phonemic cues, and the response latency. This test works well for children ages 5-13. An additional language test is the Controlled Word Association Test, which assesses verbal fluency, but may also be used as a measure of executive function. To assess grammatical and pragmatic aspects of language development, the Clinical Evaluation of Language Fundamentals, 4th Ed. (CELF-4) can be used. This also has a Spanish language version.

Generative language fluency is important not only to language but also to executive function. One way to test this is phonemic fluency, which requires asking the child to generate as many words as possible that start with a specific letter of the alphabet. This is done in three 60-second trials. Because the most common letters used are F, A, and S, this test is often called the FAS test. The Spanish version of this test uses the letters PMR, to adjust for the more common frequency of words in that language. In cases involving temporal lobe dysfunction, semantic memory in language may be more affected. The most common fluency task is animal naming, or alternatively naming fruits and vegetables. An optional language task is the CELF-4, used from 5-21 years of age. It is a stepwise approach that allows for flexibility and decreases assessment time. The first level is a screen for language disorders, and subsequent levels are more specific for affected modalities and content areas, working memory, and phonological awareness, with testing of more applied aspects of language. This test is available in Spanish. Interrater reliability is good, and sensitivity and specificity for language disorders is high. However, the CELF-4 has not been demonstrated to identify epilepsy-specific language disorders and the incremental value for naming and expressive vocabulary beyond the Boston naming test and the WISC-IV vocabulary subtest is not demonstrated.

Executive function

An important element of the pediatric evaluation is executive function. This includes a diverse set of cognitive processes such as planning, initiation, inhibition, sustained attention, working memory, and task alteration. These depend primarily on the functional integrity of the frontal lobes but impairments can be seen in other brain lesions. The best test for this is Trail Making, A and B, which test visual attention and mental flexibility. Trails B is considered more sensitive to executive function deficits but should not be given alone because that alters the task demands without getting the practice effects associated with first completing trails A. Both take less than 10 minutes to administer. Administering both parts is recommended, and there is a Spanish version. This task is widely used and it is sensitive not only to diffuse dysfunction but also to the effects of AEDs. In one study, completion time of this test was sensitive to the tapering of topiramate, which has known cognitive side effects (Kockelmann et al., 2003). A parent questionnaire that assesses executive function in children in the home is the behavior rating inventory of executive function (BRIEF). It can be completed by parents or teachers, and has a Spanish version.

The Wisconsin Card Sorting Test (WCST) assesses the ability to abstract and shift cognitive strategies; the sorting principles shift at various points during the test. It is sensitive to frontal lobe structural lesion and in some studies has been able to discriminate between deficits in frontal and temporal lobe epilepsy (Piazzini et al., 2008). There are practice effects so use over longitudinal studies is not recommended. It takes 15-30 minutes to administer, but the 128 card version can be given in a shorter version of 64 cards. It is considered optional.

Attention

Measures of auditory attention include the digit span subtest from the WISC-IV which assess both backward (working memory) and forward (apprehension) digit spans. These take 5-7 minutes to administer. Norms are available for ages 6-16. The Connors Continuous Performance 2 Version 5 (used in the CAE trial) is a computerized version of attention and impulsivity that reflects, in part, inhibitory control. It is often used for ADHD. The test of variable attention (TOVA) may be more suitable for younger or lower functioning children as it does not use letters, but rather non language geometric forms. There are 2 types of tasks; one that assesses inhibitory processing with a frequently occurring target, and one that measures boredom with an infrequently occurring target. This requires about 22 minutes longer than the CPT-II. The WCST assesses the ability to abstract and to change cognitive strategy. It is subject to substantial practice effect.

Psychomotor speed

Slowing of cognitive speed is a common complaint in pediatric epilepsy, and with AEDs (Loring et al., 2007). It can persist even after remission of epilepsy (Berg, 2008). Part of the WISC-IV can be used to assess psychomotor speed, the Processing speed index (PSI) which has 2 subtests, coding and symbol search, and though it is part of the standard IQ test it can be used individually; it is scored as the performance on the coding and symbol search Wechsler subtest. Measures of pure motor speed such as finger tapping or reaction time are not widely used and have little normative data. The grooved pegboard test may be more sensitive to lateralized brain impairment and has been used in epilepsy studies.

Behavior rating scales

In pediatric epilepsy patients, behavioral and psychiatric comorbidity is common. The biggest problem areas are attention, internalizing disorders, and thought problems (Plioplys et al., 2007). The primary tool is the child behavior checklist (CBCL) which is filled out by parents, who rate their child for behavior in the past six months. It yields a total composite score but also has scales of competence in social and school activities, and problem behaviors such as aggression, anxiety, depression, social problems, somatic complaints, and rule breaking behavior (Barry et al., 2008).

In most clinical trials of epilepsy in children, the outcome of visuospatial skills is not of specific interest, these skills tend to remain stable with the exception of hemisphere surgery. The tests used, such as the Judgment of Line orientation test, the Beery visual motor integration test, and the Rey-Osterreith complex figure copy test, have greater variability than the language tests. In most cases, the Block Design subtest of the Wechsler IQ test can be used, or the WISC-IV perceptual reasoning index.

Adaptive behaviors are a problem in many children with intractable or catastrophic pediatric epilepsies; these provide a good estimate of functional ability when IQ is not testable, and these scales can be predictive of quality of life. Possible instruments are the Vineland adaptive behavior scales II, and the adaptive behavior assessment scale-II. Easiest to use may be the Scales of Independent behavior – revised (SIB-R).

■ Testing in the 0-5-year age range

In the youngest children with epilepsy, neurocognitive testing may be particularly challenging. Particularly when looking at evolution of skills over time, any results must be compared to the normal developmental trajectory for age. Especially under age two years, formal developmental assessment is less reliable than in older subjects and studies usually rely heavily on rating scales completed by parents. Children with epilepsy are often behaviorally challenged and/or cognitively impaired, making testing difficult and requiring skilled examiners. However, having tests available across relevant domains can facilitate comparisons across studies and even permit aggregation of data.

Developmental level

The tests recommended and most widely used in this age range are the Wechsler preschool and primary scale of intelligence (WPPSI-III) age range 2 years 6 months to 7 years 3 months, with time of administration from 30-50 minutes; the Mullen scales of early learning (MSEL) birth up to 68 months, with time to administer 15 minutes at age one year and up to 40-60 minutes by age 5 years, and the Bayley scales of infant and toddler development (Bayley-III), ages 1-42 months. The WPPSI-III is a comprehensive measure of general cognitive ability with verbal and nonverbal measures and including processing speed. This test is the younger version of the WISC, which is recommended for older children. Thus it is useful for longitudinal studies in which the age threshold may be crossed for the WPPSI-III. The disadvantage is that there is no short form. The Mullen scales include measures of gross motor, visual reception, fine motor expressive language, and receptive language. In the Bayley-III, fine and gross motor function, receptive and expressive language, and cognitive development are assessed. The time range is 30-90 minutes. There is no Spanish version for any of these three tests.

Learning and memory

In the California verbal learning test, children's version (CVLT-C), verbal learning is tested with 5 learning trials of 15 words. There is then a distractor trial of a list of 15 words, then free recall of the initial word list. This yields a learning score and delayed free recall measure. This test takes about 25 minutes and there is a Spanish version. There are no tests in this age range for visual memory.

Language

The Peabody picture vocabulary test- 4 can be used from a 30-month old developmental level up, to assess receptive vocabulary, and takes 10-20 minutes to administer. A Spanish version is reportedly under development.

Visuospatial function

If the WPPSI-III is being used, the Block Design module can be used to assess non-verbal spatial perception and reasoning; this takes 15 minutes.

Executive function

In the very young child, questionnaires completed by family members may be used to assess executive function. In the 2.5-5 years range, the behavior rating inventory of executive function and BRIEF-Preschool version (Gioia et al., 2000) is completed by parents and teachers, and takes about 10-15 minutes. It provides scores in emotional control, planning, organizing, inhibitory self-control, flexibility, inconsistency and negativity.

Processing speed

The lower limit of testing for processing speed is age 4 years. To generate scores for this domain, the WPPSI-III coding and symbol search are timed non-linguistic tests that are used to transcribe symbols paired with numbers and to scan symbols to assess the presence or absence of a target. Together this takes about 10 minutes.

Motor speed

Motor speed can be assessed using the Purdue pegboard for ages 2 1/2 years and older, however, the grooved pegboard is recommended for children over age 5 years. The Purdue pegboard does not require the child to rotate slotted pegs to fit into the pegboard. The primary measure is dominant hand time to completion; this takes 5-10 minutes. This is a nonlinguistic test and Spanish directions can be used.

Sustained attention

In small children ages 4-5 years it is possible to measure sustained visual attention and inhibition of impulsivity over time by using the Conners Kiddie CPT. This is a computerized measure using pictures rather than letters. A version of the TOVA may be used for low functioning or preliterate children that involves pressing the spacebar in response to geometric forms on the screen. Both tests take 10 minutes or less.

Behavioral rating scales

There is a version of the child behavior checklist that is appropriate for as low as an 18 month developmental level. It is the CBCL 1 and 1/2 to 5 and takes about 10-15 minutes for parents to do; there is a Spanish version. For adaptive behavior, the Scales of independent behavior-revised (SIB-R) is recommended because of its ease of use; it can be a questionnaire format or an interview, and parents rate their children on domains that include motor skills, communication skills, social interactions and personal and community living skills. Other adaptive scales that can be used at this age are the Vineland-II and the Adaptive behavior assessment scale Infant and preschool kit for ages birth to 5 years.

Assessing quality of life outcomes

The NINDS CDE website addresses quality of life outcome measures for pediatric epilepsy. The following information is taken from the NINDS Epilepsy CDE website and the excellent section on Pediatric QOL measures that was written by Joan Austin, Avital Cnaan, and Christine O'Dell, available at: http://www.commondataelements.ninds.nih.gov/epilepsy.aspx#tab=Data_Standards). They reviewed all relevant literature, and four epilepsy specific scales and three generic quality of life scales were selected. Of the generic scales reviewed, one has an epilepsy module and the other two have been used in research with children with epilepsy. In the 2012 re-review of the literature, no additional instruments were found that were being used frequently enough to be added to their recommendations.

In general, the pediatric quality-of-life scales are newer and thus less well developed than the scales for adults. No one scale was recommended over the others for more general use (*e.g.*, in clinical trials). All of the scales they described are relatively easy to use and involve parent-report and/or self-report. Because the epilepsy-specific instruments have primarily been developed relatively recently, additional information is especially needed on subpopulations of children with epilepsy.

Health Related Quality of Life (HRQOL) (Ronen *et al.*, 2003)

Developed in Canada, this covers interpersonal/social consequences; worries and concerns; intrapersonal/emotional; secrecy; and quest for normality. There is both a child (8-15 years) self-report and a parent proxy scale; each takes approximately 15 minutes. If both the child and parental scales are used, a comparison of perceptions can be made. The subscales could discriminate between children with few versus more health problems related to their epilepsy. There is only an English version (copyright 2003, International League Against Epilepsy).

Impact of Childhood Neurologic Disability Scale (ICND) (Camfield, 2003)

This questionnaire has 11 items related to the child's or family's life during the past 3 months for epilepsy, cognition, behavior and physical/neurologic condition. It takes about 12 minutes to complete. The scale expands on the Impact of Pediatric Epilepsy Scale (IPES), which was developed by the same authors and published in 2001. This parent-report scale can be used for a wide age range (ages 2 to 18 years) of children. It is only available in English.

Quality of Life in Childhood Epilepsy (QOLCE) (Sabaz, 2000)

This instrument developed in Australia is specific for children with epilepsy and covers 5 domains; physical function (12 items), emotional well-being (19 items), cognitive function (23 items), social function (12 items) and behavior (23 items). Two subscales cover overall quality of life and general health. Questions are answered by the parents about the previous 4 week time period. It takes 30 minutes to complete. It is sensitive to differences in seizure severity and medication effects. Most QOL subscales were ranked worse as seizure severity increased. Memory and language subscales were adversely affected by number of antiepileptic medications: It is available in English and for parental report only. One recent multicenter prospective study of children with newly diagnosed epilepsy collected data using this questionnaire at time of diagnosis and at 6, 12, and 24 months thereafter (Speechley et al., 2012). From 456 potentially eligible children, parents returned all 4 questionnaires at a rate of 62%. At least one questionnaire was completed by 283/374 (82%). They found absence of cognitive problems, fewer AEDs and better family environment as baseline factors that predicted better quality of life 2 years after diagnosis.

Quality of Life in Epilepsy Inventory for Adolescents (QOLIE-AD-48) (Cramer et al., 1999)

This is a survey for adolescents, ages 11 to 17 years, with epilepsy. It contains 48 items in 8 subscales: epilepsy impact (12 items); memory/concentration (10 items); attitudes toward epilepsy (4 items); physical functioning (5 items); stigma (6 items); social support (4 items); school behavior (4 items); health perceptions (3 items). A higher total summary score (0-100 points) indicates better HRQOL. Questions pertain to the 4 weeks prior to taking the survey. It takes 20 minutes to complete. This scale has been widely used and has been translated into a number of other languages including Chinese, Portuguese, Serbian, and Spanish.

DISABKIDS: a chronic generic module (DCGM-37) with an Epilepsy Module (Simeoni et al., 2007)

This quality of life in chronic disease tool for children 8 to 16 years was developed in seven European countries (Austria, France, United Kingdom, Netherlands, Sweden, Greece and Germany), it has seven disease-specific modules, including epilepsy and has been validated for use in the following languages: English, French, German, Dutch, Greek, and Swedish. It has a short version with only 12 questions, covering the same domains, which can be used for screening. The DISABKIDS Smiley form is available for children 4-7 years old or children who have not reached reading ability. It takes approximately 5 minutes to complete. An epilepsy module includes two scales – impact, which is anxiety about having seizures and the potential public stigma (5 items) and social, which assesses self-esteem (5 items), in both child and parent versions for the 8-16 year olds and a proxy/parent version for the 4-7 year olds. This tool is not used or validated in the US.

Child Health Questionnaire (CHQ) (Landgraf et al., 1996)

This comprehensive quality of life scale has been tested in children with a variety of chronic conditions including 31 children with epilepsy. There were ceiling effects found for four subscales and test-retest reliability problems found for five subscales thus its use is limited for testing effects of interventions. There are no items specific to epilepsy.

Pediatric Quality of Life Inventory (PedsQL™) (Varni et al., 2001)

This modular approach to measuring health-related quality of life (HRQOL) can be used in children and adolescents with acute and chronic health conditions. The PedsQL™ Measurement Model covers 4 domains: physical (8 items), emotional (5 items), social (5 items) and school (5 items). The instrument takes 4 minutes to complete and is translated in multiple international languages including Spanish. There are versions for parents/guardians of children between the ages of 2 to 18 years (in 4 age groups) and child versions for all age groups except the 2-4 years old. This does not have an epilepsy specific module and it is likely that the PedsQL™ will not be sensitive to change as a result of treatment of epilepsy.

Neuro-QOL

Neuro-QOL is a multi-site NINDS funded project that has been developing clinically relevant and psychometrically robust health-related quality of life (HRQL) assessment tools for adults and children: www.neuroqol.org. Neuro-QOL seeks to incorporate patient reported outcomes of functioning, such as social, psychological, and mental well-being in clinical research and to develop psychometrically robust instruments that will be accepted by neurology clinical trials community. Domains and items have been validated for pediatric epilepsy in subjects and caregivers; these can be found on the website and can be used in clinical studies.

■ Concluding remarks

Consideration must be taken in clinical trial design that epilepsy in children encompasses many diverse syndromes, with developmental implications and different symptoms and severities of impact on behavioral and cognitive function and quality of life. Design of prevention and intervention trials will vary with the population examined and the specific questions addressed. However, having a platform of common elements for selection of entry criteria and outcome will allow for more meaningful results and comparisons across studies when this is possible based on populations and questions under study.

References

- Achenbach T, Edelbrock C. *Manual for the Child Behavior Checklist and 4-18 and 1991 Profile*. Department of Psychiatry, University of Vermont; 1991.
- Achenbach TM, Rescorla LA. *Manual for ASEBA school age forms and profiles*. Burlington, University of Vermont, Research Center for Children, Youth and Families, 2001.
- Barry JJ, Ettinger AB, Friel P, et al. Consensus statement: The evaluation and treatment of people with epilepsy and affective disorders. *Epilepsy Behav* 2008; 13: S1-S29.
- Beery KE, Buktenica NA, Beery NA. Beery-Buktenica. *Developmental Test of Visual-Motor Integration*. Cleveland: Modern Curriculum Press; 1997.
- Benedict RHB. *Brief Visuo-spatial Memory Test-Revised*. Odessa, FL: Psychological Assessment Resources, Inc., 1997.
- Berg AT, Langfitt JT, Testa FM, et al. Residual cognitive effects of uncomplicated idiopathic and cryptogenic epilepsy. *Epilepsy Behav* 2008; 13: 614-9.
- Brown L, Sherbenou RJ, Johnson SK. *Test of Nonverbal Intelligence. 3*. Austin, TX: Pro-Ed; 1997.
- Camfield C, Breau L, Camfield P. Assessing the impact of pediatric epilepsy and concomitant behavioral, cognitive, and physical/neurologic disability: Impact of Childhood Neurologic Disability Scale. *Dev Med Child Neurol* 2003; 45: 152-9.
- Conners CK. *Conners' Continuous Performance Test II: Technical Guide and Software Manual*. North Tonawanda, NY: Multi-Health Systems; 2002.
- Cramer J, Westbrook L, Devinsky O, Perrine K, Glassman MB, Camfield C. Development of the Quality of Life in Epilepsy Inventory for Adolescents: the QOLIE-AD-48. *Epilepsia* 1999; 40: 1114-21.
- Dunn LM, Dunn LM. *Peabody Picture Vocabulary Test-III*. Circle Pine, MN: American Guidance Services; 1997.

- Engel J, McDermott UP, Wiebe S, et al. Design considerations for a multicenter randomized controlled trial of early surgery for mesial temporal lobe epilepsy. *Epilepsia* 2010; 51: 1978-86.
- Fertig E, Fureman B, Bergey GK, et al. *Inclusion/Exclusion Criteria for Epilepsy Clinical Trials Recommendations*. NINDS workshop, April 30, 2011: in press.
- Glauser TA, Cnaan A, Shinnar S, et al. Ethosuximide, valproic acid and lamotrigine in childhood absence epilepsy. *N Eng J Med* 2010; 362: 790-9.
- Gioia GA, Isquith PK, Guy SC, Kenworthy L. Behavior rating inventory of executive function. *Child Neuropsychol* 2000; 6: 235-8.
- Heaton KR, Chelune GJ, Talley JL, Kay GG, Curtis G. *Wisconsin card Sorting Test Manual: Revised and Expanded*. Odessa, Fl.: Psychological Assessment Resources. 1993.
- Kalviainen R, Nousiainen I. Visual field defects with vigabatrin: epidemiology and therapeutic implications. *CNS Drugs* 2001; 15: 217-30.
- Kaplan E, Goodglass H, Weintraub S. *The Boston Naming Test, 2nd ed*. Philadelphia: Lippincott, Williams and Wilkins, 2001.
- Kaufman J, Birmaher B, Brent D, et al. Schedule for affective disorders and schizophrenia for school-age children – present and lifetime version (K-SADS-PL): initial reliability and validity data. *J Am Acad Child Adolesc Psychiatry* 1997; 36: 980-8.
- Kockelmann E, Elger CE, Helmstaedter C. Significant improvement in frontal lobe associated neuropsychological functions after withdrawal of topiramate in epilepsy patients. *Epilepsy Res* 2003; 54: 171-8.
- Kwan P, Arzimanoglou A, Berg AT, et al. Definition of drug resistant epilepsy: Consensus proposal by the ad hoc Task Force of the ILAE Commission on Therapeutic Strategies. *Epilepsia* 2009; 50: 3-11.
- Landgraf JM, Abetz LN. Measuring Health Outcomes in Pediatric Populations: Issues in Psychometrics and Application. In: Spilker B (ed). *Quality of Life and Pharmacoeconomics in Clinical Trials*. Philadelphia: Lippincott-Raven Publishers, 1996, pp. 793-802.
- Loring DW, Marino S, Meador KJ. Neuropsychological and behavioral effects of antiepilepsy drugs. *Neuropsychol Rev* 2007; 17: 413-25.
- Loring DW, Hermann BP. Neuropsychology and the Epilepsy Common Data Element Project. In: Helmstaedter C, Lassonde M, Hermann B, Kahane P, Arzimanoglou, A (eds). *Neuropsychology in the Care of People with Epilepsy*. Montrouge: John Libbey Eurotext, 2011.
- Loring DW, Lowenstein DH, Barbaro NM, et al. Common Data Elements in Epilepsy Research: Development and Implementation of the NINDS Epilepsy CDE Project. *Epilepsia* 2011; 52: 1186-91.
- Pellock JM, Faught E, Leppik IE, Shinnar S, Zupanc ML. Felbamate: consensus of current clinical experience. *Epilepsy Res* 2006; 71: 89-101.
- Piazzini A, Turner K, Vignoli A, Canger R, Canevini MP. Frontal cognitive dysfunction in juvenile myoclonic epilepsy. *Epilepsia* 2008; 49: 657-62.
- Plioplys S, Dunn DW, Caplan R. 10-year research update review: psychiatric problems in children with epilepsy. *J Am Acad Child Adolesc Psychiatry* 2007; 46: 1389-402.
- Ronen GM, Ronen DL, Streiner PR; the Canadian Pediatric Epilepsy Network. Health-related Quality of Life in Children with Epilepsy: Development and Validation of Self-report and Parent Proxy Measures. *Epilepsia* 2003; 44: 598-612.
- Sabaz M, Cairns DR, Lawson JA, Nheu N, Bleasel AF, Bye AM. Validation of a new quality of life measure for children with epilepsy. *Epilepsia* 2000; 41: 765-74.
- Schmidt M. *Rey Auditory Verbal Learning Test*. Los Angeles: Western Psychological Services, 1996.
- Sheehan DV, Lecrubier Y, Janavs J, et al. *Mini International Neuropsychiatric Interview* (MINI). Tampa, Florida: Paris, France: University of South Florida Institute for Research in Psychiatry; Inserm-Hôpital de la Salpêtrière, 1994.

- Sheslow D, Adams W. *Wide Range Assessment of Memory and Learning, 2.* Wilmington, DE: Western Psychological Services, 2003.
- Simeoni MC, Schmidt S, Muehlan H, Debensason, D, Bullinger M, Group TD. Field testing of a European quality of life instrument for children and adolescents with chronic conditions: the 37-item DISABKIDS Chronic Generic Module. *Quality of Life Research* 2007; 16: 881-93.
- Speechley KN, Ferro MA, Camfield CS, *et al*. Quality of life in children with new-onset epilepsy: A 2-year prospective cohort study. *Neurology* 2012; 79: 1548-55.
- Strauss E, Sherman EMS, Spreen O. *A Compendium of Neuropsychological Tests; Administration, Norms and Commentary*, 3rd ed. New York: Oxford Press, 2006.
- Varni JW, Seid M, Kurtin PD. PedsQL 4.0: Reliability and validity of the pediatric quality of life inventory Version 4.0 generic core scales in healthy and patient populations. *Medical Care* 2001; 38: 800-12.
- Wechsler D. *Wechsler Memory Scale-Revised.* San Antonio: Psychological Corporation, 1987.
- Wechsler D. *Wechsler Adult Intelligence Scales – III.* San Antonio: Psychological Corporation; 1997.
- Wechsler D. *Wechsler Intelligence Scale for Children – IV.* San Antonio: Psychological Corporation; 2003.
- Wilkinson GS. *The Wide Range Achievement Test. 3.* Wilmington, DE: Jastak; 1993.
- Woodcock RW, McGrew KS, Mather N. *Woodcock-Johnson III Tests of Achievement.* Itasca, IL: Riverside Publishing; 2007.

Is it possible to predict the outcome of childhood epilepsy?

Peter Camfield, Carol Camfield

Department of Pediatrics, Dalhousie University and the IWK Health Centre, University Ave, Halifax, Nova Scotia, Canada

---

On the day that a child is diagnosed with epilepsy, after several months or even years later, it would be highly desirable to predict what will happen for seizure control and social outcome. Prediction is a complex concept. Obviously the first question is: *What is to be predicted?* – Is it seizure control, remission with or without ongoing AED treatment, intractability, social outcome or a combination? The second question is: *What is the purpose of attempting prediction and who will use the information?* The third question is: *How accurate is the prediction?*

Statistical modelling allows identification of risk factors for outcome. Usually risk factors are deemed important if they are associated with the outcome of interest with a probability of < 0.05 in univariate analysis. If several risk factors are inter-related then multivariate modelling can reveal which factors have the strongest association with the outcome and by default which risk factors from univariate analysis are not such powerful predictors.

Many important health issues for populations of people are associated with statistically significant risk factors; however, it is less clear how such risk factors should be applied to individual patients. It may be complex to distinguish between statistical and clinical significance. For example, hypertension is a significant risk factor for stroke, but not all people with hypertension will go on to have a stroke and not all people with stroke have a history of hypertension. Considering epilepsy, a striking example of the tension between statistical and clinical significance is the risk of epilepsy after a febrile seizure. A simple febrile seizure has only a 2% of chance of leading to epilepsy (Nelson & Ellenberg, 1976; Annegers *et al.*, 1987; Verity & Golding, 1991). A complex febrile seizure imparts a high statistical risk for subsequent epilepsy – yet the absolute risk is only 10-15% (Nelson & Ellenberg, 1976; Annegers *et al.*, 1987). Most children who develop epilepsy after a febrile seizure do so after a simple febrile seizure, because simple febrile seizures are more common than complex febrile seizures (Nelson & Ellenberg 1976; Verity, 1991). The great majority of children with complex febrile seizures do not develop epilepsy. Obviously family anxiety will be increased if parents are told that their child is at high risk for epilepsy. This would not be such an important issue if complex febrile

+ febrile seizures. The recursive tree model came to different conclusions – the epilepsy syndromes of cryptogenic generalized, symptomatic generalized and symptomatic partial were identified as having a poor outcome while the syndromes of idiopathic generalized, idiopathic partial, cryptogenic partial and unknown were predicted to remit provided the age of onset was ≤ 12 years. When the onset in this latter group was > 12 years, the outcome was predicted as poor.

These predictive factors were not unexpected based on previous studies but the novel feature of our study was the assessment of accuracy. Two types of error may occur with prediction of outcome for an individual patient. Some patients will be predicted to remit but fail to do so – their epilepsy will persist. Others will be predicted not to remit, but somehow their clinical course is more optimistic and remission occurs. Overall, at the end of follow up of the Dutch and Nova Scotia cohorts about 60% of patients were in remission and 40% were not. Based on our statistically robust modeling exercise, we were correct in our predictions in 70% of children but incorrect in 30%. Errors were nearly equal in both directions – incorrect prediction for good outcomes and bad outcomes. Prediction was incorrect for about one-third of individual patients, which represents disappointing accuracy for clinical practice involving an individual patient.

We conclude that based on currently available clinical data, accurate prediction of outcome for most children with epilepsy is impossible on the day of diagnosis or after 6 months of treatment.

There are few exceptions based on epilepsy syndrome diagnosis. The outcome is virtually 100% remission for benign rolandic epilepsy and Panayiotopoulos syndrome (Bouma *et al.* 1997, Ferrie *et al.*, 2006). The outcome is virtually 0% remission for syndromes such as Lennox-Gastaut, Ohtahara, epilepsy of infancy with migrating focal seizures, Dravet syndrome, epilepsy with myoclonic absences, Rasmussen syndrome, gelastic seizures with hypothalamic hamartoma, progressive myoclonus epilepsies (PME) and autosomal-dominant nocturnal frontal lobe epilepsy (ADNFLE). However, note that this collection of syndromes includes no more than 30% of childhood epilepsy (Camfield & Camfield, 2003). All other syndromes have an intermediate prognosis – some remit, some do not.

Prediction of social outcome also remains elusive. In the Nova Scotia study we were unable to find a useful statistical model for social outcome (Camfield *et al.*, 1993). Children with specific learning disorders seemed to be at higher risk of poor social outcome, while those with only simple partial seizures were more likely to have a good outcome. However, most of the statistical variance was not accounted for by either of these factors. In the population-based study from Finland of Matti Sillanpaa, we assisted in the analysis of a 30-year follow up of 100 patients with "epilepsy only" compared with two carefully chosen control groups (Jalava *et al.* 1997). Patients had "epilepsy only" if seizures were thought to be their only neurological problem. In this special group those with persistent seizures and/or AED treatment were less likely to be socially successful than those in remission and off AED treatment. However, there were many exceptions.

Should we abandon our attempts to predict outcome?

- No, these efforts are informative for future studies that may further refine risk. For example, we know that 15% of children with childhood absence epilepsy will develop juvenile myoclonic epilepsy (Wirrell et al., 1996). Learning how to predict this outcome by whatever means probably would be useful.
- No, these efforts may guide families somewhat. We need to continue to be aware that our predictions at the time of presentation are not very good. Families will continue to ask about the outcome, although it remains unclear if they will be happier with a more exact prediction. In our experience, families with a child diagnosed with Benign Rolandic Epilepsy usually seem to benefit from knowing about the good outcome – but this "sense" has never been formally studied. Some families remain persistently anxious and "over-protective" even though we had explained that SUDEP would not occur, that there would be few seizures and no brain injury, and that remission would occur in adolescence and that social outcome should be good (Peters et al., 2001).
- No, some outcomes are disastrous – surely we should continue to try to identify those at risk for epileptic encephalopathies and intractable focal epilepsy.
- No, a more integrated effort to predict social outcome would be very valuable – after all what could be more important?

What will it take to find our way to accurate predictions?

It is clear that the currently available clinical factors and results from investigations are very unlikely to be the source of more accurate prediction. Brain imaging needs more study but this is difficult because MRI techniques in particular are changing rapidly. The magnet field strength is increasing and specific sequences reveal more lesions. The sophistication of interpretation of MRI also varies a great deal (Sørensen et al. 2001). Currently available data indicate that the prediction of outcome is not certain even if there is a single lesion on MRI that is convincingly the cause of the epilepsy. Studies from both Olmstead County Minnesota and Connecticut indicate that children with focal, "causative" MRI lesions still have a 30% chance of long-term remission with medical (non-surgical) treatment (Berg et al., 2010; Wirrell et al., 2011).

Genetic investigations are unlikely by themselves in the near future to be sufficiently predictive to be useful for most patients. Perhaps one of the best examples to support this contention occurs in a family with a dominantly inherited GEFS+ syndrome from an SCN1A mutation. Approximately 20% of those inheriting the SCN1A mutation have no seizures at all, 30% have only febrile seizures, and 30% have a variety of mild epilepsy types; however an occasional family member has catastrophic Dravet syndrome (Singh et al., 1999). The modifying factors remain obscure for the variable phenotypes that result from a single SCN1A mutation.

Moving ahead

Our opinion is that prediction schemes that will be useful for individual patients will combine seizure type + epilepsy syndrome + neurological/intellectual status along with MRI results and genetic findings. The number of variables in these models may be very large, so big cohorts will be needed.

For directing further research and tightening hypotheses, we will need to continue to pay attention to traditional statistical models. It will continue to be of great value to identify disorders that never remit and disorders that always remit. We are quite pessimistic that useful models to predict social outcome will be developed in the foreseeable future. Social outcome studies are particularly challenging because they require long follow up into adulthood, so an individual researcher can only do one study in a lifetime.

We do not know if our predictions for epilepsy outcome are better or worse than for many other diseases - the application of statistical risk factors for the prediction of outcome of an individual patient with many conditions is challenging. We urge clinicians caring for an individual patient with epilepsy to be wary of prognostic schemes. These schemes offer broad guidelines but exceptions are common.

References

- Annegers JF, Hauser WA, Shirts SB, Kurland LT. Factors prognostic of unprovoked seizures after febrile convulsions. *N Engl J Med* 1987; 316: 494-8.
- Arts WFM, Brouwer OF, Peters ACB, *et al.* Course and prognosis of childhood epilepsy: 5-year follow-up of the Dutch study of epilepsy in childhood. *Brain* 2004; 127: 1774-84.
- Berg A, Shinnar S. The risk of seizure recurrence following a first unprovoked seizure: a quantitative review. *Neurology* 1991; 41: 965-72.
- Berg AT, Testa FM, Levy SR, Complete remission in nonsyndromic childhood-onset epilepsy. *Ann Neurol* 2011; 70: 566-73.
- Bouma PA, Bovenkerk AC, Westendorp RG, Brouwer OF. The course of benign partial epilepsy of childhood with centrotemporal spikes: a meta-analysis. *Neurology* 1997; 48: 430-7.
- Camfield CS, Camfield PR, Gordon KE, Dooley JM, Smith BS. Predicting the outcome of childhood epilepsy – a population based study yielding a simple scoring system. *J Pediatr* 1993; 122/6: 861-8.
- Camfield CS, Camfield PR, Gordon KE, Dooley JM, Smith BS. Biologic Factors as predictors of social outcome in epilepsy in intellectually normal children: A population based study. *J Pediatr* 1993; 122/6: 869-73.
- Camfield PR, Camfield CS, Dooley JM, Tibbles J, Fung T, Garner B. Epilepsy after a first unprovoked seizure in childhood. *Neurology* 1985; 35: 1657-60.
- Camfield PR, Camfield CS. Childhood Epilepsy: What is the evidence for what we think and what we do? *J Child Neurol* 2003; 18: 272-87.
- Commission on Classification and Terminology of the International League Against Epilepsy. Proposal for revised classification of epilepsies and epileptic syndromes. *Epilepsia* 1989; 30: 389-99.
- Ferrie C, Caraballo R, Covanis A, *et al.* Panayiotopoulos syndrome: a consensus view. *Dev Med Child Neurol* 2006; 48: 236-40.
- Fisher RS, Leppik I. Debate: When does a seizure imply epilepsy? *Epilepsia* 2008; 49 (Suppl 9): 7-12.
- Geelhoed M, Boerrigter AO, Camfield P, *et al.* The accuracy of outcome prediction models for childhood-onset epilepsy. *Epilepsia* 2005; 46: 1526-32.
- Geerts A, Arts WF, Stroink H, *et al.* Course and outcome of childhood epilepsy: a 15-year follow-up of the Dutch Study of Epilepsy in Childhood. *Epilepsia* 2010; 51: 1189-97.
- Gordon K, MacSween J, Dooley J, Camfield C, Camfield P, Smith B. Families are content to discontinue antiepileptic drugs at different risks than their physicians. *Epilepsia* 1996; 37: 557-62.

- Gordon KE, Dooley JM, Camfield PR, Camfield CS, MacSween J. Treatment of febrile seizures: the influence of treatment efficacy and side-effect profile on value to parents. *Pediatrics* 2001; 108: 1080-8.
- Hauser WA, Rich SS, Lee JR, Annegers JF, Anderson VE. Risk of recurrent seizures after two unprovoked seizures. *N Engl J Med* 1998; 338: 429-34.
- Jalava M, Sillanpaa M, Camfield C, Camfield P. Social adjustment and competence 35 years after onset of childhood epilepsy: a prospective controlled study. *Epilepsia* 1997: 38; 708-15.
- Nelson KB, Ellenberg JH. Predictors of epilepsy in children who have experienced febrile seizures. *N Engl J Med* 1976; 295: 1029-33.
- Peters J, Camfield PR, Camfield CS. Benign rolandic epilepsy can be safely managed without medication: A population-based study. *Neurology* 2001; 57: 537-9.
- Pohlmann-Eden B, Beghi E, Camfield C, Camfield P. The first seizure and its management in adults and children. *BMJ* 2006: 332: 339-42.
- Shinnar S, Berg AT, O'Dell C, et al. Predictors of multiple seizures in a cohort of children prospectively followed from the time of their first unprovoked seizure. *Ann Neurol* 2000; 48: 140-7.
- Sillanpää M, Camfield P, Camfield C. Predicting long-term outcome of childhood epilepsy in Nova Scotia, Canada, and Turku, Finland. Validation of a simple scoring system. *Arch Neurol* 1995; 52: 589-92.
- Sillanpää M, Jalava M, Kaleva O, Shinnar S. Long-term prognosis of seizures with onset in childhood. *New Eng J Med* 1998; 338: 1715-22.
- Singh R, Scheffer IE, Crossland K, Berkovic SF. Generalized epilepsy with febrile seizures plus: a common childhood-onset genetic epilepsy syndrome. *Ann Neurol* 1999; 45: 75-81.
- Sørensen JS, Jensen FT, Andersen PB, Nielsen MS, Pedersen B, Christensen T. Is visual assessment of MRI adequate in the investigation of patients with temporal lobe epilepsy? Evaluation of the diagnostic accuracy of the visual assessment of MRI in mesial temporal sclerosis. *Ugeskr Laeger* 2001; 163: 6271-4.
- Verity CM, Golding J. The accuracy of outcome prediction models for childhood-onset epilepsy. Risk of epilepsy after febrile convulsions: a national cohort study. *BMJ* 1991; 303: 1373-6.
- Wirrell EC, Camfield CS, Camfield PR, Gordon K, Dooley J. Long-term prognosis of typical childhood absence epilepsy. *Neurology* 1996: 47: 912-8.
- Wirrell EC, Grossardt BR, So EL, Nickels KC A population-based study of long-term outcomes of cryptogenic focal epilepsy in childhood: Cryptogenic epilepsy is probably not symptomatic epilepsy. *Epilepsia* 2011; 52: 738-45.

Prognostic factors for recurrence after a first unprovoked seizure in childhood

Shlomo Shinnar

Departments of Neurology, Pediatrics and Epidemiology and Population Health and the Comprehensive Epilepsy Management Center, Montefiore Medical Center, Albert Einstein College of Medicine, Bronx New York, USA

There have been a large number of studies addressing the risk of recurrence following a first seizure in childhood (Annegers et al., 1986; Camfield et al., 1985, 1989; Hauser et al., 1982; Hirtz et al., 1984; Shinnar et al., 1990, 1996; Stroink et al., 1998; van Donselaar et al., 1997). The range of recurrence risk has been variable but if one examines the studies that have prospectively examined recurrence risk after a first unprovoked seizure in largely untreated populations and have excluded those with a history of prior events at presentation, the best estimates of recurrence are 40-45% (Berg & Shinnar, 1991; Shinnar et al., 1990, 1996). In this chapter we will examine the time course to recurrence and risk factors for recurrence. In accordance with the International League Against Epilepsy (ILAE) guidelines for epidemiologic research in epilepsy, a first unprovoked seizure is defined as a seizure or flurry of seizures all occurring within 24 hours in a person older than 1 month of age with no prior history of unprovoked seizures (Commission on Epidemiology and Prognosis, 1993). The latter phrase of no history of prior unprovoked seizures is of particular importance as a substantial proportion of children who first present to medical attention with a convulsion or other seizure have a history of prior events (Hirtz et al., 2000). In this chapter we focus on those who after careful evaluation, in fact presented with a first unprovoked seizure.

■ Overall recurrence risk following a first unprovoked seizure

There is a wide variability in the recurrence risk reported in different studies of recurrence risk after a first unprovoked seizure in children and adults ranging from 27% to 71% (Berg & Shinnar, 1991). The highest recurrence risk comes from a study that defined those with multiple seizures in one day as recurrent (Elwes et al., 1985). Other high recurrence risks are from studies that did not exclude those with prior seizures. When one limits the studies to those which used the ILAE definition of multiple seizures in one day being a single seizure and excluded those with prior events, the recurrence risks are 27% to 52%

(Berg & Shinnar, 1991). If one examines largely untreated populations including the untreated group in the randomized clinical trials of treatment following a first seizure (Camfield *et al.*, 1989; First Seizure Trial Group, 1993; Marson *et al.*, 2005), then recurrence risks are largely in the 40% to 50% range and this is supported by a metanalysis of the available studies up to 1990 (Berg & Shinnar, 1991).

Interestingly, despite the wide range of absolute recurrence risks reported, there is a strong agreement across studies in both the time course to recurrence and the risk factors for recurrence. The majority of recurrences occur in the first 2 years. We have followed patients for up to 20 years following a first seizure (Shinnar *et al.*, 2000) and approximately half of the recurrences will happen in the first 6 months and 80% within the first 2 years. Late recurrences do occur but are quite rare (Shinnar *et al.*, 1996; 2000). Most studies have followed subjects for considerably shorter periods of time but report a similar proportion of the recurrences occurring over the first two years whether their absolute recurrence risk is high or low (Annegers *et al.*, 1986; Berg & Shinnar, 1991; Camfield *et al.*, 1985, 1989; Hauser *et al.*, 1982, 1990; Shinnar *et al.*, 1990, 1996, 2000).

Similar to the agreement on the timing of recurrence, there is reasonable agreement about risk factors for recurrence. Individual factors are discussed in detail below but the most important ones are the etiology of the seizure and the presence of an epileptiform electroencephalogram (EEG) (Berg & Shinnar, 1991; Camfield *et al.*, 1985; Shinnar *et al.*, 1990, 1996; Hirtz *et al.*, 2000). Whether the seizure occurred while the child was awake or asleep also influences recurrence risk (Shinnar *et al.*, 1993) but this has only been addressed in one pediatric study. When we address the risk factors, it should be noted that factors that affect recurrence risk may or may not be the same factors that influence the risk of multiple recurrences or long term prognosis. For example, a remote symptomatic etiology increases recurrence risk after a first or second seizure and also carries with it a worse long term prognosis than having an idiopathic/cryptogenic etiology. The presence of an epileptiform EEG increases the risk of recurrence after a first unprovoked seizure but not after a second one (Shinnar *et al.*, 2000) and depending on the epilepsy syndrome associated with that EEG (*e.g.*, benign rolandic) may actually have a favorable prognosis on long term outcomes. Selected risk factors of interest are presented in more detail below.

■ Risk factors for recurrence

Etiology

In the older ILAE classification (Commission on Epidemiology and Prognosis, 1993), the etiology of seizures is classified as remote symptomatic, cryptogenic, or idiopathic. Remote symptomatic seizures are those without an immediate cause but with an identifiable prior brain injury or the presence of a static encephalopathy such as mental retardation or cerebral palsy, which are known to be associated with an increased risk of seizures. In contrast, idiopathic and cryptogenic seizures occur in children who were otherwise normal and had no clear etiology other than a possible genetic predisposition. The new classification system (Commission on Classification and Terminology, 2010) has changed the criteria for cryptogenic and idiopathic and has renamed cryptogenic as "of unknown etiology". However, essentially all the published studies on recurrence risk following a first unprovoked seizure were done prior to the new classification and so, for purposes of this discussion, we will retain the old classification and combine cryptogenic and idiopathic, as was done in the original studies by Hauser and colleagues (1982) and carried on in other studies since. This has little to no effect on the results of the analysis.

Children with a remote symptomatic first seizure have a higher recurrence risk than those with a cryptogenic first seizure. In our first seizure study (Shinnar et al., 1996) 44 of 65 (68%) with a remote symptomatic etiology recurred compared with 127 of 342 (37%) with a cryptogenic etiology. This effect is consistently seen in studies of recurrence including both children and adults. In a meta-analysis of studies prior to 1990 (Berg & Shinnar, 1991), we found that the relative risk of recurrence comparing patients with a remote symptomatic first seizure to those with a cryptogenic first seizure was 1.8 (95% confidence interval, 1.5-2.1). The effect of etiology on recurrence persists after a second seizure (Shinnar et al., 2000). More recent studies confirm the effect of etiology on recurrence risk (Hirtz et al., 2000; Stroink et al., 1998).

Electroencephalogram (EEG)

While in adults the data are more controversial, in children, studies have consistently shown that an epileptiform EEG is a significant risk factor for recurrence, especially if the etiology is not known to be remote symptomatic (Berg & Shinnar, 1991; Camfield, 1985; Shinnar et al., 1990, 1994, 1996; Stroink et al., 1998; Hirtz et al., 2000). The magnitude of the effect in children is similar to the effect of etiology (Berg & Shinnar, 1991; Shinnar et al., 1990, 1996). Furthermore, an abnormal EEG is a common finding in children with a first unprovoked seizure older than age 3 with the most common epileptiform abnormality being centrotemporal spikes associated with benign rolandic epilepsy (Shinnar et al., 1994). There are conflicting data on whether non-epileptiform abnormalities modestly increase recurrence risk or not (Shinnar et al., 1990, 1994, 1996; Camfield et al., 1985), but clearly the effect is not nearly as strong as that of an epileptiform EEG. Despite minor discrepancies, it is clear that, in children with cryptogenic/idiopathic seizures, the EEG is the most important factor in predicting recurrence. In 2000, the American Academy of Neurology published a guideline on the diagnostic evaluation of a first unprovoked seizure in children and the EEG is considered a standard of care (Hirtz et al., 2000). It is considered a standard of care not only because it carries implications about recurrence risk, but it also may predict long term prognosis and the need for an imaging study. The optimal timing of the EEG is unclear though for logistical reasons, the vast majority of the EEGs in first seizure studies were done electively and not in the immediate post ictal period. In children with remote symptomatic etiology, an abnormal EEG is more common but does not carry with it additional prognostic information on recurrence risk (Shinnar et al., 1990; 1994; 1996). It may still have implications for long term prognosis.

Sleep state

Only one study has examined whether seizures occurring in sleep are more likely to recur than seizures occurring while awake (Shinnar et al., 1993, 1996). We found that children whose initial seizure occurred during sleep were more likely to recur than those whose first seizure occurred while awake. Furthermore, if the first seizure happeneed during sleep and there was a recurrence, it tended to also occur in sleep. The same held true if the first seizure occurred while awake (Shinnar et al., 1993). While some epilepsy syndromes are more associated with night time seizures, this did not explain the effect as when we limit the analysis to children with centrotemporal spikes, those with an initial seizure in sleep had a higher risk of recurrence than those with an initial seizure while awake (Shinnar et al., 1993). On multivariable analysis, in children with cryptogenic/idiopathic seizures, both an abnormal EEG and a first seizure occurring while asleep are predictors of recurrence (Shinnar et al., 1993, 1996). While there are no other pediatric studies that have specifically examined this topic, a study of first unprovoked seizures in adults reported that an initial seizure occurring at night was associated with a higher recurrence risk than if occurred during the day (Hopkins et al., 1988) which offers further evidence for this finding. From a therapeutic point of view, the implications remain unclear as seizures occurring at night when the child is in bed are less likely to be associated with injury than those occurring in the daytime and SUDEP is not a major concern in this population (Shinnar et al., 2005; Sillanpaa & Shinnar, 2010).

Seizure type

The effect of seizure type on recurrence risk is very unclear. It should be noted that absence and myoclonic seizures essentially never present with an isolated seizure. So effectively, for a first seizure, as distinct from new onset epilepsy population, we are dealing with the distinction between what clinically appear to be generalized tonic clonic seizures and partial onset seizures (with or without secondary generalization). The results in the literature are mixed (Berg & Shinnar, 1991). Those studies that do find the association usually find it in univariate analysis. In our first seizure study (Shinnar et al., 1990, 1996) we found that a partial first seizure is associated with a higher risk of recurrence. However, partial seizures were more common in children with remote symptomatic etiology and in those with epileptiform EEGs and the effect did not remain significant in multivariable analysis.

Duration

There is little evidence that duration of the initial seizure is associated with a change in recurrence risk in children (Shinnar et al., 1996; 2001). A duration of 30 minutes or more meeting the older definitions of status epilepticus is not uncommon, occurring in 12% of children and 11% of adults (Hauser et al., 1990; Shinnar et al., 2001). While a prolonged initial seizure is not associated with an increased risk of recurrence, if a recurrence does occur, it is likely to also be prolonged (Shinnar et al., 2001). This may also be true for febrile seizures (Berg & Shinnar, 1996). This carries therapeutic implications, as while this author does not usually initiate chronic antiepileptic drug therapy following an isolated prolonged seizure, these children may benefit from having abortive therapy available at home (Shinnar, 2007).

Number of seizures in 24 hours

In approximately one quarter of cases, the initial presentation in children consists of 2 or more seizures within 24 hours (Shinnar et al., 1996). Prospective studies in both children and adults have shown no difference in recurrence risk in those whose initial presentation was an isolated seizure compared with those whose initial presentation was two or more seizures within 24 hours (Kho et al., 2006; Shinnar et al., 1996). This is consistent with the ILAE definition that considers a flurry within 24 hours to be s single event (Commission on Epidemiology and Prognosis, 1993). When one defines a second seizure within 24 hours to be a recurrence as was done in one adult study (Elwes et al., 1985), this increases the reported recurrence risk by over 20% resulting in the highest recurrence risk of any first seizure study. The epidemiologic data support continuing to consider a flurry of seizures in one day as a single event with little impact on recurrence risk.

Effect of treatment on recurrence risk

Treatment is not a predictive factor but does have an impact on recurrence risk. The effect of treatment following a first unprovoked seizure has now been examined in several randomized clinical trials (Camfield et al., 1989; First Seizure Trial Group, 1993; Hirtz et al., 2003; Kim et al., 2006; Marson et al., 2005; Musicco et al., 1997) most of which have included children. The two large well designed randomized clinical trials of treatment versus no treatment following a first unprovoked seizure, one of which included children, found that treatment reduced recurrence risk by about 50% from approximately 50% to 25%, but did not alter long term outcome (First Seizure Trial Group, 1993; Kim et al., 2006; Marson et al., 2005; Musicco et al., 1997). The chances of attaining remission were similar on the treated and untreated groups in both the Italian first seizure study (First Seizure Trial Group 1993; Musicco et al., 1997) and the British Multicenter Trial for Early Epilepsy and Single Seizures (MESS) (Kim et al., 2006; Marson et al., 2005). These data, that early treatment, while reducing recurrence risk does not affect long term outcome, led to the practice parameter of the American Academy of Neurology that states that treatment following a first seizure is not indicated to prevent epilepsy but is only indicated in those cases where the benefits of preventing an additional seizure outweigh the pharmacologic and psychological side effects associated with chronic antiepileptic drug therapy (Hirtz et al., 2003).

Prognostic factors after a second seizure

After two seizures, the child meets criteria for having epilepsy. However, the group of children who present with a single seizure are different than children who present with newly diagnosed epilepsy rather than with the initial seizure. The recurrence risk is approximately 70% in both children and adults (Hauser et al., 1998; Shinnar et al., 2000) and there is no group with a very low risk of recurrence. Etiology continues to be an important risk factor for predicting further seizures as well as long term prognosis. An abnormal EEG and a seizure occurring in sleep, which increased the recurrence risk after a first seizure, no longer have predictive value for the risk of further seizures (Shinnar et al., 2000). The occurrence of the second seizure within 6 months of the first increases recurrence risk compared to a second seizure occurring more than 6 months after the initial seizure. Treatment after a second seizure reduces recurrence risk by half similar to what was seen in the randomized clinical trials (Shinnar et al., 2000). It should be noted that many of these children have self-limited epilepsy syndromes (van Donselaar et al., 1997) which some have argued may not need treatment even after several seizures (Ambrosetto & Tassinari, 1990; Freeman et al., 1987) and that, as a group, the children who initially present with a first unprovoked seizure have a very low seizure frequency and are very unlikely to develop medically refractory epilepsy (Shinnar et al., 2000; van Donsellar et al., 1997). They have a very different distribution of epilepsy syndromes than if we look at all newly diagnosed epilepsy in childhood (Shinnar et al., 1999; Sillanpaa et al., 1999; Berg et al., 1999).

Conclusion

In children with a first unprovoked seizure, approximately 40-45% will recur with most recurrences occurring soon after the initial seizure. Etiology, the EEG and sleep state at the time of the first seizure are the key risk factors associated with a differential risk of seizure recurrence. Age at first seizure, duration of first seizure and number of seizures in

Newly diagnosed epilepsies: clinically relevant conclusions from global studies on outcome

Willem F. Arts

Department of Paediatric Neurology, Erasmus Medical Center – Sophia Children's Hospital, Rotterdam, The Netherlands

---

Several large, prospective cohort studies (both hospital and population based) of children with a solitary unprovoked seizure and with newly diagnosed epilepsy have been performed in the past four decades. However, no one has combined the available data in an all-encompassing overview or meta-analysis. Methodological differences severely impair such efforts. Nevertheless, comparing the available datasets could help to increase our understanding of the course, outcome and comorbidities after the diagnosis of new onset childhood epilepsy.

Table I details cohort size, study nature, age at onset of epilepsy and at start of inclusion, duration of follow-up and aetiology for four studies on which I propose to concentrate in this chapter. Here, they are called "global", because they encompass the entire field of childhood epilepsy and do not focus on specific types or syndromes. These studies are the Finnish study (Sillanpää *et al.*, 1993, 1998, 2006, 2009), the Nova Scotia study (Camfield & Camfield, 1993, 1997, 2007, 2010), as the population based studies; and the Connecticut study (Berg *et al.*, 1999, 2000, 2001a-c, 2006) and the Dutch study (1999, 2004, 2010), as the hospital-based studies. A number of other studies will be mentioned in passing, but not dealt with systematically. These include the Wirrell *et al.* (2011) study, the Oskoui *et al.* (2005) study and the Wakamoto *et al.* (2000) study. They are population based, but case ascertainment was mainly retrospective. The prognosis after a first solitary seizure (Shinnar *et al.*, 1999) will be dealt with elsewhere. Kwong *et al.* (2001, 2003) studied a pure prevalence cohort; it seems to me better to avoid the selection bias caused by this method (see below). Casetta *et al.* (1997, 1999) deal only with idiopathic and cryptogenic epilepsies, while Kokkonen *et al.* (1997) only present data about the psychosocial outcome. Finally, Chin *et al.* (2012) described the follow-up after 33 years of the children with epilepsy out of the 1958 British National Child Development Study (NCDS; Chin *et al.*, 2011), also with a special focus on psychosocial outcome.

After a discussion of methodological issues, I will compare the results of the various studies. This will hopefully yield the opportunity to formulate some cautious conclusions about the long-term prognosis of childhood epilepsy, the variables related to the outcome, the role of treatment and the clinical relevance of the global outcome studies. This review will focus on the seizures and epilepsy. Data on the cognitive and emotional development, school performance and psychosocial outcome will be discussed elsewhere.

■ Criteria defining the quality of a cohort study

Epidemiological research is commonly divided into three categories: cohort, case-control and cross-sectional studies. A number of requirements for such studies and the way of reporting about them have been presented in various guidelines (ILAE, 1993, 2010; Hirtz et al., 2000; Von Elm et al., 2007). For the purely observational cohort studies, a prospective study of patients, all from the same population, with a clearly established diagnosis, recruited in a consecutive and non-selective manner, with one or more clear question(s), preferably in the form of hypotheses formulated in advance, and with an adequate sample size to answer these questions are minimally required. However, the guidelines lack recommendations for the answers to be given and the choices to be made after these conditions have been fulfilled. Examples are: How should one deal with the problem of classification of the epilepsy, especially in view of the changing nature of the seizures when the child grows older? Should we prefer a population-based or a hospital-based cohort? How long should the cohort be followed? Should duration of follow-up be the same for every patient in the cohort, or can it be left to statistics to deal with the varying duration of follow-up at the fixed endpoint date? Which hypothesis is the starting point of the study? Can it be falsified? Which variables should be registered at intake? Is it worthwhile to collect determinants describing the early course of the epilepsy? How do we define the outcome parameters? By necessity, the definitions of the determinants and outcome parameters contain arbitrary components (e.g., an individual is considered in remission if the terminal remission is more than five years: why not four or six?). Does the arbitrary character of these definitions significantly influence the results of the analyses? These questions should be answered before the study starts, and the answers should be available in the protocol. If the answer cannot be given, e.g., for outcome parameters with an arbitrary component such as intractability or treatment resistance, it is best to adhere to generally applied definitions, agreed upon by epidemiological experts in authoritative societies like the ILAE.

None of the studies in *Table I* completely fulfils all requirements. Many methodological choices had to be made according to the local situation and the preferences of the investigators. I suggest that the accuracy and reliability of the diagnosis of epilepsy and of its classification should be enhanced by discussing every patient at intake and after follow-up in an expert panel, as we and others have demonstrated (Stroink et al., 2003, 2004; Middeldorp et al., 2002; Berg et al., 2000). But even then, systematic classification discrepancies between various groups of investigators may explain otherwise unexplainable differences in the aetiological classification of the patients (see *Table I*). Especially the distinction between "cryptogenic" and "idiopathic" seems to have been liable to misinterpretation and misunderstanding.

Further, an incidence cohort is better suited for a prospective follow-up study than a prevalence cohort, because collecting all active epilepsy cases in a population at a certain day or in a certain period of time may lead to overestimation of the more serious cases of epilepsy, and omit the benign and short-lived cases. The Finnish study contains more remote symptomatic cases and shows a greater mortality rate than the other studies

Table I. Basic information about the studies to be discussed

	Cohort size	Nature of the study	Age at inclusion	Year(s) of inclusion	Mean FU (years)	Aetiology
Finland	150 incident 95 prevalent	Population based until 1972 retrospective after 1972 prospective, partly incident, partly prevalent cohort	< 15 years	1961-1964	37.0 (SD 7.1, median 40.0, range 11-42) for 144 of the 150 incident cases	Incident cases: 31% idiopathic, 25% cryptogenic, 44% remote symptomatic
Nova Scotia	693 incident	Largely prospective population based, incident cohort	1 month to 16 years	1977-1985	13 (median 13.9, range 0-22.5) for 660 remaining subjects	31% idiopathic, 35% cryptogenic, 34% remote symptomatic
Connecticut	613 incident	Prospective hospital based with high recruitment rate, incident cohort	1 month to 16 years	1993-1997	Median 10.5	30% idiopathic, 52% cryptogenic, 18% remote symptomatic
Netherlands	493 incident	Prospective hospital based, ≈ 75% recruitment rate, incident cohort	1 month to 16 years	1988-1992	14.8 (11.6-17.5) for 413 remaining subjects	51% idiopathic, 21% cryptogenic, 28% remote symptomatic

(Sillanpää & Shinnar, 2010). This might be attributable to the more prevalent character of this study as compared with the others. The same applies to population-based cohorts as compared with hospital-based cohorts. Although the figures are not significantly different (see *Table I*), a bias might occur because a hospital-based cohort may contain relatively more serious cases compared with a population-based cohort. Here, history may illustrate my argument. The studies discussed in this chapter were in my view all initiated with the following hypothesis: epilepsy in children is to a large extent a more benign condition than current knowledge (that is: the knowledge of the sixties and seventies of the last century) holds. The knowledge of those days was mainly coming from epilepsy hospitals, institutions and wards that had the most serious epilepsy patients as their inhabitants, causing a lot of misunderstanding about the severity of the affection in the average epilepsy patient.

The discussion on the outcome parameters centres around the concept of intractability, as the ILAE 1993 definitions of remission and active epilepsy are, although somewhat arbitrary, relatively straightforward, and accepted by most investigators in the field. There is no consensus on the definition of intractable or difficult-to-treat epilepsy, although recently the ad hoc taskforce of the ILAE commission on therapeutic strategies has tried to lift the fog (Kwan *et al.*, 2010). The approach chosen by the task force was to define drug resistance, and they did so by looking at the length of the seizure-free period in any treated patient. To be successful, any given medical treatment should yield a seizure-free period of at least three times the longest pre-treatment seizure-free period, or one year, whichever is longest. However, apart from the practical difficulties in applying this definition in large groups of patients, it may include patients who are not really intractable. Patients might be considered drug-resistant when they have only sporadic seizures and are themselves satisfied with their degree of control. The same holds true for patients who have one or more incidental seizure(s) shortly before the follow-up moment, or have had long periods of remission in-between periods with seizures. This will be discussed in the next paragraph. Overall, drug resistance could be both a quality of the epilepsy of that patient, but also a quality of the prescribed treatment. In the opinion of our group, really intractable epilepsy is something more serious than the situations outlined above, and it is without any doubt a quality of the epilepsy itself. Therefore, while a definition based upon resistance to (medical) treatment can be used in individual cases to justify other treatment modalities (*e.g.*, surgery), a definition based upon lack of remission of a certain duration appears to be better suited for epidemiological research. For that reason, we defined intractability as not having a remission of more than three months during the last year of follow-up despite adequate treatment (Geerts *et al.*, 2012). Berg *et al.* (2006) used a similar definition, while Sillanpää and Schmidt (2006) defined drug resistance as having no remission of at least five years during ten or more years of follow-up despite continuous and adequate AED therapy. It can be added that a comparison of the taskforce approach with ours in the Dutch cohort reveals similar results, our definition being indeed more restrictive (Geerts *et al.*, 2012). Finally, we would certainly agree with the suggestion by Kwan *et al.* (2010) that, in addition to clinical criteria for the concept of intractability, clinicians should be encouraged to use a rating scale measuring patient (and parental) satisfaction in the assessment of their intervention and in clinical decision making.

The global prognosis studies: course and outcomes

According to the ILAE Commission (2011), terminal remission (TR) is still the best parameter to distinguish between good and poor outcome of epilepsy. Depending on the duration of follow-up, TR is defined as a period of 2 or 5 years without seizures and off AEDs. Most studies report TR numbers and percentages both on and off AEDs, however. *Table II* details 5-year terminal remissions for the four studies that present these data and deal exclusively with children. It should be remembered that the remission status at the time of follow-up represents only a static snapshot image, whereas the course of epilepsy really is a dynamic process. Nevertheless, it appears from the table that the proportions of patients in five-year remission are quite comparable despite differences in the duration of long-term follow-up. After shorter follow-up, the two- and one-year remission percentages are similar, too, as appears from a comparison of the short-term results of the Connecticut and the Dutch studies, illustrated in *Table III* (Berg et al., 2001c; Arts et al., 1999; Arts et al., 2004). From this table, it also becomes apparent that remission percentages tend to increase with longer follow-up.

Table II. Five-year terminal remission after long-term follow-up in four cohort studies

	Finland, incident cases only	Netherlands	Mayo Clinics	Japan
No. of patients	144	413	115	155
Follow-up (years)	37 (11-42)	15 (12-18)	20	19 (6-38)
TR ≥ 5 yrs, all	97 (67%)	293 (71%)	81 (70%)	93 (60%)
TR ≥ 5 yrs, off AED	58 (40%)	256 (62%)	52 (45%)	81 (52%)
Reference	Sillanpää, 2006	Geerts, 2010	Annegers, 1979	Wakamoto, 2000

Table III. One-year terminal remission after two years and two-year terminal remission after four or five years of follow-up in two prospective, hospital-based studies (n.a.: not available)

	Connecticut	Netherlands
TR2 ≥ 1 year	314/595 (53%)	264/466 (57%)
TR4 ≥ 2 years	261/390 (67%)	n.a.
TR5 ≥ 2 years	n.a.	290/453 (64%)

On the reverse side of the coin, the persistence of active epilepsy in about one third of the patients does not mean in the opinion of most investigators that these are all necessarily intractable. This is true for all durations of follow-up. Berg et al. (2001c) reported persisting epilepsy in 46%, but intractability in only 8% at the two-year follow-up, and at four years these numbers were 33% and 10%, respectively. In the Dutch study, 24% did not attain a one-year terminal remission at five years of follow-up, but only 6% fulfilled the criteria for intractability (Arts et al., 2004). After 15 years, the results were comparable, 9% being intractable and 29% still having active epilepsy (Geerts et al., 2010). Sillanpää and Schmidt (2006) considered 19% drug resistant, while 33% still had active epilepsy after very long-term follow-up. The greater proportion of intractable epilepsy in the latter study might again be attributed to the more prevalent character of the Finnish cohort, but the studies are difficult to compare as Sillanpää and Schmidt defined outcome in two categories: remission or not in remission, whereas the Connecticut and Dutch studies used three outcome categories: good, poor and in-between. In addition, the varying definitions of intractability and drug resistance could explain some of the differences found.

To get a better idea of prognosis and outcome in terms of remission, active epilepsy and intractability, focus should be shifted to the course of the epilepsy during the follow-up period. The reason for this is twofold. First, it has been demonstrated that an early poor course is strongly associated with a poor outcome after long-term follow-up. This can be illustrated in several ways. A poor response to the first AED trials (Carpay et al., 1998; Oskoui et al., 2005), or the repeated occurrence of seizures during the first months of follow-up without any significant period of remission (Arts et al., 2004; Sillanpää & Schmidt, 2009; Geerts et al., 2010) are both predictive of a poor outcome (see below). It also appears that early intractability is a strong predictor for late intractability, and this especially in combination with structural brain anomalies (Wirrell, personal communication). Secondly, as stated above, the course of epilepsy is a dynamic process. Both remission as well as active epilepsy and even intractability may be temporary phenomena of variable duration and frequency during the course of the epilepsy (Sillanpää and Schmidt 2006, Geerts et al., 2010, 2012). The variations of the course of the epilepsy during follow-up have led to a classification of the four possible categories: continuously favourable with a stable and long-lasting remission from the first year of treatment; improving, with a late but from then on stable remission of at least five years after a period with a poor or variable course; persistently poor, with continuing seizures during the entire follow-up; and variable and/or deteriorating, with early remission followed by alternating relapses and remissions but not attaining a five-year terminal remission (Sillanpää & Schmidt, 2006; Geerts et al., 2010). Table IV gives the corresponding percentages for the Finnish and Dutch cohort (Dutch data revised to fit the definitions used by Sillanpää) after 37 and 15 years of follow-up, respectively. It should be stressed that 66% of the Finnish and 45% of the Dutch cohort reached their endpoint through a process during which remission(s) and relapse(s) alternated. It cannot be stated with certainty that the follow-up of these patients was sufficiently long to be sure that the patient had reached his or her final result. Generally, though, the picture is again positive: two thirds of the cases in both cohorts have a favourable or improving course and one third a poor, deteriorating or variable course. It should be added that many investigators have the impression that intractability diminishes with a small percentage (1-2%) each year, although the long-term follow-up in the Dutch and Connecticut studies does not support this.

Table IV. Four types of possible clinical course and their frequency, expressed as numbers (percentages) with the specified course in two cohorts. For definitions of the categories of clinical course, see text

	Favourable	Improving	Poor	Deteriorating or variable
Finland (n = 144)	23 (16)	74 (52)	27 (19)	20 (14)
Netherlands (n = 413)	186 (45)	107 (26)	41 (10)	79 (19)

▪ Predictive variables

All studies have tried to identify predictors of the outcome available at the intake or start of treatment. Some (Camfield *et al.*, 1993; Camfield & Camfield, 2003; Ozkoui *et al.*, 2005) chose to focus on determinants for a good outcome; most, however, looked for determinants of a poor outcome. A few studies (Wakamoto, 2000; Sillanpää & Schmidt, 2006; Geerts *et al.*, 2010) have additionally examined the relation between the early course after the start of treatment and the eventual outcome. All studies agree that symptomatic epilepsy is the most important determinant for a poor outcome. Relative risks of symptomatic *vs.* idiopathic aetiology are surprisingly similar, varying between 3.6 and 4.3 (Sillanpää & Schmidt, 2006; Geerts *et al.*, 2010). Symptomatic epilepsy interacts with epilepsy type (symptomatic generalized [Camfield & Camfield, 2007] or localization-related symptomatic, notably complex partial epilepsy [Sillanpää & Schmidt, 2006; Camfield & Camfield, 2013]), with mental retardation (Wakamoto *et al.*, 2000; Camfield & Camfield, 2003; Sillanpää & Schmidt, 2006), and with the presence of structural brain anomalies (Wirrell *et al.*, submitted).

The early course of the epilepsy is also statistically relevant for the later course and outcome. Geerts *et al.* (2010) found in their multivariable analysis that not achieving a 3-month remission in the first six months of follow-up increased the odds for a poor outcome (OR 2.3, 95% CI 0.9; 5.6), and that a period of intractability in the first five years of follow-up was associated with an immensely increased risk for a poor outcome on the long run (OR 12.9, 95% CI 5.1; 32.4). Sillanpää & Schmidt (2009) found that having weekly seizures during the first year of treatment carried an eight-fold risk of developing drug-resistant epilepsy later. But in a slightly contradictory fashion, the same authors in the same cohort but a different publication (Sillanpää & Schmidt, 2006) concluded that initial success or failure of AED therapy to induce remission was not a reliable indicator for later remission or persisting active epilepsy. Early unresponsiveness to AEDs was usually associated with a poor or deteriorating course, but persisting remission could also be attained after many years of active epilepsy. And on the other hand, early remission could be followed by a persisting relapse and eventually a poor outcome in rare, almost all symptomatic cases. In my opinion, this illustrates the continuing struggle between the statistical probabilities in a cohort *vs.* the individual exceptions that always occur, impairing the use of statistical conclusions for clinical practice.

I will not deal with specific epilepsy types and syndromes here, as they will be discussed in several chapters elsewhere in this book. Camfield & Camfield (2003) gave a comprehensive overview of studies that examined the prognosis of various specific syndromes. They had to conclude that for most studies, the level of evidence was only class 3. In most publications on cohort studies, a survey of syndrome diagnoses and their outcomes was given (Berg *et al.*, 2001c; Sillanpää & Schmidt, 2006; Camfield & Camfield, 2007; Geerts *et al.*, 2010). Usually, only the more frequent syndromes were represented in the cohorts in sufficient numbers to draw conclusions about long-term remission or not. For the rarer syndromes, cohort studies are not the best way to study their prognosis.

▪ Treatment effects

Most global cohort studies were pragmatic studies, meaning that the treating physician was free to prescribe the individual patient the treatment of his choice. Moreover, methodologically a cohort study may not be the best way to evaluate the effect of specific antiepileptic drugs. And in the third place, most AEDs show comparable results in randomized clinical trials. Therefore, it is justifiable that most cohort studies only describe the effects of treatment in general. With that in mind, the following issues can be addressed: starting AED treatment, yes or no; response to AEDs; the effect of AED therapy on the long-term prognosis of epilepsy and the prevention of intractable or chronic epilepsy. In the past, a number of studies have in addition dealt with the issue of withdrawal of AEDs in children after years of remission. This will not be discussed here.

Only two studies presented data about the number of children in which the decision to withhold treatment was taken. Berg et al. (2001) mentioned that 20% of the children in the Connecticut cohort were not treated initially, half of which remained untreated after one year. Of these 10%, more than half had a two-year remission of more than one year. No data about longer follow-up of this cohort are available. In the Dutch study (Arts et al., 1999, 2004; Geerts et al., 2010), 74 out of 466 children were not treated during the first two years of follow-up. At that time, 12 of them (16%) had not succeeded in attaining at least a 6-month terminal remission (overall 31%). In most of them, the decision not to start treatment was maintained because of the type of epilepsy (e.g., benign rolandic) or the low frequency of the isolated seizures. After five years of follow-up, 65 of the above 74 (14% of the 453 children remaining in the follow-up) were still not treated, with 61 of them (94%) having a TR5 of at least one year. After 15 years, 57 out of the remaining 413 children (14%) had never used AEDs, a terminal remission of more than five years was attained by 53 of them. Apparently, not all children with epilepsy will need treatment, and physicians experienced in the treatment of childhood epilepsy are capable of identifying them (Arts & Geerts, 2009). It is our impression that this group consists mainly of children with benign rolandic epilepsy or with idiopathic generalized epilepsy with sporadic generalized tonic-clonic seizures. As a group, they are comparable with children who are treated, but successfully stop treatment relatively early during their follow-up because they remit early and remain seizure-free thereafter, and both groups can be labelled together as "smooth-sailing epilepsy" (Camfield et al., 1990). In the Nova Scotia study, this group comprised 21% of the cohort, in the Dutch study 26% (128 children, of which 42 untreated and 86 with a fast and stable remission following treatment, i.e., within two months). In the Dutch study, 47 of these 128 children (10.4% of the cohort) had sporadic generalized tonic-clonic convulsions (30 only afebrile, 17 in combination with febrile seizures). Their excellent outcome (TR > 5 years at long-term follow-up in 84%, in combination with the smooth-sailing course) made us suggest that this might be a separate epileptic syndrome.

Most children with definitely diagnosed epilepsy are treated with AEDs, usually first in mono-, and if necessary later in polytherapy. Literature data suggest that many children go in remission while on their first AED, and that this first remission is permanent for most of them. However, even from this group some develop later intractability, while on the other hand, a considerable proportion of those with a terminal remission reach their remission only with the second or higher AED regime (Table V).

Table V. Results of AED treatment in three cohorts.

Note that the composition of the cohorts, the duration of follow-up and the definitions of terminal remission and intractability / drug resistance vary between these studies. The table is, therefore, only able to indicate trends. Numbers (%)

Result of first AED	Camfield et al., 1997 (n = 417)	Sillanpää & Schmidt, 2006 (n = 144)	Arts et al., 2004 (n = 388)
Positive on 1st AED	345 (83)	45 (31)	206 (53)
Terminal remission	210 (50)	37 (26)	178 (46)
Intractable	14 (3)	8 (6)	15 (4)
Negative on 1st AED	72 (17)	99 (69)	182 (47)
Terminal remission	30 (7)	60 (42)	109 (28)
Intractable	21 (5)	39 (27)	12 (3)

In addition to these data, Carpay et al. (1998) and Berg et al. (2001c) noted that non-compliance and other reasons not to take AEDs could explain only a relatively small part of the patients who did not respond well to the initial treatment. All this suggests that the response to treatment is part of the disease process, and that treatment has only a limited effect on the long-term course of the epilepsy while it is often able to suppress seizures. This may also be concluded from studies in third-world countries, where the availability of AED is limited. In a cross-sectional study of 1029 patients with epilepsy in Ecuador (Placencia et al., 1994), only 12% took AED, while 37% had taken AED at least some time in the past. Of the seizure-free patients (44% of the cohort), two thirds had never used AED. In a 10-year prospective follow-up study of 118 untreated patients with "active" epilepsy in Bolivia, data on 71 patients were of sufficient quality to draw conclusions (Nicoletti et al., 2009). Of these 71, 31 (44%) had been seizure-free for more than five years, despite the fact that only 3 of them received regular AED therapy during at least part of the follow-up period.

Progress in this field is hampered by the fact that we do not know much about the natural history of a chronic disorder like epilepsy. The concept of smooth-sailing epilepsy, its predictability and the need to collect knowledge about the course of untreated epilepsy convinced the Halifax and Dutch groups that we should start a study of omitting treatment in children with epilepsy with a good to excellent prognosis. Unfortunately, we did not succeed in making this a randomized trial, since parents refused their child to be randomized for AED treatment. Once they knew what we were up to, they decided for themselves that they wanted the no-treatment option. Therefore, the study developed into an observational prospective study of an initially untreated cohort with a supposedly good prognosis. We agreed to start treatment when 10 or more seizures had occurred (Camfield et al., 1996), after a status epilepticus or when the parents, patient and treating physician agreed that treatment should be started. Children up to 12 years with a history of not more than five unprovoked seizures, who had not yet been treated, without neurologic signs, developmental delay, imaging abnormalities, and not having a history of neonatal seizures, status epilepticus, absences, myoclonic jerks or any sign of a malignant epilepsy syndrome were included. We recruited 176 children and could follow 151 (64 female; age at onset 6.7 + 0.4 years) for three years. After three years, 97 children (64%) remained untreated, among which were 14 who had had more than 10 seizures. On the other hand,

- Kwong KL, Sung WY, Wong SN, So KT. Early predictors of medical intractability in childhood epilepsy. *Pediatr Neurol* 2003; 29: 46-52.
- Middeldorp CM, Geerts AT, Brouwer OF, et al. Nonsymptomatic generalized epilepsy in children younger than six years: excellent prognosis, but classification should be reconsidered after follow-up: the Dutch Study of Epilepsy in Childhood. *Epilepsia* 2002; 43: 734-9.
- Nicoletti A, Sofia V, Vitale G, et al. Natural history and mortality of chronic epilepsy in an untreated population of rural Bolivia: a follow-up after 10 years. *Epilepsia* 2009; 50: 2199-206.
- Oskoui M, Webster RI, Zhang X, Shevell MI. Factors predictive of outcome in childhood epilepsy. *J Child Neurol* 2005; 20: 898-904.
- Placencia M, Sander JW, Roman M, et al. The characteristics of epilepsy in a largely untreated population in rural Ecuador. *J Neurol Neurosurg Psychiatry* 1994; 57: 320-5.
- Shinnar S, O'Dell C, Berg AT. Distribution of epilepsy syndromes in a cohort of children prospectively monitored from the time of their first unprovoked seizure. *Epilepsia* 1999; 40: 1378-83.
- Sillanpää M. Remission of seizures and predictors of intractability in long-term follow-up. *Epilepsia* 1993; 34: 930-6.
- Sillanpää M, Jalava M, Kaleva O, Shinnar S. Long-term prognosis of seizures with onset in childhood. *N Engl J Med* 1998; 338: 1715-22.
- Sillanpää M, Schmidt D. Natural history of treated childhood-onset epilepsy: prospective, long-term population-based study. *Brain* 2006; 129: 617-24.
- Sillanpää M, Schmidt D. Early seizure frequency and aetiology predict long-term medical outcome in childhood-onset epilepsy. *Brain* 2009; 132: 989-98.
- Sillanpää M, Shinnar S. Long-term mortality in childhood-onset epilepsy. *N Engl J Med* 2010; 363: 2522-9.
- Stroink H, Van Donselaar CA, Geerts AT, Peters AC, Brouwer OF, Arts WF. The accuracy of the diagnosis of paroxysmal events in children. *Neurology* 2003; 60: 979-82.
- Stroink H, Van Donselaar CA, Geerts AT, et al. Interrater agreement of the diagnosis and classification of a first seizure in childhood. The Dutch Study of Epilepsy in Childhood. *J Neurol Neurosurg Psychiatry* 2004; 75: 241-5.
- Von Elm E, Egger M, Altman DG, Pocock SJ, Götzsche PC, Vandenbroucke JP, for STROBE. Strengthening the reporting of observational studies in epidemiology (STROBE) statement: guidelines for reporting observational studies. *Brit Med J* 2007; 335: 806-8.
- Wakamoto H, Nagao H, Hayashi M, Morimoto T. Long-term medical, educational, and social prognoses of childhood-onset epilepsy: a population-based study in a rural district of Japan. *Brain Dev* 2000; 22: 246-55.
- Wirrell EC, Camfield CS, Camfield PR, Dooley JM, Gordon KE, Smith B. Long-term psychosocial outcome in typical absence epilepsy. Sometimes a wolf in sheeps' clothing. *Arch Pediatr Adolesc Med* 1997; 151: 152-8.
- Wirrell EC, Grossardt BR, Wong-Kisiel LC, Nickels KC. Incidence and classification of new-onset epilepsy and epilepsy syndromes in children in Olmsted County, Minnesota from 1980 to 2004: a population-based study. *Epilepsy Res* 2011; 95: 110-8.

Does treatment with antiepileptic drugs influence the long-term outcome of newly diagnosed epilepsies?

Alexis Arzimanoglou

Epilepsy, Sleep and Paediatric Neurophysiology Department, University Hospitals of Lyon (HCL), Lyon, France

The term "newly diagnosed epilepsy" refers to a number of epilepsies and epilepsy syndromes, some often requiring life-long treatment with antiepileptic drugs (AEDs). For the majority of these disorders or diseases, natural evolution and outcome are either still poorly known or mainly seem to depend upon the underlying aetiology. Furthermore, patients with epilepsy, most particularly children, are at risk not only for seizures, but also for a number of comorbid health conditions, including cognitive dysfunction (memory, attention, and concentration problems) and other mental health conditions, such as depression or anxiety (2012 IOM Report: Epilepsy Across the Spectrum). Consequently, the question to be treated in this chapter is expected to cover not just control of one symptom (seizures) but a complex algorithm of symptoms referring to different disorders or diseases (epilepsies). A different formulation could be: *do currently available AEDs modify the natural evolution of each epilepsy disorder and if "yes", how?*

It is however difficult to define the limits of the most appropriate answer to such a question in the absence of a consensus definition of *"disease modification"*. It could be required, for example, that the intervention, in our case AEDs, addresses the underlying neurobiological processes leading and/or sustaining epileptogenesis. A broader definition could be two-fold: halting, slowing, or preventing the development of epilepsy in susceptible individuals and/or having an impact on clinically relevant milestones once epilepsy is present.

Unresolved issues remain regarding the definition of "clinically relevant" milestones. From a patient's point of view a "simple" control of seizures is often considered as a sufficiently strong disease modification factor. However, patients also hope for a more global control of their disease, usually expressed as a questioning on when AEDs could be discontinued, a strong sign that they are cured from their disease.

The whole issue of disease modification becomes even more multifactorial when aspects related to the causes of the epilepsies have to be considered. Disease onset and progression are variable, with survival ranging from months to decades. Factors underlying this variability may represent targets for therapeutic intervention.

For the sake of space issues related to disease modification by treating the underlying causal aetiology, for example the medical treatment of a metabolic epilepsy or the surgical/curative treatment of a focal lesional epilepsy will not be discussed in this chapter.

■ What can we conclude from the currently available studies on AEDs?

In spite of the development and the availability of more than 20 AEDs, labelled as effective and efficacious based on large, double blind, randomized clinical trials, it is estimated that still at least 25-40% of newly diagnosed patients will remain refractory and continue to have seizures (Schmdit & Sillanpää, 2012). Regulatory approval has been based on clinical trial designs that measure responder rate (> 50% seizure reduction). These many trials do not permit a distinction to be made between an effect of the drug on seizure frequency and eventual effects on other symptoms of a given epilepsy syndrome. They also do not allow any evaluation of the effects on the pathophysiological mechanisms that underlie the disorder. Most of the available trials are also of too short duration (6 months to one year), thus not designed to provide clues on long-term outcome (Arzimanoglou et al., 2010).

Consequently all currently available trials designed to assess seizure reduction, cannot provide evidence-based data about the influence of AED treatment on long-term outcome.

Quality of life (QOL) is an important outcome measure for which validated scales are available; however, it does not directly reflect seizure reduction or other efficacy measures. QOL is most strongly influenced by AED tolerability, but is also modestly influenced by other parameters, including seizure frequency, seizure severity, and convenience. Change in mood appears to be the second most important influence on QOL, and may be relevant to some AEDs. As there is a weak correlation between seizure frequency and QOL, use of QOL alone may be insufficient (Ben-Menachem et al., 2010). A drug might improve mood and, by doing so, enhance QOL without reducing the seizure load. AED use may impact a patient's health-related QOL (HRQOL) substantially (Jacoby et al., 2007). Because individuals with epilepsy report significant reductions in HRQOL compared with healthy individuals (Centers for Disease Control and Prevention, 2001; 2005) complete seizure control with AEDs should improve HRQOL, contingent upon AED tolerability.

The exact causes of cognitive impairment in epilepsy have not been explored fully, but three factors clearly are involved: aetiology, the seizures, and the "central" side effects of drug treatment (Aldenkamp & Bootsma, 2005). When evaluating the unwanted effects of antiepileptic medication separately, it is imperative to realize that in clinical practice most cognitive problems have a multifactorial origin and that, for the most part, the three aforementioned factors combine and become responsible for the cognitive problem of an individual patient. Moreover, the factors are related, which causes a therapeutic dilemma in some patients when seizure control can only be achieved with treatments that are associated with cognitive side effects. A general conclusion that may be derived from most of the meta-analyses (Vermeulen & Aldenkamp, 1995) is that polypharmacy shows a relatively severe impact on cognitive function when compared with monotherapy, irrespective of the type of AEDs included. Possibly the most remarkable finding is that, although the severity of cognitive side effects is generally considered to be mild to moderate for most AEDs (Vermeulen & Aldenkamp, 1995), all commonly used AEDs have some impact on cognitive function. Such mild impact may be amplified in specific conditions and may become substantial in some patients when crucial functions are involved, such as learning in children or driving capacities in adults (often requiring millisecond precision), or when functions are impaired that are already vulnerable, such as memory function. The effects may increase with prolonged therapy, which contributes to the impact on daily life functioning in refractory epilepsies.

In summary, studies on adverse events of AEDs, particularly those evaluating cognitive effects or Quality of Life (QOL) assessments do provide some data on long-term outcome. However, extrapolation from these studies is not possible when evaluating the impact of AEDs on long-term outcome and prognosis for each epilepsy syndrome.

■ What can we conclude from clinical practice and studies on global outcome?

When discussing outcome in clinical practice it is apparent that patients need to be considered by their specific epilepsy diagnosis and/or syndrome. By definition, outcome as related to AED treatment cannot be discussed when considering all types of epilepsy together. The reason is that each epileptic syndrome or epilepsy disease has its own characteristics; types of seizures are not the same and the drugs to be used differ.

Focal idiopathic epilepsies

In terms of seizure control, outcome of rolandic and occipital epilepsies (both the Gastaut and the Panayiotopoulos types), have an age-dependent natural evolution not directly related to the AEDs chosen and/or to early treatment with AEDs, when treated. As an example, the mean duration of active rolandic epilepsy is estimated to be of 3 years only (Bouma et al., 1977). This is regardless of initial resistance to treatment (approximately 20%), the presence or absence of a Todd's paralysis and probably independently of treatment or no treatment with AEDs. Long-term cohort studies reached similar conclusions (Callenbach et al., 2010) since, all children in this cohort, both those with typical and atypical rolandic epilepsy, had a very good prognosis with 100% entering remission by age 12-17 years.

However, the above facts need to be tempered when evaluating educational and societal aspects. As recent studies clearly suggest the educational, social and professional achievements of patients with rolandic epilepsy *as a group* may not differ from those of the general population, no matter what treatment was used and when. But at an *individual level*, a diversity of educational deficits, behavioural impairments, language delay and other neuropsychological deficits have been reported. One interpretation could be that AED treatments, even when appropriately chosen, do not influence long-term outcome of these epilepsy syndromes. Another consideration would be the value of treating (how?) interictal EEG abnormalities, especially in sleep. In this case the "clinically meaningful" factor to evaluate should be short and long-term cognitive and behavioural parameters, rather than seizure frequency.

Generalized idiopathic epilepsies (IGE)

The great majority of children and adolescents with epilepsy syndromes corresponding to this large category (benign myoclonic epilepsy; childhood or adolescence absence epilepsy; juvenile myoclonic epilepsy) respond rather easily to a number of the currently available broad spectrum AEDs. Drugs like sodium valproate, lamotrigine, levetiracetam, topiramate and the benzodiazepines are usually efficacious, although at a variable degree, for the control of typical absence seizures, generalized tonic-clonic seizures or myoclonic seizures while ethosuximide can be used for the control of absences or myoclonic seizures. In terms of prognosis all entities concerned are *age-related syndromes*, both in terms of age at onset and seizure outcome (Duron et al., 2005).

Long-term outcome of *childhood absence epilepsy* (CAE) is considered favourable with one study finding only 7% still having seizures after 12-17 years of age (Callenbach et al., 2009). Other studies have been somewhat less optimistic (Wirrell et al., 1996). Remission cannot be accurately predicted on the basis of baseline and EEG characteristics but the early clinical course has some predictive value with respect to the total duration of absence epilepsy. *Juvenile myoclonic epilepsy* (JME) seems to be a life-long disorder for most patients. In many case series, only a small percent (about 10%) of children with clear-cut JME can discontinue AEDs and enter a very long (if not permanent) remission (Panayiotopoulos et al., 1994). However, a lifetime of daily medication is difficult to justify if it is not clearly needed. A highly individual decision has to be made, with the consequences of another seizure weighed against years of unnecessary medication. According to the Camfields (2005) and to our personal experience, most patients choose to continue with daily AEDs, often at a lower dose to what is needed during adolescence. Better markers for those who will succeed without medication are sorely needed.

As is the case for focal idiopathic epilepsies, control of seizures in IGE syndromes appears to be independent of the interval between the first seizure and the beginning of AED treatment. This is not surprising for age dependent syndromes. Consequently, it could be argued that AED treatment is not disease-modifying in this setting at least from the perspective of seizure control. What is much more difficult to evaluate is global outcome, both educational and social. Controlled studies are lacking on the importance of controlling (how?) or failing to control interictal bilateral spike-wave discharges. The long-term effects of transient cognitive impairment from spike-wave bursts are unknown. Social integration is often unsatisfactory in IGE syndromes. Even in patients with CAE that has remitted, up to 30% have serious social problems (Loiseau et al., 1983). The social outcome of JME patients has also not been extensively evaluated. According to Camfield and Camfield (2009), after a follow-up of 25 to 43 years, 31% were unemployed, 61% had taken a psychotropic drug, and overall 74% had at least one measure of negative social outcome.

As above, one interpretation could be that AED treatments, even when appropriately chosen, do not influence long-term outcome of IGE epilepsy syndromes. However, such an extrapolation is rather risky in the absence of controlled studies comparing treated with non-treated patients. We personally find it difficult to accept that untreated IGE patients with persisting seizures and abundance of EEG abnormalities during the crucial period, in terms of education and learning, of childhood and adolescence would have the same social integration as those controlled by currently available AEDs. The simple fact that uncontrolled seizures in a patient with JME would deprive him/her of a driving licence supports the argument that when approached in terms of global outcome, current AEDs have a disease-modifying effect in the broadest sense of this term.

Epileptic encephalopathies (EE)

For the purposes of this chapter we included in this category epilepsy syndromes like West syndrome, Lennox-Gastaut syndrome, Dravet syndrome and encephalopathy with status epilepticus during sleep (ESES). Epilepsies with predominantly myoclonic-astatic seizures could be included in the previous section on IGE. They will be briefly discussed in this section because in our opinion they represent, together with West syndrome, the best examples suggesting at least some degree of disease modification by the currently available AEDs.

West syndrome is probably the best example. The global prognosis for children with infantile spasms is strongly influenced, if not entirely determined, by the pathologic process underlying the syndrome (for an extensive review see Arzimanoglou et al., 2004). The influence of treatment lag has been variously reported. Most authors, however, believe that the earlier the treatment, whether medical or surgical, the better the ultimate outcome. The association between a short treatment lag and a good prognosis is not necessarily one of *cause and effect* as the effect of prompt treatment is difficult to separate from the effect of the intrinsic severity of the disorder. A rapid response to medical therapy, with disappearance of the spasms and the hypsarrhythmic pattern within a week, probably has a favourable prognostic significance.

The role of treatment on global outcome of *Lennox-Gastaut syndrome* (LGS) is more difficult to evaluate. The term LGS is often loosely used to denote severe epilepsy syndromes of childhood featuring several types of intractable seizures, including falls. However, such a broad definition encompasses several types of epilepsy, including some of the epilepsy disorders that have predominantly myoclonic-astatic seizures, for which the outcome and therapy can differ (Arzimanoglou et al., 2004). The nosological uncertainty is accentuated by the fact that the core seizures (*i.e.*, tonic, atonic, and atypical absences) are not always present at onset and the interictal EEG pattern of slow spike-waves that is associated with LGS is not pathognomonic (Arzimanoglou et al., 2009).

Controlled studies on treatment of LGS with new AEDs were, unfortunately, not designed to assess the overall value of early treatment. To be included in these studies a child had to present the full clinical and EEG picture of the syndrome. As a result, and in the absence of biological markers that could confirm the diagnosis at its early stages, young patients had to be excluded in favour of patients with a long history of drug-resistant LGS. Aetiology, as in West syndrome, remains one of the most determinant factors. Nevertheless, clinical experience and anecdotal reports during the last 10-15 years strongly suggest that in a number of cases treated early in the course of the disorder, *i.e.*, before the development of the full clinical picture, with appropriately chosen large spectrum AEDs, global outcome is better than in the past. It remains possible that some of these children with favourable outcome in fact have one of the relatively benign disorders in the spectrum of epilepsies with predominantly myoclonic-astatic seizures. This introduces a bias when discussing response and overall effect of treatment. However, there is a strong impression that the number of cases of so-called typical (and severe) LGS has reduced in recent years even in tertiary centers that deal with severe epilepsies. Novel endpoints and measurements

- Camfield C, Camfield P. Management guidelines for children with idiopathic generalized epilepsy. *Epilepsia* 2005; 46 (Suppl 9): 112-6.
- Camfield CS, Camfield PR. Juvenile myoclonic epilepsy 25 years after seizure onset: a population-based study. *Neurolog.* 2009; 73: 1041-5.
- Centers for Disease Control and Prevention. Health-related quality of life among persons with epilepsy-Texas, 1998. *MMWRMorb Mortal Wkly Rep* 2001; 50: 24-6, 35.
- Centers for Disease Control and Prevention. Prevalence of epilepsy and healthrelated quality of life and disability among adults with epilepsy, South Carolina, 2003 and 2004. *MMWR Morb Mortal Wkly Rep* 2005; 54: 1080-2.
- Dravet C, Bureau M, Oguni H, Cokar O, Guerrini R. Dravet syndrome (severe myoclonic epilepsy in infancy). In: Bureau M, Genton P, Dravet C, et al. (eds). *Epileptic Syndrome Infancy, Childhood and Adolescence, SH ed.* Montrouge: John Libbey Eurotext, 2012, pp. 125-56.
- Durón RM, Medina MT, Martínez-Juárez IE, et al. Seizures of idiopathic generalized epilepsies. *Epilepsia* 2005; 46 (Suppl 9): 34-47.
- Geerts A, Arts WF, Stroink H, et al. Course and outcome of childhood epilepsy: a 15-year follow-up of the Dutch Study of Epilepsy in Childhood. *Epilepsia* 2010; 51: 1189-97.
- Geerts A, Brouwer O, Stroink H, et al. Onset of intractability and its course over time: the Dutch study of epilepsy in childhood. *Epilepsia* 2012; 53: 741-51.
- Haut SR, Velísková J, Moshé SL. Susceptibility of immature and adult brains to seizure effects. *Lancet Neurol* 2004; 3: 608-17.
- Helmstaedter C, Hermann B, Lassonde M, Kahane P, Arzimanoglou A. *Neuropsychology in the Care of People with Epilepsy.* Paris: John Libbey Eurotext, 2011.
- Holthausen H, Fogarasi A, Arzimanoglou A, Kahane P. Structural (symptomatic) focal epilepsies of childhood. In: Bureau M, Genton P, Dravet C, et al. (eds). *Epileptic Syndromes in Infancy, Childhood and Adolescence, 5th edition.* Paris: John Libbey Eurotext, 2012, pp. 455-505.
- Jacoby A, Gamble C, Doughty J, et al. Quality of life outcomes of immediate or delayed treatment of early epilepsy and single seizures. *Neurology* 2007; 68: 1188-96.
- Loiseau P, Pestre M, Dartigues JF, Commenges D, Barberger-Gateau C, Cohadon S. Long-term prognosis in two forms of childhood epilepsy: typical absence seizures and epilepsy with rolandic (centrotemporal) EEG foci. *Ann Neurol* 1983; 13: 642-8.
- Panayiotopoulos CP, Obeid T, Tahan AR. Juvenile myoclonic epilepsy: a 5-year prospective study. *Epilepsia* 1994; 35: 285-96.
- Schmidt D, Sillanpää M. Evidence-based review on the natural history of the epilepsies. *Curr Opin Neurol* 2012; 25: 159-63.
- Veggiotti P, Termine C, Granocchio E, Bova S, Papalia G, Lanzi G. Long-term neuropsychological follow-up and nosological considerations in five patients with continuous spikes and waves during slow sleep. *Epileptic Disord* 2002; 4: 243-9.
- Vermeulen J, Aldenkamp AP. Cognitive side-effects of chronic antiepileptic drug treatment: a review of 25 years of research. *Epilepsy Res* 1995; 22: 65-95.
- Wirrell EC, Camfield CS, Camfield PR, Gordon KE, Dooley JM. Long-term prognosis of typical childhood absence epilepsy: remission or progression to juvenile myoclonic epilepsy. *Neurology* 1996; 47: 912-8.

relationship of aetiology and other outcomes within this cohort described above, it was surprising that aetiology rather than CSE was not significant in multivariable analysis especially since it was more significant on univariable analysis compared to a history of CSE. This may be related to the high attrition with resulting modest sample size at follow-up and the characteristics of the remaining participants compared to those lost to follow-up.

1958 British Birth Cohort Study (Chin et al., 2011)

In this study, a subgroup of 101 children with epilepsy who were previously identified and validated amongst 17,414 children born in one week in Britain in the 1958 National Child Development Study (NCDS), a national UK birth cohort study, were studied. 51 (50%) were male, 34 (34%) required special needs schooling by age 7 years, 65 (65%) were seizure free by age 23 years, and there were no reported deaths (95% CI 0-4%) by age 16 years, although 6 were reported as having died between ages 16 and 23 years. Eighteen had CSE by age 23 years. At age 23 years, 77 were available for follow up and 65 at age 33 years. In multivariable analysis, CSE was not an independent predictor for seizure freedom by age 23 years. Having had CSE was not independently associated with increased mortality, lower educational attainments, being a parent, being married, or being employed.

Nova Scotia, Canada (Camfield & Camfield, 2012)

All children with newly diagnosed epilepsy were identified by EEG requests, review of medical records, and direct interview by two paediatric neurologist in Nova Scotia between 1977 and 1985. They were seen intermittently by the two original neurologists from initial enrollment to 2009-2011 (24-34 year follow up) when the effect of unprovoked CSE on the prognosis for otherwise normal children with focal epilepsy was investigated.

One hundred and eighty eight cases with focal epilepsy, normal intelligence, and neurologic examination and follow-up ≥ 10 years had a mean follow-up of 27 ± 5 years with no deaths from CSE. Thirty-nine (20%) had CSE. The remission rate (seizure-free without AEDs at the end of follow-up) for CSE patients was 24 of 39 (61%) *versus* 99 of 149 (66%) who had no CSE (P = .5). At follow-up, 11 (28%) CSE and 49 (33%) no-CSE patients had learning disorders (not statistically significant). Grades repeated, high school graduation, and advanced education did not differ between CSE and non-CSE children. Together, these results suggest that CSE has little influence on long-term seizure outcome and educational level in normally intelligent children with focal epilepsy.

Japan (Wakamoto et al., 2000)

One hundred and forty eight children who developed epilepsy before age 16 years between 1961-1992 within the prefecture of Ehime were followed up for a mean period of 18.9 years (range 6-37.5 years). Of these, 93% were followed up at a mean age of 26 years through medical record review and telephone interviews. They were compared to age matched controls from the same geographic area. Forty percent were idiopathic, 14% were cryptogenic and 46% were remote symptomatic. Twenty nine (20%) had a history of CSE. No multivariable analysis was done but on univariable analysis a lower proportion of those who had a high frequency of CSE (7/29 = 24%) achieved 5YTR compared to those who had a low frequency or absence of CSE (83/119 = 70%). Three quarters of patients who had idiopathic or cryptogenic epilepsy attained 5YTR compared to 46% of those who had remote symptomatic epilepsy. No analysis of the effect of CSE on other outcomes were reported.

■ Convulsive status epilepticus in recent longitudinal hospital based studies of childhood onset epilepsy

Dutch study of epilepsy (Stroink et al., 2007)

Stroink and colleagues developed a hospital-based cohort of 494 children aged 1 month to 15 years with newly diagnosed epilepsy (defined as two or more unprovoked seizures within a 1-year period) recruited from August 1988 to August 1992. Children were recruited from two University hospitals in Rotterdam and Leiden, and two hospitals in The Hague – a children's hospital and a general hospital. The cohort comprised about 75% of the expected incidence in their referral areas. In this study, the cohort was followed prospectively for 5 years to investigate terminal remission at 5 years and mortality in children having had CSE as the presenting sign or after the diagnosis.

Two hundred and fifty (51%) children had idiopathic epilepsy, 96 (19%) had cryptogenic epilepsy, and 148 (30%) had remote symptomatic epilepsy. Forty seven (10%) children had CSE. Forty-one of them had CSE when epilepsy was diagnosed. Mortality was not significantly increased for children with CSE: 4.9% of children who had CSE versus 1.6% in those who had not had CSE. Terminal remission at 5 years (TR5) was not significantly worse for these 41 children. On multivariable analysis, aetiology was the strongest predictor for poor outcomes; CSE was not an independent risk factor for poor outcomes.

■ Population-based studies of childhood convulsive status epilepticus

North London, United Kingdom (Chin et al., 2006; Pujar et al., 2011)

The north London Convulsive status epilepticus in childhood surveillance study (NLSTEPSS) was the first population-based study focused on childhood status epilepticus. Two hundred and twenty six children with CSE, of which 176 had lifetime first episodes were enrolled between 2002 and 2004. Follow up investigating morbidity at a mean follow up of 8.5 years is currently ongoing but preliminary results suggest that the underlying aetiology and not CSE itself is predictive of poor outcomes. It will be interesting to compare the results from the population-based NLSTEPSS with those from hospital based studies, including the work by Maytal et al. (Maytal et al., 1989) and Aicardi and Chevrie (Aicardi & Chevrie, 1970). Maytal et al. recruited 193 children (97 prospectively) and followed them up for a mean of 8.1 months. At follow up, 4% had died (which is similar to the 30 day survival reported in NLSTEPSS below), and amongst survivors 9% had new motor or cognitive deficits, and 29% had afebrile seizures. In Aicardi and Chevrie's retrospective study of 239 children with at least 60 minutes of seizure activity defining status epilepticus (Aicardi & Chevrie, 1970), fatality 5 to 10 years after CSE was 11% (which is similar to the long term fatality in NLSTEPSS below) and morbidity in excess of 50%.

Overall case fatality at a mean follow up of 7.7 years in NLSTEPSS was 11% (95% confidence interval 7.5-16.2%); seven children died within 30 days of their episode of convulsive status epilepticus and 16 during follow-up (Pujar et al., 2011). The overall mortality was 46 times greater than expected in the UK childhood reference population, and was predominantly due to higher mortality in children who had pre-existing clinically significant neurological impairments when they had their acute episode of convulsive status epilepticus. No child with prolonged febrile seizures died.

The authors had no comparison group of children with epilepsy in the study to assess the direct effect of CSE. However, the authors indirectly analysed the attributive role of CSE by comparing mortality in idiopathic CSE in their cohort with the published mortality in children with idiopathic epilepsy, and mortality in children with neurological impairments in their cohort with that of remote symptomatic epilepsy and cerebral palsy. The latter groups were chosen because they were the main groups that made up the subcategory of children with pre-existing neurological problem in their cohort.

There were no deaths in children who had idiopathic CSE in the NLSTEPSS cohort (SMR 0, 95% CI 0.0-3.68), an observation similar to the low mortality reported in children with idiopathic epilepsy (Camfield et al., 2002; Berg et al., 2004; Geerts et al., 2010, Sillanpaa & Shinnar, 2010). The SMR for children with significant neurological impairment prior to their episode of CSE in NLSTEPSS was 91.4 (95% CI 53.2-146.3). In comparison, reported SMRs in children with symptomatic epilepsies range between 22.9 (95% CI 7.9-37.9) and 49.7 (95% CI 31.7-77.9) (Callenbach et al., 2001; Geerts et al., 2010; Berg et al., 2004). The mortality in the NLSTEPSS cohort with significant neurological impairment prior to CSE was higher than that reported for remote symptomatic epilepsy. Children with remote symptomatic epilepsy do not necessarily have major neurological impairments and therefore direct comparison with the NLSTEPSS cohort is not very robust. The mortality in the NSLTEPSS cohort is probably more comparable with the reported mortality in children with cerebral palsy, a cohort likely to have similar neurological impairments (SMR 36.4 for mild and 102.8 for severe cerebral palsy) (Strauss et al., 1999).

Kenya, Africa (Sadarangani et al., 2008)

Three hundred and eighty eight episodes of CSE, 155 (40%) confirmed and 233 probable cases were identified through review of case notes of all children between 1 months and 13 years of age with a history of seizures, epilepsy, febrile seizures or encephalopathy who were admitted between Jan 1, 2002 and Dec 31, 2003 to the main district level hospital serving Kilifi. Confirmed cases had been observed directly whilst probable cases was inferred from arrival to hospital convulsing and requiring treatment with phenytoin or phenobarbitone with a recent history of seizures. The hospital was situated within a demographic surveillance system (DSS) area mapped in 2000 by fieldworkers on motorcycles and on foot. Every building was registered by its global positioning system coordinates, and a census defined the resident population. All subsequent births, deaths, changes in housing and migration events were monitored by fieldworkers who visited participating household every 4 months. Enrolled children were followed up between March and to June 2006 with neuropsychological/neurological assessment. Seventy one percent of CSE were caused by infection. Using confirmed cases only, the incidence of CSE was 3.5 times that reported in NLSTEPSS, but if probable cases were included, the incidence may be as much as at least 8 times higher. The fatality was higher than that reported in London: 15% of children died within their acute hospitalization and 21% died during the following 3 years. Acute bacterial meningitis and focal onset seizures were the only significant risk factors for death in multivariable analysis. As they were not able to accurately assess the interval between onset of seizures and arrival to hospital, the authors were not able to assess whether delayed treatment was associated with increased mortality; previous studies in Kenya show that children can have a history of CSE for many hours before treatment.

Data were available for 138 of the 154 (90%) children who were discharged from hospital who resided within the DSS area during their admission. 15 (11%) had neurological sequelae, with motor and speech impairments each affecting 11 (7%) children. 16 (12%) children from this cohort had active epilepsy (at least one unprovoked seizure within 1 year of admission).

■ Summary and concluding remarks

The available data analysed at the group level suggest that in children, timely treated CSE does not apparently influence the outcome of their epilepsy; aetiology is the main determinant. These findings should not detract away from prompt treatment of CSE, which should include treating possible underlying aetiology, because there is undisputed evidence of individuals with severe and irreversible brain damage associated with prolonged CSE. Clinicians can be more reassuring to parents and caregivers that children who were previously normal prior to their CSE and survive the acute episode of CSE, can have a good outcome.

References

- Aicardi J, Chevrie, JJ. Convulsive status epilepticus in infants and children. A study of 239 cases. *Epilepsia* 1970; 11: 187-97.
- Berg AT, Shinnar S, Testa FM, Levy SR, Smith SN, Beckerman, B. Mortality in childhood-onset epilepsy. *Arch Pediatr Adolesc Med* 2004; 158: 1147-52.
- Callenbach PM, Westendorp RG, Geerts AT, *et al*. Mortality risk in children with epilepsy: the Dutch study of epilepsy in childhood. *Pediatrics* 2001; 107: 1259-63.
- Camfield CS, Camfield PR, Veugelers PJ. Death in children with epilepsy: a population-based study. *Lancet* 2002; 359: 1891-5.
- Camfield P, Camfield C. Unprovoked status epilepticus: the prognosis for otherwise normal children with focal epilepsy. *Pediatrics* 2012; 130: E501-6.
- Chin RF, Cumberland PM, Pujar SS, Peckham C, Ross EM, Scott RC. Outcomes of childhood epilepsy at age 33 years: a population-based birth-cohort study. *Epilepsia* 2011; 52: 1513-21.
- Chin RF, Neville BG, Peckham C, Bedford H, Wade A, Scott RC. Incidence, cause, and short-term outcome of convulsive status epilepticus in childhood: prospective population-based study. *Lancet* 2006; 368: 222-9.
- Geerts A, Arts WF, Stroink H, *et al*. Course and outcome of childhood epilepsy: a 15-year follow-up of the dutch study of epilepsy in childhood. *Epilepsia* 2010; 51: 1189-97.
- Logroscino G, Hesdorffer DC, Cascino G, Annegers JF, Hauser WA. Short-term mortality after a first episode of status epilepticus. *Epilepsia* 1997; 38: 1344-9.
- Logroscino G, Hesdorffer DC, Cascino GD, Annegers JF, Bagiella E, HauserWA. Long-term mortality after a first episode of status epilepticus. *Neurology* 2002; 58: 537-41.
- Maytal J, Shinnar S, Moshe SL, Alvarez LA. Low morbidity and mortality of status epilepticus in children. *Pediatrics* 1989; 83: 323-31.

- Pujar SS, Neville BG, Scott RC, Chin RF. Death within 8 years after childhood convulsive status epilepticus: a population-based study. *Brain* 2011; 134: 2819-27.
- Raspall-Chaure M, Chin RF, Neville BG, Scott RC. Outcome of paediatric convulsive status epilepticus: a systematic review. *Lancet Neurol* 2006; 5: 769-79.
- Sadarangani M, Seaton C, Scott JA, *et al*. Incidence and outcome of convulsive status epilepticus in kenyan children: a cohort study. *Lancet Neurol* 2008; 7: 145-50.
- Sillanpaa M, Schmidt D. Long-term employment of adults with childhood-onset epilepsy: a prospective population-based study. *Epilepsia* 2010; 51: 1053-60.
- Sillanpaa M, Shinnar S. Status epilepticus in a population-based cohort with childhood-onset epilepsy in finland. *Ann Neurol* 2002: 52: 303-10.
- Sillanpaa M, Shinnar S. Long-term mortality in childhood-onset epilepsy. *N Engl J Med* 2010; 363: 2522-9.
- Strauss D, Cable W, Shavelle R. Causes of excess mortality in cerebral palsy. *Dev Med Child Neurol* 1999; 41: 580-5.
- Stroink H, Geerts AT, Van Donselaar CA, *et al*. Status epilepticus in children with epilepsy: Dutch study of epilepsy in childhood. *Epilepsia* 2007; 48: 1708-15.
- Wakamoto H, Nagao H, Hayashi M, Morimoto T. Long-term medical, educational, and social prognoses of childhood-onset epilepsy: a population-based study in a rural district of Japan. *Brain Dev* 2000; 22: 246-55.

Mortality in children with epilepsy

Oebele F. Brouwer

Department of Neurology, University Medical Center Groningen, University of Groningen, Groningen, The Netherlands

In most children with newly diagnosed epilepsy, long-term prognosis is favorable, and in particular, patients with idiopathic etiology will eventually reach remission. Still, epilepsy remains active in 30% and even becomes intractable in 10% (Geerts et al., 2010). It has also been shown that patients with epilepsy, including children, have an increased mortality risk when compared to the general population (Hauser et al., 1980, Cockerell et al., 1994). Reasons for this include complications from an underlying static or progressive neurological disorder, and from the epilepsy itself or its treatment. Except for this, there still remains a proportion of patients whose death cannot be adequately explained.

In studying mortality in children with epilepsy epidemiological data on incidence, causes of death and risk factors involved are of utmost importance to get insight into the mechanisms involved. They may also help clinicians with giving adequate information to patients and their families about the risk of early death and certain measures that might be taken to prevent it. This paper reviews the actual knowledge on this subject with an emphasis on epidemiological data from some large cohort studies.

■ Definitions

To understand the meaning of some often used epidemiologic terms it is essential to know how they are defined (Logroscino & Hesdorffer, 2005). Case fatality (CF) is the proportion of subjects dying within a cohort during a specific time period and is calculated as the number of deaths divided by the number of subjects with the disease in the cohort. Mortality rate (MR) indicates the incidence rate of death in a cohort and is calculated as the number of deaths in a specific time period divided by the person-years at risk. Standardized mortality ratio (SMR) is the ratio of the observed number of deaths in the study group divided by the expected number of deaths. The expected number of deaths is calculated by applying the death rate of a general or external population to the gender, age, and calendar-period distribution of the study population. Both CF and MR are measures using internal comparisons, the denominator being given by the group at risk for death in the study. In contrast, SMR uses an external comparison relating to the expected deaths derived from the general population (Logroscino & Hesdorffer, 2005). Sudden unexpected death in epilepsy (SUDEP) is a category of death in people with epilepsy occurring in the absence of a known structural cause of death and is most

In 2002, Camfield et al. reported on mortality in a population-based pediatric cohort from Nova Scotia (Canada) who developed epilepsy between 1977 and 1985 (Camfield et al., 2002). Data were retrieved in 1999, 14-22 years after inclusion. Twenty-six (3.8%) of 692 children had died, the rate of death being 5.3 and 8.8 times higher than in the reference populations in the 1980s and 1990s, respectively. Notably, the difference in survival between the childhood epilepsy cohort and the reference population increased with time since onset of seizures. In 22 patients death was not unexpected and resulted from severe disorders sufficient to cause functional neurological deficit. Four deaths were unexpected, all young adults (18-30 years) without severe neurological deficits. The cause of death was documented by necropsy as suicide in two, homicide in one, and as definite SUDEP in a 21-year-old woman with tuberous sclerosis who was poorly compliant with antiepileptic medication. On the day she died she had several seizures during sleep and was found dead in bed a few hours later. Mortality rate of patients with epilepsy without severe neurological deficits was estimated to be approximately 0.7/1,000 person-years, which was no different from the reference, non-epileptic population, but approximately 15/1,000 person-years for those with epilepsy and severe neurological deficits.

In 2004, data on mortality were published from a prospective community-based cohort study in Connecticut (U.S.A.) of 613 children with newly diagnosed epilepsy, after a median follow-up of 7.9 years (Berg et al., 2004). Thirteen (2.1%) children had died, implying a mortality rate of 2.7/1,000 person-years: 0.52/1,000 for the non-symptomatic patients and 12.6/1,000 person-years for the symptomatic group. In 10 patients, death was associated with the underlying cause of the epilepsy; in two, with the occurrence or probable occurrence of seizures. In one patient death was considered a definite SUDEP with autopsy confirmation. On multivariable analysis symptomatic etiology (rate ratio, 10.2; 95% CI, 2.1-49.6) and epileptic encephalopathy (rate ratio, 13.3; 95% CI, 3.4-51.7) were associated with mortality. The overall SMR for the cohort was 7.54 (95% CI, 4.38-12.99); for those with symptomatic and non-symptomatic epilepsy SMR was 33.46 (95% CI, 18.53-60.43) and 1.43 (95% CI, 0.36-5.73), respectively.

In 2010, mortality was reported in a Finnish population-based cohort of 245 children who were diagnosed with epilepsy before 1964 and prospectively followed for 40 years (Sillanpaa & Shinnar, 2010). Apart from the extraordinary long-term follow-up, this study was characterized by the high percentage (70-80%) of autopsies. The cohort included 150 incident cases of epilepsy (first seen between 1961 and 1964) and 95 prevalent cases (first seen before 1961; seen again between 1961 and 1964 for active epilepsy). Sixty subjects (24.5%) had died with a death rate of 6.9/1,000 person-years among all subjects. The age- and sex-adjusted rates of death were 7.2/1,000 person-years, with SMR of 6.4 (95% CI, 5.9-7.0) in the overall cohort. The highest rate of death occurred among subjects who were not in 5-year terminal remission: 51 deaths in 107 subjects (15.9/1,000 person-years). Lower death rates were found in those with 5-year terminal remission receiving medication (5 deaths in 35 subjects; 11.8/1,000 person-years) or without medication (4 deaths in 103 subjects; 1.5/1,000 person-years). A remote symptomatic cause of epilepsy was also associated with an increased risk of death as compared with an idiopathic or cryptogenic cause (11.1/1,000 person-years *versus* 3.5/1,000 and 2.9/1,000 person-years, respectively; P < 0.001). In 26 (43%) of the 60 patients who died, the cause of death was not directly related to the seizure disorder but to the underlying neurological problem or another disease. In 33 (55%) patients it was related to the epilepsy, including SUDEP in 18 (30%), probable or definite seizure in 9 (15%), and accidental drowning in 6 patients (10%). In 15 of the 18 SUDEP cases autopsy was performed. Seven SUDEP cases had idiopathic or cryptogenic epilepsy, 11 had remote symptomatic epilepsy. Remarkably, median age at death among SUDEP cases was 27 years (range, 13 to 48) in the non-symptomatic group and 23 years (range, 4 to 49) in the symptomatic group. The authors noticed that if they used the Nashef SUDEP definition, which includes possible or definite seizures but not status epilepticus, 23 (38%) instead 18 (30%) of the deaths would have been due to SUDEP (Nashef, 1997).

Although the cohorts show some differences with respect to methodology and composition of patient groups, the main outcome data regarding mortality are comparable and even rather similar. Despite the fact that the Finnish cohort has a relatively high proportion of symptomatic cases and a considerably higher case fatality and mortality rate compared to the other cohorts, its standardized mortality ratio lies within the same range.

Recently, data were published on mortality in a population-based incidence cohort from Minnesota (USA) of 467 children who had been diagnosed with epilepsy over a 30-year period (1980-2009) and followed for a median of almost 8 years (Nickels et al., 2012). Data were collected retrospectively. Sixteen children (3.4%) had died, amounting a MR of 3.5/1,000 person-years. Two deaths (12.5%) were epilepsy related (0.44/1,000 person-years); one died of probable SUDEP, and the other died of aspiration during a seizure. The remaining 14 deaths (87.5%) were caused by other complications of underlying disease, including respiratory failure related to profound neurologic impairment (n = 9) and progressive metabolic disease (n = 4). Therefore, despite its retrospective nature, this study generated mortality data that are quite similar to those from the other cohorts.

■ Risk factors

The most important risk factor for epilepsy-related death is a symptomatic etiology and associated neurological deficit *(Table II)*. Children who have symptomatic epilepsy have a 20- to 30-fold increased mortality risk compared to the general population (Camfield et al., 2002; Berg et al., 2004; Geerts et al., 2010). The majority of deaths in this group are due to complications, most often respiratory, of the underlying neurologic disease which do not seem to be directly related to epilepsy. On the other hand, in children who are neurologically normal, mortality is only minimally, if at all, elevated. Camfield et al. suggested that the presence of a severe neurological deficit better indicates children who are at increased risk of death than the diagnosis of remote symptomatic epilepsy. In fact, some children with remote symptomatic etiology of their epilepsy do not have any neurological deficit and are very unlikely to die from their epilepsy (Camfield et al., 2002). In one study epileptic encephalopathy was independently associated with mortality (Berg et al., 2004). Similarly, in one cohort study abnormal neurologic examination, abnormal cognitive function, status epilepticus, poorly controlled epilepsy and structural or metabolic etiology were identified as risk factors for mortality (Nickels et al., 2012). Using a multivariable regression model, abnormal neurologic examination was the only risk factor that remained statistically significant.

Seizure-related death occurs infrequently *(Table I)*. In one cohort study the cause of death in two children was attributed to the occurrence or probable occurrence of seizures. One of these children died during a witnessed seizure that may have been status epilepticus, although there is incomplete confirmation of the seizure's duration (Berg et al., 2004). Although this study found evidence suggesting an independent role of seizure control in the risk of mortality (adjusted RR for intractable epilepsy, 4.1; 95% CI, 0.9-17.5), this was not the most important factor in this age group. In the Canadian cohort study one child died in status epilepticus and he had a severe neurological disorder (Camfield et al., 2002).

Many epilepsy related risk factors for mortality identified such as onset of seizures in the first year of life, status epilepticus before diagnosis and poor seizure control, seem to be merely markers of the severity of the underlying neurologic disease.

Table II. Statistically significant risk factors identified in the four cohorts for all deaths and SUDEP

All deaths	Uni-/bivariate analysis: RR (95% CI)	Multivariate analysis: RR (95% CI)
Early age at onset – < 1 yr – < 2 yr	+[1] 7.9 (2.3-30.1)[2]	
Epilepsy type – secondary generalized – epileptic encephalopathy	+[1] 24.1 (6.3.-109.4)[2]	13.3 (3.4-51.7)[2]
Etiology – remote symptomatic – severe neurological disorder	20.6 (4.4-134.0)[2]; 3.4 (1.9-6.1)[3] 22.19 (8.33-59.15)[1]	10.2 (2.1-49.6)[2]; 1.9 (0.7-4.8)[3] 22.03 (6.97-69.65)[1]
Early intractability	16.0 (4.5-62.1)[2]	
Early status epilepticus – at diagnosis of epilepsy – prior to diagnosis	5.8 (1.7-18.9)[2] 1.9 (1.2-3.2)[3]	
Absence of 5-year terminal remission	5.3 (2.6-11.0)[3]	4.7 (1.5-14.9)[3]
SUDEP		
Absence of 5-year terminal remission	5.2 (1.4-18.5)[3]	5.0 (1.2-20.1)[3]
Prior status epilepticus	2.8 (1.1-7.0)[3]	

[1] Canadian cohort; [2] Connecticut cohort; [3] Finnish cohort.
In the Dutch cohort remote symptomatic etiology was by far the most important risk factor, but no formal analysis was done.

■ Sudden unexpected death

The overall rate of sudden unexpected death in people with epilepsy is more than 20 times higher than in the general population. The lowest incidence rates, 0.9 to 3.5 per 10,000 person-years, were reported from unselected cohorts of incident cases; in general epilepsy populations, incidence rates ranged from 9 to 23 per 10,000 person-years, and 63 to 93 per 10,000 person-years in epilepsy surgery candidates (Shorvon & Tomson, 2011).

From the large pediatric cohort studies discussed earlier one may conclude that the risk of SUDEP is much lower in children with epilepsy (1.1-3/10,000 person-years). Only the Finnish study reported a higher SUDEP rate of 20.7/10,000 person-years (Sillanpaa & Shinnar, 2010) (Table I). This might be explained by the longer follow-up as most cases of sudden death occurred after subjects had reached adulthood with a median age at death among the 18 subjects with SUDEP of 25 years (range 4-49). Another reason for the higher prevalence of SUDEP in the Finnish cohort might be the relatively high proportion of patients with profound neurologic impairment. However, from the 18 SUDEP deaths reported, 7 had idiopathic or cryptogenic epilepsy (median age at death 27 years; range 13 to 48), and 11 had remote symptomatic epilepsy (median age at death 23 years; range 4 to 49). This means that also patients with a diagnosis of idiopathic or cryptogenic epilepsy at young age may be at risk for SUDEP in adolescence or adulthood. Long-term follow-up data of the Dutch study of epilepsy in childhood have shown that intractability may occur only after many years of follow-up, even in patients with idiopathic and cryptogenic childhood-onset epilepsy (Geerts et al., 2012).

In adults, the most important risk factor for SUDEP is the presence of generalized tonic-clonic seizures, the risk increasing with higher seizure frequency (Hessdorfer et al., 2011). In the Finnish study, the absence of terminal remission and a history of status epilepticus, but not a remote symptomatic cause or a localization-related epilepsy syndrome, were associated with an increased risk of SUDEP. On multivariate analysis, only the absence of 5-year terminal remission was significantly associated with SUDEP *(Table II)*.

A population-based study in the province of Ontario (Canada) identified 27 cases of SUDEP in children less than 18 years of age occurring over a 10-year period: 14 had symptomatic epilepsy (46%), five cryptogenic (18%), and eight idiopathic (30%). Low serum AED levels at time of death and AED polytherapy, both previously described as risk factors for SUDEP in adults, did not appear to be a significant risk factor in children (Donner et al., 2001).

It is extremely important to keep in mind that SUDEP by definition is unexplained. So it is not a specific cause of death, but a clinical entity with different pathophysiological mechanisms. An adequate autopsy should therefore be considered in every patient with epilepsy who died from an unknown cause, specifically in those who are otherwise healthy.

■ Informing families about risk of early death and prevention

There seems to be a general feeling amongst pediatric neurologists that discussing the possibility of death with the families of children in whom a diagnosis of epilepsy has been made should not be avoided. The question is how to balance such information without causing unnecessary anxiety. This is a challenge that clinicians obviously often have to deal with in daily practice, not only with regard to epilepsy and its possible complications (Green, 2000). One might argue that the issue of early death should be only spontaneously raised in cases with symptomatic epilepsy and in those with non-symptomatic epilepsy with drug-resistant tonic-clonic seizures (Appleton, 2003). In addition, it should also be discussed with the families of those patients who are specifically at risk for early death such as children with Dravet syndrome (Sakauchi et al., 2011).

The most important aspect of prevention is good seizure control. This implies giving information on the importance of minimizing avoidable seizures by adequate medication intake and discussing the risks of acute withdrawal or non-compliance. In some patients with intractable seizures it even might justify the risks of experimental drugs or surgery. A difficult topic is in which children monitoring and resuscitation facilities should be used, especially during periods without personal observation. At present, there are no data to support the idea that such devices might prevent early death including SUDEP. Therefore the benefit of some reassurance for the parents should be outbalanced against the stress of intrusive monitoring including frequent false alarms during the night.

■ Concluding remarks and suggestions

In the last decade some large prospective cohort studies of incident cases of childhood-onset epilepsy have supplied important information about the incidence of early death and risk factors involved. Mortality risk in children with epilepsy is only minimally, if at all, elevated in children who are neurologically normal. Almost all of the excess risk is in children with severe neurological conditions, due to infections and other complications of the underlying disorder. Seizure-related death and SUDEP do occur in children, and the risk factors for this – primarily the underlying neurologic disease – are not preventable. Despite this low risk, it is important to counsel patients and families adequately. Mortality risk in patients with childhood-onset epilepsy, whether idiopathic or symptomatic, is still present, if not getting even higher, when they reach adolescence and adulthood, especially in those who are not entering terminal remission. Autopsy should be considered in any patient with epilepsy who dies unexpectedly, especially in those who are otherwise healthy.

References

- Annegers JF. United States perspective on definitions and classifications. *Epilepsia* 1997; 38 (Suppl.11): 9-12.
- Annegers JF, Coan SP. SUDEP: overview of definitions and review of incidence data. *Seizure* 1999; 8: 347-52.
- Appleton RE. Mortality in paediatric epilepsy. *Arch Dis Child* 2003; 88: 1091-4.
- Berg AT, Shinnar S, Testa FM, Levy SR, Smith SN, Beckerman B. Mortality in childhood-onset epilepsy. *Arch Pediatr Adolesc Med* 2004; 158: 1147-52.
- Callenbach PMC, Westendorp RGJ, Geerts AT, *et al*. Mortality risk in children with epilepsy: the Dutch study of epilepsy in childhood. *Pediatrics* 2001; 107: 1259-63.
- Camfield CS, Camfield PR, Veugelers PJ. Death in children with epilepsy: a population-based study. *Lancet* 2002; 359: 1891-5.
- Cockerell OC, Johnson AL, Sander JWS, *et al*. Mortality from epilepsy: results from a prospective population-based study. *Lancet* 1994; 344: 918-21.
- Donner EJ, Smith CR, Carter Snead O. Sudden unexplained death in children with epilepsy. *Neurology* 2001; 57: 430-4.
- Geerts AT, Arts WFM, Stroink H, *et al*. Course and outcome of childhood epilepsy: a 15-year follow-up of the Dutch study of epilepsy in childhood. *Epilepsia* 2010; 51: 1189-97.
- Geerts AT, Brouwer OF, Stroink H, *et al*. Onset of intractability and its course over time: the Dutch study of epilepsy in childhood. *Epilepsia* 2012; 53: 741-51.
- Green S. Risk and advice in child neurology. *Dev Med Child Neurol* 2000; 42: 795.
- Hauser WA, Annegers JF, Elveback LR. Mortality in patients with epilepsy. *Epilepsia* 1980; 21: 399-412.
- Hesdorffer DC, Tomson T, Benn E, *et al*. Combined analysis of risk factors for SUDEP. *Epilepsia* 2011; 52: 1150-9.

- Logroscino G, Hesdorffer. Methodologic issues in studies of mortality following epilepsy: measures, types of studies, sources of cases, cohort effect, and competing risks. *Epilepsia* 2005; 46 (Suppl 11): 3-7.
- Nashef L. Sudden unexpected death in epilepsy: terminology and definitions. *Epilepsia* 1997; 38 (Suppl 11): 6-8.
- Nashef L, So EL, Ryvlin P, Tomson T. Unifying the definitions of sudden unexpected death in epilepsy. *Epilepsia* 2012; 53: 227-33.
- Nickels KC, Grossardt BR, Wirrell EC. Epilepsy-related mortality is low in children: a 30-year population-based study in Olmstedt County, MN. *Epilepsia* [Epub ahead of print].
- Sakauchi M, Oguni H, Kato I, *et al*. Retrospective multiinstitutional study of the prevalence of early death in Dravet syndrome. *Epilepsia* 2011; 52: 1144-9.
- Shorvon S, Tomson T. Sudden unexpected death in epilepsy. *Lancet* 2011; 378: 2028-38.
- Sillanpaa M, Shinnar S. Long-term mortality in childhood-onset epilepsy. *N Engl J Med* 2010; 363: 2522-9.

Immune-related mechanisms of seizures: insights from experimental models

Teresa Ravizza, Silvia Balosso, Valentina Iori, Federica Frigerio, Annamaria Vezzani

Department of Neuroscience, Istituto di Ricerche Farmacologiche "Mario Negri", Milano, Italy

Inflammation is a tissue response to noxious stimuli leading to the production of inflammatory mediators. It represents the prototypical response to pathogens which is instrumental for their recognition (*i.e.*, pathogen associated molecular patterns, PAMPs), and for their killing and removal, thereafter promoting tissue healing by activating homeostatic programs (Ulevitch & Tobias, 1995). In the last decade, a specific form of inflammation has been described in brain tissue, named "sterile" inflammation. This type of inflammation is a response to tissue injury, such as cell damage, chronic stress or aberrant neuronal excitability, in the absence of pathogens (Tsan & Gao, 2004; Bianchi, 2007).

While the response to pathogens engages both the innate and the adaptive arms of the immune system, sterile inflammation is predominantly driven and sustained by the activation of innate immunity cells, pivotally represented in the brain by microglia and astrocytes. These cells recognize *danger signals* released following a tissue threat (danger associated molecular patterns, DAMPs), and activate inflammatory pathways in part overlapping with those activated by infection (Maroso et al., 2011b; Vezzani et al., 2011b). Both PAMPs and DAMPs are recognized by Toll-like receptors (TLR), a class of receptors instrumental for the activation of the innate immune system (Bianchi, 2007; Lee & Kim, 2007).

In the context of epilepsy, besides glial cells, inflammatory molecules are also produced and released by neurons and endothelial cells of the blood brain barrier (BBB). Leukocytes can also contribute to the inflammatory responses in epilepsy (Iyer et al., 2010; Vezzani et al., 2011a).

A notable finding is that the inflammatory mediators characterized in epileptic brain specimens are not only effector molecules of the immune system apt at promoting local inflammation and tissue recruitment of peripheral immune cells, but they possess the properties of neuromodulators (Vezzani et al., 2011a). In fact, they activate their cognate receptors expressed by neurons, thus directly affecting neuronal function and excitability (Viviani et al., 2007; Vezzani et al., 2011b).

This chapter will describe the salient evidence of innate immunity activation in human epilepsy, the consequences of this activation for seizures and epileptogenesis in adult and immature brain, the mechanisms activated by inflammatory molecules in target cells and their relevance for the pathology, and finally the envisaged therapeutic perspectives for controlling pharmacoresistant seizures.

■ Inflammation in human epilepsy

A role of inflammation in human epilepsy has been first recognized in Rasmussen's encephalitis (RE) where cytotoxic T cells were described in close apposition with neurons and astrocytes, releasing Granzyme B and provoking cell apoptosis (Bien et al., 2002; Bauer et al., 2007; Pardo et al., 2004). Recent evidence highlighted the presence of interleukin (IL)-1β in microglia nodules, which are also hallmark of tissue pathology in this syndrome (Wirenfeldt et al., 2009; Bauer et al., personal communication). This evidence supports the activation of innate immunity in RE, and the release of inflammatory molecules not only from T cells by also from microglia. Interestingly, overexpression of TLR2, TLR3 and TLR4 in glia and neurons was also recently described in RE (Pardo et al., personal communication). These receptors recognize gram+, viral, and gram– infections respectively, but they are also activated by endogenous DAMPs (e.g., extracellular matrix proteins, fibrinogen, double stranded RNA, heat shock proteins) (Piccinini & Midwood, 2010).

In addition to cytotoxic T cells, adaptive immunity may contribute to brain pathology by producing auto-antibodies against neuronal proteins, as recognized in limbic encephalitis as well as in systemic and neurological autoimmune disorders often associated with seizures (Vincent et al., 1999; Bien et al., 2012).

In the last decade, however, increasing evidence showed a prominent role of glial cells in the induction and perpetuation of inflammatory processes linked to epilepsy. These findings have been obtained by analyzing brain tissues resected at surgery from patients with pharmacoresistant forms of epilepsy, such as mesial temporal lobe epilepsy (mTLE) or epilepsies associated with malformations of cortical development (including focal cortical dysplasia (FCD) type 2b, ganglioglioma, dysembrioplastic neuroepithelial tumors, tuberous sclerosis) (Vezzani et al., 2011a). In particular, in these forms of epilepsy there is immunohistochemical evidence of activation of innate immune signaling: IL-1 receptor type 1 (IL-1R1), TLR4 and Receptor for Advanced Glycation End products (RAGE) are induced together with their endogenous ligands, namely IL-1β, High Mobility Group Box1 (HMGB1) and S100β (Griffin et al., 1995; Vezzani et al., 2011a; Zurolo et al., 2011). Activated astrocytes, microglia and neurons chiefly express these inflammatory molecules and their receptors; in MCD also dysmorphic neurons and balloon cells contribute to the activation of these inflammatory signals (Boer et al., 2006; Ravizza et al., 2006a; Iyer et al., 2010; Aronica et al., 2012). Additionally, microvessels express markers of inflammation in epilepsy tissue, including upregulation of various adhesion molecules (Librizzi et al., 2007; Fabene et al., 2008; Morin-Brureau et al., 2011; Zattoni et al., 2011).

The inflammatory cascade is complex and comprises various molecules and their signaling pathways, including COX-2, TNF-alpha, IL-6, chemokines and the complement cascade (Vezzani et al., 2011a). The IL-1R/TLR signaling is chiefly involved in the induction of these molecules by mediating transcriptional upregulation of their genes (O'Neill & Bowie, 2007). Notably, IL-1R/TLR signaling is the pivotal activator of innate immune mechanisms not only following brain injury but also during infections (Lee & Kim, 2007).

As far as peripheral immune cells are concerned, counting of lymphocytes and dendritic cells in brain tissues in common forms of epilepsy (thus excluding RE, viral and limbic encephalitis and autoimmune disorders) revealed a significant number of cells only in FCD type 2b and tumor cases (Iyer *et al.*, 2010). In FCD type 1 or mTLE only minor tissue extravation was observed; peripheral immune cells were predominantly located perivascularly, rather than in brain parenchyma (Ravizza *et al.*, 2008a; Iyer *et al.*, 2010). In all these forms of epilepsy, T cells even if detected in brain tissue, did not typically showed close apposition to neurons or glia, or release of cytotoxic granules, differently from RE tissue.

The evidence of prominent activation of innate immunity and related inflammatory molecules in epilepsies of differing etiologies opens up two important questions: 1) which are the triggers of this inflammatory response; and 2) which are the consequences for tissue excitability and neuropathology. These questions have been addressed using experimental models of seizures in rats and mice.

■ What causes inflammation in experimental models of epilepsy?

Experimental studies have highlighted two classes of crucial triggers of brain inflammation in epilepsy, namely *seizures* and *cell injury*, which includes stressor events not necessarily related to cell degeneration. These events that typically promote epilepsy development in animal models (*e.g.*, status epilepticus, febrile seizures, traumatic brain injury), trigger glutamate and ATP, as well as DAMPs, release from brain cells which in turn activate their cognate receptors on neurons and glial cells (Vezzani *et al.*, 2011b). Importantly, intracellular decrease in K^+ and elevation in Ca^{2+}, which characterize neuronal and glial cells activation, are important determinants of inflammasome activation, the multiproteins cell constituent responsible for the release of IL-1β, IL-18 and HMGB1 (van de Veerdonk *et al.*, 2011).

Experimental models of TLE induced by status epilepticus in adult rats have been mostly used to characterize the inflammatory process triggered by seizures, and its temporal evolution. These studies showed that the inflammatory response is among the biological processes most prominently induced by brain injury (Becker *et al.*, 2003; Gorter *et al.*, 2006; Lukasiuk *et al.*, 2006). This injury-driven inflammatory response has a rapid onset time (within 30 min), outlasts the initial precipitating event (it is maintained during the epileptogenesis phase preceding onset of spontaneous seizures) and is chronically activated in brain tissue from which recurrent spontaneous seizures originate in epileptic animals (Voutsinos-Porche *et al.*, 2004; Dhote *et al.*, 2007; Ravizza *et al.*, 2008a; Kuteykin-Teplyakov *et al.*, 2009; Marcon *et al.*, 2009). The inflammatory molecules and their cell sources and targets described in experimental epilepsy models are remarkably similar to those described in human mTLE (Aronica & Crino, 2011; Vezzani *et al.*, 2011a; Aronica *et al.*, 2012). Moreover, the same classes of inflammatory molecules are measured in different forms of human and experimental epilepsy (Aronica & Crino, 2011, Vezzani *et al.*, 2011a; Aronica *et al.*, 2012).

Studies specifically addressing the inflammatory response in infantile rat models of seizures, established that seizure-induced brain inflammation is developmentally regulated. Moreover, the seizure type (focal or generalized) and the initial trigger of seizures (*e.g.*, chemoconvulsants such as kainic acid or pilocarpine, flurothyl ether, heat-induced seizures) are important determinants of the age of onset, extent and duration of brain inflammation

(Dubé et al., 2010; Rizzi et al., 2003; Marcon et al., 2009; Riazi et al., 2010). In kainate-injected pups, brain inflammation develops after the first two post-natal weeks (P14) and resembles the adult response only in P21 rats (Rizzi et al., 2003). This inflammatory response precedes the onset of seizure-induced cell loss and matches the age-dependent susceptibility of rats to develop epilepsy after status epilepticus (Rizzi et al., 2003; Marcon et al., 2009). The inflammatory response induced in models of febrile seizures is instead anticipated as compared to kainate, and occurs already at P7 (Riazi et al., 2010; Notably, this response outlasts for a few days the end of febrile seizures, and is concomitant with the development of epilepsy in a subgroup of animals (Dubé et al., 2010, 2011a).

■ What are the functional consequences of brain inflammation?

Activation of the IL-1R/TLR signaling significantly contributes to the mechanisms of ictogenesis. Thus, anticonvulsive effects in animal models arise using specific drugs blocking either IL-1R1 with IL-1 receptor antagonist (IL-1Ra/anakinra) or TLR4, or using drugs blocking IL-1β biosynthesis (pralnacasan and VX-765), or peptides inactivating HMGB1 (such as BoxA) (Vezzani et al., 2010; Vezzani et al., 2011b). In particular, these treatments delay the onset of seizures and decrease their frequency in kainate and biculline injected rats and mice (Vezzani et al., 2000; Ravizza et al., 2006b; Maroso et al., 2010; Maroso et al., 2011a). The same treatments also reduce chronic seizure recurrence in a mTLE mouse model (Maroso et al., 2010, 2011a). Similarly, IL-1Ra/anakinra delays kindling development in immature rats primed with the TLR4 agonist lipopolysaccharide (Auvin et al., 2010) and arrests seizure generalization in adult rodents (Vezzani et al., 2000; Ravizza et al.; 2008b). Moreover, systemic administration of IL-1Ra decreases the incidence of status epilepticus and reduced its duration in adult pilocarpine-injected rats (Marchi et al., 2009). Notably, VX-765 also reduces the frequency of spike-and-wave discharges in a rat model of absence seizures (Akin et al., 2011).

Other inflammatory mediators such as cytokines, prostaglandins and the complement system have been implicated in seizure mechanisms in animal models (Xiong et al., 2003; Kulkarni & Dhir, 2009; Aronica et al., 2012).

Importantly, on the one hand a proconvulsive event activates inflammatory pathways in brain cells which in turn contribute to neuronal hyperexcitability, thus reducing seizure threshold and favoring ictogenesis (Vezzani et al., 2011a). On the other hand, the induction of inflammation in brain using lipopolysaccharide or Poly I:C, prototypical activators of TLR4 and TLR3 respectively, is sufficient per se to decrease seizure threshold both acutely (Sayyah et al., 2003) and long-term (Riazi et al., 2010). In immature rats and mice aged P7-14, which rougthly corresponds to early infancy in children, either lipopolysaccharideor PolyI:C permanently changes brain excitability. In fact, these pups develop increased seizure susceptibility to various convulsant drugs in their adulthood (Galic et al., 2008; Riazi et al., 2008; Galic et al., 2009). Moreover, rats pre-exposed to brain inflammation show increased cell loss following seizures (Auvin et al., 2007; Galic et al., 2008; Riazi et al., 2008; Galic et al., 2009; Riazi et al., 2010).

Importantly, an inflammatory challenge in adult or immature rodents induces lasting behavioral deficits reminiscent of comorbities (impaired cognitive function, autism-like behavior, anxiety) often associated with epilepsy (Mazarati et al., 2010, 2011; Harré et al., 2008; Galic et al., 2009). The same phenomenon is observed in the offspring of pregnant rodents injected with inflammatory molecules during gestation (Hagberg & Mallard, 2005;

Rees et al., 2008). This phenomenon may be explained by considering that cytokines affect neuronal stem cells proliferation/migration, axonal guidance, synaptic connections and function (Carpentier & Palmer, 2009). Moreover, early life infection primes immune responses in adulthood making microglia cells more prone to activation and release of inflammatory mediators following a second-hit (Bilbo & Schwarz, 2009). The immature brain, therefore, can be permanently modified after a single inflammatory episode (Carpentier & Palmer, 2009; Riazi et al., 2010).

Is brain inflammation a promising target for anti-epileptogenesis strategies?

One demanding challenge for pharmacotherapy is to develop disease-modifying drugs which may interfere with the progression of the disease or prevent the development of epilepsy after a precipitating event in individuals at risk. Experimental studies in models of stroke, traumatic brain injury, febrile or non febrile status epilepticus, and CNS infection have shown that the inflammatory response induced by these epileptogenic events is long lasting and precedes the development of spontaneous seizures (Vezzani et al., 2011a). Intervention with anti-inflammatory drugs (e.g., NSAID such as celecoxib, parecoxib; anti-integrin antibodies; inhibitors of glia activation such as minocycline, resveratrol, fingolimod) after the initial injury, which in most cases is experimentally reproduced by status epilepticus, has shown some promising results (Pitkanen & Lukasiuk, 2011, Ravizza et al., 2011; Gao et al., 2012). Although the onset of the disease has not been prevented by these treatments, the epileptic animals developed less severe epilepsy. In particular, the successful interventions reduced the frequency of seizures in epileptic animals, modified the type of seizures by decreasing their generalization, reduced the neuropathology, and attenuated the behavioral deficits associated with epilepsy (Pitkanen & Lukasiuk, 2011; Ravizza et al., 2011). In this regard, inhibition of microglia activation with minocycline after TBI was shown to improve neuropathology and promote functional recovery, although the impact on post-traumatic epilepsy has not been addressed yet (Sanchez Mejia et al., 2001; Bye et al., 2007; Crack et al., 2009; Homsi et al., 2010).

The available evidence, therefore, indicates that the severity of epilepsy may be alleviated by anti-inflammatory treatments given post-injury, and brain inflammation contributes to neuropathology, spontaneous seizures and comorbidities.

Mechanisms underlying the effects of inflammation in epilepsy

Insights into the mechanisms by which inflammatory molecules can contribute to seizures have highlighted either direct effects on neuronal function, or indirect effects mediated by alterations of endothelial and astrocytic cells physiology. Direct effects on neurons have been demonstrated for an array of pro-inflammatory cytokines and prostaglandins, as well as for danger signals such as HMGB1 (Stellwagen et al., 2005; Viviani et al., 2007; Vezzani et al., 2011b; Vezzani et al., 2012a; Vezzani et al., 2012b). In particular, IL-β interaction with neuronal IL-1R1 activates within minutes the Src-dependent phosphorylation of the NR2B subunit of the NMDA receptor, thus promoting Ca^{2+} influx into neurons (Viviani et al., 2003; Balosso et al., 2008). The same signaling is activated by TLR4 activation by HMGB1 (Maroso et al., 2010). Increased neuronal Ca^{2+} influx is a molecular event pivotally involved in the pro-ictogenic effects of IL-1β and HMGB1 (Balosso et al., 2008; Maroso et al., 2010). Recently, activation of the IL-1R/TLR4 signaling has been shown to reduce the levels and function of HCN1 channels (Flynn et al., submitted). These channels are important regulators of the filtering properties of hippocampal pyramidal cell dendrites, their responses to excitatory inputs, and they are involved in theta rhythms, which have been linked to cognitive functions. These channels are downregulated in experimental and human epilepsy tissue, and may contribute to seizures (Brewster et al., 2002; Bender et al., 2003).

Among the indirect effects of inflammatory molecules on neuronal excitability, a prominent role is played by their ability to compromise the BBB permeability properties (Del Maschio et al., 1996; Ferrari et al., 2004; Allan et al., 2005). BBB opening is one of the hallmark of epilepsy tissue and appears to contribute to the generation of neuronal hyperexcitability. A positive correlation between the extent of BBB opening and the number of spontaneous seizures was shown in epileptic rats (van Vliet et al., 2007). Moreover, focal opening of the BBB in the rat neocortex, recapitulated by exposing the rat brain cortex to serum albumin, resulted in the delayed development of paroxysmal hypersynchronous activity (Seiffert et al., 2004; Ivens et al., 2007). Extravasation of serum albumin into the brain following BBB breakdown activates a TGF-β receptor type 2 in astrocytes inducing both local tissue inflammation and astrocytic dysfunction (Cacheaux et al., 2009). In particular, albumin induces transcriptional activation of inflammatory genes in astrocytes, and the concomitant downregulation of Kir4.1 potassium channels and the glutamate transporter (Seiffert et al., 2004; Ivens et al., 2007; David et al., 2009; Friedman et al., 2009). The resulting tissue inflammation, higher extracellular K^+ and glutamate promote hyperexcitability in surrounding tissue (Seiffert et al., 2004), and a long lasting decrease in seizure threshold (Frigerio et al., 2012).

Notably, inflammatory molecules released by perivascular glia have a prominent role in BBB breakdown by provoking the downregulation of tight junctions on microvasculature (Morin-Brureau et al., 2011; Librizzi et al., 2012). Interaction of circulating leukocytes with upregulated adhesion molecules on endothelial cells may also contribute to BBB dysfunction (Fabene et al., 2008).

■ Role of leukocytes in seizure models

There is evidence of the involvement of peripheral immune cells in some forms of epilepsy. In experimental models of mTLE, leukocytes contribution to tissue inflammation differs depending on the nature of the epileptogenic trigger. For example, $CD4^+$ and $CD8^+$ lymphocytes in perivascular location have been reported in the mouse hippocampus after status epilepticus induced by systemic pilocarpine (Fabene et al., 2008), or intrahippocampal administration of kainic acid (Zattoni et al., 2011), two convulsant drugs promoting cholinergic and glutamatergic neurotransmission, respectively. This phenomenon may reflect passive cell extravasation due to leakage of BBB induced by injury or seizures. Alternatively, lymphocytes may be primed to pass into the perivascular space by glial cells or vessels releasing cytokines after cell injury or during seizures (Librizzi et al., 2007; Zattoni et al., 2011; Librizzi et al., 2012). Active brain extravasation of these cells has been proposed to contribute to alter BBB permeability (Fabene et al., 2008). The presence of circulating antigens that may activate T cells has not been demonstrated so far. Whatever the mechanism possibly involved is, the crucial question remains if this phenomenon has some relevance for tissue hyperexcitability or neuropathology. Two divergent sets of data have been presented in mouse models of TLE. In pilocarpine-treated mice, neurotrophils, macrophages and T cells appear to play a detrimental role in epileptogenesis. Thus, mice lacking key adhesion molecules or treated with anti-integrin antibodies develop a milder form of epilepsy characterized by less recurrent seizures and decreased neuropathology as compared to control epileptic mice (Fabene *et al.*, 2008). In contrast, in kainic acid-treated mice, macrophages and T cells play a protective role by preventing neurotrophils to enter the brain tissue, and by delaying the onset and reducing the recurrence of spontaneous seizures (Zattoni *et al.*, 2011). A key to interpret these discrepant findings is to consider that pilocarpine has a primary mode of action which involves muscarinic receptors expressed by circulating leukocytes. This activation induces IL-1β release into the blood stream (Marchi *et al.*, 2009), and this event is required for inducing BBB damage and the subsequent entry of pilocarpine into the brain at convulsive concentrations, which otherwise would not be reached with an intact BBB (Vezzani & Janigro, 2009). This epilepsy model, therefore, uses a peculiar mechanism reminiscent of a systemic infection favoring seizure precipitation. On the contrary, intracerebral kainic acid more closely represents a sterile-type of brain injury leading to spontaneous seizures.

■ Conclusions

The available experimental and clinical evidence suggest that brain inflammation is both a contributing factor and a consequence of seizures (Vezzani *et al.*, 2011a). The presence of activated inflammatory cells (microglia, astrocytes and leukocytes), the consequent release of inflammatory molecules (*e.g.*, cytokines, chemokines, DAMPs, complement factors, prostaglandins) and the upregulation of their receptors have been demonstrated in brain tissue from epilepsy of differing etiologies. In some instances, cytokines have been also measured in CSF or blood of some of the affected individuals. These findings, together with the identification of subsets of auto-antibodies against neuronal proteins in some forms of epilepsy or seizure disorders, highlight a pathogenetic role of both innate and adaptive immunity in epilepsy. While activation of innate immunity, which chiefly involves glial cells, is commonly observed in epilepsy, the presence of activated T cells, or circulating auto-antibodies, is restricted to more specific cases.

What causes brain inflammation and which are the pivotal mechanisms promoting chronic inflammation in epilepsy are still open questions. Experimental findings indicate that brain inflammation predisposes animals to develop seizures, and in turn seizure recurrence can both induce and perpetuate brain inflammation. In this regard, although there is no evidence that the adaptive immune system can predispose to seizures directly, there is experimental evidence that innate immunity is directly involved in the generation of seizures. Clinical reports have shown that anti-inflammatory or immunosuppressive treatments have anticonvulsive efficacy in some forms of drug-refractory seizures, thus supporting the possible etiopathogenic role of inflammation. Since activation of immunity and inflammation are endogenous homeostatic mechanisms, the challenge is to understand which inflammatory cells and related molecules instead compromise brain physiology and promote seizure generation. The evidence-based hypothesis, therefore, suggests that dysfunction of the immune system is a pivotal component of the etiopathogenesis of seizures in human epilepsy. In this context, the development of anti-inflammatory drugs interfering with the specific inflammatory signaling underlying ictogenesis and epileptogenesis might represent a promising therapeutic approach for inhibiting drug-resistant seizures, and delay or arrest the development of epilepsy in individuals at risks.

- Kuteykin-Teplyakov K, Brandt C, Hoffmann K, Loscher W. Complex time-dependent alterations in the brain expression of different drug efflux transporter genes after status epilepticus. *Epilepsia* 2009; 50: 887-97.
- Lee MS, Kim YJ. Signaling pathways downstream of pattern-recognition receptors and their cross talk. *Annu Rev Biochem* 2007; 76: 447-80.
- Librizzi L, Noè F, Vezzani A, de Curtis M, Ravizza T. Seizure-induced brain-borne inflammation sustains seizure recurrence and blood-brain barrier damage. *Ann Neurol* 2012; 72: 82-90.
- Librizzi L, Regondi MC, Pastori C, Frigerio S, Frassoni C, de Curtis M. Expression of adhesion factors induced by epileptiform activity in the endothelium of the isolated guinea pig brain *in vitro*. *Epilepsia* 2007; 48: 743-51.
- Lukasiuk K, Dabrowski M, Adach A, Pitkanen A. Epileptogenesis-related genes revisited. *Prog Brain Res* 2006; 158: 223-41.
- Marchi N, Fan Q, Ghosh C, et al. Antagonism of peripheral inflammation reduces the severity of status epilepticus. *Neurobiol Dis* 2009; 33: 171-81.
- Marcon J, Gagliardi B, Balosso S, et al. Age-dependent vascular changes induced by status epilepticus in rat forebrain: implications for epileptogenesis. *Neurobiol Dis* 2009; 34: 121-32.
- Maroso M, Balosso S, Ravizza T, et al. Interleukin-1beta biosynthesis inhibition reduces acute seizures and drug resistant chronic epileptic activity in mice. *Neurotherapeutics* 2011a; 8: 304-15.
- Maroso M, Balosso S, Ravizza T, et al. Toll-like receptor 4 and high-mobility group box-1 are involved in ictogenesis and can be targeted to reduce seizures. *Nat Med* 2010; 16: 413-9.
- Maroso M, Balosso S, Ravizza T, Liu J, Bianchi ME, Vezzani A. Interleukin-1 type 1 receptor/Toll-like receptor signalling in epilepsy: the importance of IL-1beta and high-mobility group box 1. *J Intern Med* 2011b; 270: 319-26.
- Mazarati AM, Maroso M, Iori V, Vezzani A, Carli M. High-mobility group box-1 impairs memory in mice through both toll-like receptor 4 and receptor for advanced glycation end products. *Exp Neurol* 2011; 232: 143-8.
- Mazarati AM, Pineda E, Shin D, Tio D, Taylor AN, Sankar R. Comorbidity between epilepsy and depression: role of hippocampal interleukin-1beta. *Neurobiol Dis* 2010; 37: 461-7.
- Morin-Brureau M, Lebrun A, Rousset MC, et al. Epileptiform activity induces vascular remodeling and zonula occludens 1 downregulation in organotypic hippocampal cultures: role of VEGF signaling pathways. *J Neurosci* 2011; 31: 10677-88.
- O'Neill LA and Bowie AG. The family of five: TIR-domain-containing adaptors in Toll-like receptor signalling. *Nat Rev Immunol* 2007; 7: 353-64.
- Pardo CA, Vining EP, Guo L, Skolasky RL, Carson BS, Freeman JM. The pathology of Rasmussen syndrome: stages of cortical involvement and neuropathological studies in 45 hemispherectomies. *Epilepsia* 2004; 45: 516-26.
- Piccinini AM, Midwood KS. DAMPening inflammation by modulating TLR signalling. *Mediators Inflamm*; 2010: 1-21.
- Pitkanen A, Lukasiuk K. Mechanisms of epileptogenesis and potential treatment targets. *Lancet Neurol* 2011; 10: 173-86.
- Ravizza T, Balosso S, Vezzani A. Inflammation and prevention of epileptogenesis. *Neurosci Lett* 2011; 497: 223-30.
- Ravizza T, Boer K, Redeker S, et al. The IL-1beta system in epilepsy-associated malformations of cortical development. *Neurobiol Dis* 2006a; 24: 128-43.
- Ravizza T, Gagliardi B, Noé F, Boer K, Aronica E, Vezzani A. Innate and adaptive immunity during epileptogenesis and spontaneous seizures: evidence from experimental models and human temporal lobe epilepsy. *Neurobiol Dis* 2008a; 29: 142-60.
- Ravizza T, Lucas SM, Balosso S, et al. Inactivation of caspase-1 in rodent brain: a novel anticonvulsive strategy. *Epilepsia* 2006b; 47: 1160-8.

- Ravizza T, Noé F, Zardoni D, Vaghi V, Sifringer M, Vezzani A. Interleukin Converting Enzyme inhibition impairs kindling epileptogenesis in rats by blocking astrocytic IL-1beta production. *Neurobiol Dis* 2008b; 31: 327-33.
- Rees S, Harding R and Walker D. An adverse intrauterine environment: implications for injury and altered development of the brain. *Int J Dev Neurosci* 2008; 26: 3-11.
- Riazi K, Galic MA, Kuzmiski JB, Ho W, Sharkey KA, Pittman QJ. Microglial activation and TNFalpha production mediate altered CNS excitability following peripheral inflammation. *Proc Natl Acad Sci USA* 2008; 105: 17151-6.
- Riazi K, Galic MA, Pittman QJ. Contributions of peripheral inflammation to seizure susceptibility: cytokines and brain excitability. *Epilepsy Res* 2010; 89: 34-42.
- Rizzi M, Perego C, Aliprandi M, *et al.* Glia activation and cytokine increase in rat hippocampus by kainic acid-induced status epilepticus during postnatal development. *Neurobiol Dis* 2003; 14: 494-503.
- Sanchez Mejia RO, Ona VO, Li M and Friedlander RM. Minocycline reduces traumatic brain injury-mediated caspase-1 activation, tissue damage, and neurological dysfunction. *Neurosurgery* 2001; 48: 1393-9; discussion 1399-401.
- Sayyah M, Javad-Pour M, Ghazi-Khansari M. The bacterial endotoxin lipopolysaccharide enhances seizure susceptibility in mice: involvement of proinflammatory factors: nitric oxide and prostaglandins. *Neuroscience* 2003; 122, 1073-80.
- Seiffert E, Dreier JP, Ivens S, *et al.* Lasting blood-brain barrier disruption induces epileptic focus in the rat somatosensory cortex. *J Neurosci* 2004; 24: 7829-36.
- Stellwagen D, Beattie EC, Seo JY and Malenka RC. Differential regulation of AMPA receptor and GABA receptor trafficking by tumor necrosis factor-alpha. *J Neurosci* 2005; 25: 3219-28.
- Tsan MF, Gao B. Endogenous ligands of Toll-like receptors. *J Leukoc Biol* 2004; 76: 514-9.
- Ulevitch RJ, Tobias PS. Receptor-dependent mechanisms of cell stimulation by bacterial endotoxin. *Annu Rev Immunol* 1995; 13: 437-57.
- van de Veerdonk FL, Netea MG, Dinarello CA, Joosten LA. Inflammasome activation and IL-1beta and IL-18 processing during infection. *Trends Immunol* 2011; 32: 110-6.
- van Vliet EA, da Costa Araujo S, Redeker S, van Schaik R, Aronica E, Gorter JA. Blood-brain barrier leakage may lead to progression of temporal lobe epilepsy. *Brain* 2007; 130: 521-34.
- Vezzani A, Auvin S, Ravizza T, Aronica E. Glia-neuronal interactions in ictogenesis and epileptogenesis: role of inflammatory mediators. In: Noebels JL, Avoli M, Rogawski MA, Olsen RW, Delgado-Escueta A (eds). *Jasper's Basic mechanisms of the Epilepsies- Fourth Edition*, 2012.
- Vezzani A, Balosso S, Maroso M, Zardoni D, Noé F, Ravizza T. ICE/caspase 1 inhibitors and IL-1beta receptor antagonists as potential therapeutics in epilepsy. *Curr Opin Investig Drugs* 2010; 11: 43-50.
- Vezzani A, Balosso S and Ravizza T. Inflammation and epilepsy. *Handb Clin Neurol* 2012b; 107: 163-75.
- Vezzani A, French J, Bartfai T, Baram TZ. The role of inflammation in epilepsy. *Nat Rev Neurol* 2011a; 7: 31-40.
- Vezzani A, Janigro D. Leukocyte-endothelial adhesion mechanisms in epilepsy: cheers and jeers. *Epilepsy Curr* 2009; 9: 118-21.
- Vezzani A, Maroso M, Balosso S, Sanchez MA, Bartfai T. IL-1 receptor/Toll-like receptor signaling in infection, inflammation, stress and neurodegeneration couples hyperexcitability and seizures. *Brain Behav Immun* 2011b; 25: 1281-9.
- Vezzani A, Moneta D, Conti M, *et al.* Powerful anticonvulsant action of IL-1 receptor antagonist on intracerebral injection and astrocytic overexpression in mice. *Proc Natl Acad Sci USA* 2000; 97: 11534-9.
- Vincent A, Lily O, Palace J. Pathogenic autoantibodies to neuronal proteins in neurological disorders. *J Neuroimmunol* 1999; 100: 169-80.

- Viviani B, Bartesaghi S, Gardoni F, et al. Interleukin-1beta enhances NMDA receptor-mediated intracellular calcium increase through activation of the Src family of kinases. *J Neurosci* 2003; 23: 8692-700.
- Viviani B, Gardoni F, Marinovich M. Cytokines and neuronal ion channels in health and disease. *Int Rev Neurobiol* 2007; 82: 247-63.
- Voutsinos-Porche B, Koning E, Kaplan H, et al. Temporal patterns of the cerebral inflammatory response in the rat lithium-pilocarpine model of temporal lobe epilepsy. *Neurobiol Dis* 2004; 17: 385-402.
- Wirenfeldt M, Clare R, Tung S, Bottini A, Mathern GW, Vinters HV. Increased activation of Iba1+ microglia in pediatric epilepsy patients with Rasmussen's encephalitis compared with cortical dysplasia and tuberous sclerosis complex. *Neurobiol Dis* 2009; 34: 432-40.
- Xiong ZQ, Qian W, Suzuki K, McNamara JO. Formation of complement membrane attack complex in mammalian cerebral cortex evokes seizures and neurodegeneration. *J Neurosci* 2003; 23: 955-60.
- Zattoni M, Mura ML, Deprez F, et al. Brain infiltration of leukocytes contributes to the pathophysiology of temporal lobe epilepsy. *J Neurosci* 2011; 31: 4037-50.
- Zurolo E, Iyer A, Maroso M, et al. Activation of TLR, RAGE and HMGB1 signaling in malformations of cortical development. *Brain* 2011; 134: 1015-32.

Febrile infection-related epilepsy syndrome (FIRES): pathogenesis, treatment and outcome
A large cohort and update

Uri Kramer

Pediatric Neurology Unit, Tel Aviv Sourasky Medical Center, Tel Aviv University, Tel Aviv, Israel

---

Febrile infection-related epilepsy syndrome (FIRES) is a catastrophic epileptic encephalopathy with a yet undefined etiology. Close to 300 patients were described in the literature (Ismail & Kossoff, 2011). FIRES was given many names that emphasize either the characteristics of acute refractory partial epilepsy or the presumed pathogenesis, among them "acute encephalitis with refractory, repetitive partial seizures" (AERRPS) (Sakuma et al., 2001), "severe refractory status epilepticus due to presumed encephalitis" (Sahin et al., 2001), "idiopathic catastrophic epileptic encephalopathy" (Baxter et al., 2003), "new-onset refractory status epilepticus" (NORSE) (Wilder-Smith et al., 2005), "devastating epileptic encephalopathy in school-aged children" (DESC) (Mikaeloff et al., 2006), and FIRES (van Baalen et al., 2010). Japanese authors prefer the term AERRPS while the current preferred term by European authors is FIRES.

Most of the patients described in these series share common clinical characteristics, including a known febrile infection preceding the onset of the prolonged disease and the absence of any identified infectious agent. FIRES is encountered both in adults (Wilder-Smith et al., 2005) and children, but it is more frequent in children. The mechanism underlying this prolonged state is not clear, and an immunologic source (Specchio et al., 2010; van Baalen et al., 2010), a genetic predisposition, and an inflammation-mediated process (Nabbout et al., 2011) have been hypothesized.

The seizure types at the onset of the disease are mainly partial or secondarily generalized. The partial seizures are often complex partial seizures, at times with facial myoclonia (Mikaeloff et al., 2006; Sakuma et al., 2010; Kramer et al., 2011). Except for the periods of an induced burst-suppression coma (BSC), electroencephalography (EEG) is mainly bifocal or multifocal. The origin of recorded seizures is most often temporal followed by frontal onset (Mikaeloff et al., 2006; Kramer et al., 2011). Results of the initial magnetic resonance imaging (MRI) are usually normal. Hyperintensities are detectable in some patients, predominantly in the temporal regions, but also in the insula and the basal ganglia (Sahin et al., 2001; Mikaeloff et al., 2006; van Baalen et al., 2010), probably secondary to long-lasting epileptic activity. Brain biopsies of a few FIRES patients demonstrated gliosis but no histopathologic features of encephalitis (van Baalen et al., 2010). Treatment with different antiepileptic drugs, including immunosuppressive agents, is disappointing (Sahin et al., 2001; Kramer et al., 2005; Lin et al., 2008). There are descriptions of therapeutic success with a ketogenic diet (Mikaeloff et al., 2006; Nabbout et al., 2010; Ismail & Kossoff 2011; Vaccarezza et al., 2012). The outcome of FIRES is poor, with a death rate of up to 30% in some series (Kramer et al., 2005; Lin et al., 2008; van Baalen et al., 2010), refractory epilepsy at follow-up often immediately following the acute phase (Sakuma et al., 2001), and mental retardation in 66-100% of the survivors (Kramer et al., 2005, Mikaeloff et al., 2006). The survivors with normal cognitive levels will usually present with learning disabilities (Kramer et al., 2005, Mikaeloff et al., 2006), and only a small minority survive the episode without any neurologic sequelae (Kramer et al., 2005, Lin et al., 2008). While there was no correlation between the duration of BSC and outcome in one study (Lin et al., 2008), such correlation was found in the multicenter study (Kramer et al., 2011).

■ Methods

We performed a retrospective multicenter study. The data include those of the patients from eight pediatric studies that were published between November 2001 and July 2010. (Tungs' Taichung MetroHarbor Hospital, Taichung, Taiwan; Chang Gung Children's Hospital and Chang Gung Memorial Hospital, Taoyuan, Taiwan; Bambino Gesu Children's Hospital, Rome, Italy; Children's Hospital, Boston, Massachusetts, USA; Hôpital Necker-Enfants Malades, Paris, France; Schön Klinik, Vogtareuth, Germany; Christian-Albrechts-Universität, Kiel, Germany). The authors of those series were asked to provide additional data on their reported patients as well as on new ones. The inclusion criterion was the diagnosis of acute onset catastrophic status epilepticus. The condition was defined as continuation of seizures following the first cycle of BSC, or continuation of multiple seizures per day for > 1 week despite prompt treatment, the absence of any identifiable etiology for SE despite thorough investigation, and at least 1 year of follow-up. Exclusion criteria were age younger than 2 years, children with previously reported seizures, known neurologic disease, developmental delay prior to the acute disease, structural lesion on magnetic resonance imaging (MRI), or identification of an infectious agent in blood or cerebrospinal fluid (CSF). Because more detailed information on the parameters of the EEG during a BSC was not available from the patients' records, only the duration of the BSC was included in the analysis. The detailed statistical analyses were described in our previous report (Kramer et al., 2011).

■ Results

Clinical presentation

The cohort included 77 patients that had been recruited as of January 1992, and 69 of them were recruited during the last decade. The median age at the onset of FIRES was 8 years (range 2-17 years). The male-to-female ratio was 4:3. All but two patients exhibited a nonspecific illness prior to the SE. The disease was febrile in 96% of the patients and consisted mainly of upper respiratory tract infection and, to a lesser extent, gastroenteritis. The fever preceded the onset of seizures with a median duration of 4 days (range 1-14 days). Shortly after the onset of seizures, often within 24 hours, the seizures rapidly exacerbated into either SE or became frequent (up to dozens and even hundreds of seizures per day), with loss of consciousness between the attacks that required treatment with high-dose barbiturates or midazolam accompanied by mechanical ventilation. Most patients (58 of 77) had partial seizures. Thirty-one of these 58 patients had either simple partial or complex partial with secondary generalizations, and 19 had secondarily generalized seizures only. Five had generalized seizures accompanied by generalized discharges. Nine had characteristic semiology of facial or peribuccal myoclonia suggestive of opercular extension of the temporal focus. Data on epileptic foci were available for 59 patients. Ictal and interictal electroencephalography (EEG) studies revealed a single epileptic focus in only three of them. Five patients had generalized discharges, and the rest had two to four foci each from bilateral origins. The location of the epileptic foci was temporal in 16 cases (26.7%), frontotemporal in 16 (26.7%), and frontal in 13 (21.4%). The foci were evenly spread between the other brain regions (central, parietal, and occipital) in the remaining 15 (25%). The median duration of mechanical ventilation in the surviving patients was 41 days (mean ± standard deviation (SD) 49 ± 44.5, range 4-220).

Investigations

The detailed thorough investigation for possible infectious and metabolic etiology was previously described (Kramer et al., 2011). No such cause was found in any case.

Magnetic resonance imaging (MRI) was performed at least once in all 77 patients. Details of the initial MRI were available for 63 patients and were normal in 35 (55%) of them. The abnormalities detected in the remaining 28 patients included mainly signal hyperintensities in both hippocampi (seven patients), or in the peri-insular region (three patients), or in a combination of both (two patients). Leptomeningeal or ependymal enhancement was seen in another four patients. Generalized atrophy was observed in only two patients. A second follow-up MRI was performed later in the disease course in 58 patients, and it revealed generalized atrophy in 28 patients and signal hyperintensity in an additional 17 patients. The signal hyperintensity was located in the hippocampal region bilaterally in 11 of those 17 patients.

Brain biopsy was performed in 13 patients and revealed gliosis in 7 and leptomeningeal inflammatory infiltrate in one. There were no pathologic findings in the other five patients.

Treatment

A median of 6 (SD 2.9, range 2-16) antiepileptic drugs (AEDs) were given per patient during the acute phase of FIRES. Thirty patients were treated with intravenous immunoglobulin (IVIG), and 29 patients were treated with steroids in different forms and doses, mainly with pulse methylprednisolone. The only evidence of a beneficial effect of any of those treatments was provided by Specchio et al. (2010), who reported a positive response to IVIG in two of eight patients. Both patients – who had seizure reduction of > 75% following IVIG treatment – were not treated with BSC. In both, IVIG was given following failure of three other AEDs as repeated courses of 2 g/kg, once per month for 8-9 months. CSF investigation of both patients revealed the presence of oligoclonal bands. Because of the long time until clinical improvement, the relative efficacy of this specific treatment can be debated.

Four patients were treated with ketogenic diet; one showed an immediate and sustained effect of that treatment (Mikaeloff et al., 2006). This patient, who had > 100 seizures a day, demonstrated total cessation of seizures within 2 days of starting the ketogenic diet. In addition, small numbers of patients were treated with various agents, including propofol, lidocaine, ketamine, verapamil, magnesium, B6, folinic acid, biotin, paraldehyde, dextromethorphan, and plasmapheresis, without any response.

Data on mechanical ventilation was available for 58 patients. The median period of mechanical ventilation required by those 58 patients was 41 days (mean 49, SD 44.56, range 4-220). Two of the participating centers reported not using BSC for any of their patients following earlier reports on severe adverse reactions (Shyu et al., 2008; Specchio et al., 2010). Forty-six of the study patients were treated by BSC with barbiturates (phenobarbital, pentothal, or thiopental) or midazolam. Because of the retrospective nature of the current study, details on the ratio between the bursts and the interburst silent periods are not available. The median duration of the total BSC cycles was 7 days (mean 14.3, SD 14, range 1.5-49) days. The patients were ventilated for periods that were significantly longer than the BSC itself. This is because the total ventilation period also included the time until the BSC was achieved, the time until the patient was weaned from BSC, and time of anesthesia induction by either barbiturates or midazolam for the sake of seizure control and not aiming at the depth of a BSC.

Outcome

Nine patients (11.7%) died during the acute phase of FIRES. Five of them had been treated by BSC. The cause of death was sepsis in two patients, intracranial hemorrhage in one, and undetermined in the other six. There was no correlation between the probability of death and any of the tested variables. At follow-up, 66 of the 68 survivors had epilepsy that was refractory to treatment in 63 of them. Therefore, 93% (63 of 68) survivors of FIRES were left with refractory epilepsy. The seizures either continued without interruption following the acute phase of FIRES or they appeared after a lag of a few weeks to 3 months. The seizure type was complex partial or simple partial in all patients with secondary generalizations in the minority.

Cognitive levels at follow-up of at least one year were as follows: 12 patients (18%) were diagnosed as normal (with or without attention deficit disorder and learning disabilities), 11 (16%) had a borderline cognitive level, 10 (14%) had mild mental retardation, 16 (24%) had moderate mental retardation, 8 (12%) had severe mental retardation, and 11 (16%) were in a vegetative state. Poor cognitive outcome at follow-up was significantly associated with younger age at FIRES onset (Wald chi-square = 4.83, $p = 0.02$), and higher log of BSC duration (Wald chi-square = 7.65, $p = 0.005$). In addition to the cognitive insult, some of the patients had motor dysfunction due to severe secondary peripheral neuropathy and ataxia. The exact rate of these insults and their evolution could not be ascertained in the current study because of missing data. There was no correlation between mortality or degree of cognitive insult at follow-up and number of foci in EEG during the acute phase, MRI abnormalities, and duration of mechanical ventilation.

Discussion

FIRES is a catastrophic epilepsy syndrome that represents an extreme form of epileptic disease subsequent to a febrile episode. The age at onset of this specific syndrome is clustered around the early school years, with the majority of the children (73%) presenting between the ages of 4 and 9 years.

Pathogenesis

The pathogenesis underlying the cascade leading to such severe epilepsy is still enigmatic. A number of series referred to a possible infectious encephalitis due to an unidentified agent (Sahin et al., 2001, Kramer et al., 2005, Lin et al., 2008), others considered the involvement of an immune process (Specchio et al., 2010, van Baalen et al., 2010), and an inflammation mediated process was hypothesized as well (Nabbout et al., 2011).

The typical evolution of FIRES following a non-exceptional febrile event in the presence of pleocytosis in the CSF of most patients could be suggestive for encephalitis. A thorough and extensive investigation for possible infectious agents, however, failed to identify any pathogen in the current series of patients, and so the term "presumed encephalitis" (Sahin et al., 2001; Kramer et al., 2005; Lin et al., 2008) was rejected. It is important to note that a similar course was seen in other patients from the same centers in whom an infectious agent had been identified. These latter patients had herpes simplex virus, human herpes virus type 6 (Sahin et al., 2001), parvovirus B19, rhinovirus, respiratory syncytial virus, Epstein-Barr virus, echovirus, and mycoplasma pneumonia (van Baalen et al., 2010), and thus they are not considered FIRES patients. The biphasic clinical course seen in all 77 study patients suggests a possible infection-triggered process rather than an infectious disease.

Antineuronal autoantibodies are associated with several epileptic disorders specifically implicating several autoantibodies, such as anticardiolipin antibodies, anti-nuclear antibodies, anti-GAD antibodies, anti-VGKC antibodies, anti-NMDA (N-methyl-D-aspartate) receptor antibodies, and GluR3 antibodies. Two groups of investigators suggested an immune mechanism as being the leading process in FIRES patients (Specchio et al., 2010; van Baalen et al., 2010). However, taking into account the recently published series, it seems that the rate of positive detection of antibodies is low: a summary of detected antibodies in recent series and case reports is as follows (Sakuma et al., 2010; Specchio et al., 2010; Illingworth et al., 2011; Nabbout et al., 2011; Howell et al., 2012; van Baalen et al., 2012): GluRϵ2 6/9, GAD 3/7, GluR3 1/4, VGKC 1/22, NMDA 0/15, AMPA 0/15, GABAa 0/15. It is also possible that this association may represent a secondary phenomenon and not the primary pathogenic mechanism (Majoie et al., 2006).

Inflammatory processes have also been recently hypothesized to be involved with acute aggravations of epilepsy (Nabbout et al., 2011). SE may induce a pro-inflammatory process via an increased release of glutamate (Tian et al., 2005) and other molecules, such as cytokines, prostaglandins, and complement (Vezzani et al., 2008) which, in turn, further promote the epileptic process, perhaps by modifying ion-channel function and stimulating neuronal excitability in FIRES (Nabbout et al., 2011).

A genetic predisposition was also suggested by some authors. The yield of genetic investigations was, however, negative in most tested children. Altogether, 16 patients were tested for SCN1A (Carranza et al., 2012; van Baalen et al., 2012), and five were tested for POLG1 (Van Baalen et al., 2012). In a single patient, a female with fever triggering acute onset epilepsy mimicking FIRES, a missense mutation of PCDH19 gene was found (Specchio et al., 2011). Currently some groups are investigating FIRES patients for other possible genes.

Treatment

It would appear that none of the many AEDs or the various other therapeutic agents that were tried contributed to decreasing the seizure load or shortening the duration of the disease in our cohort. The epileptic process in FIRES may, therefore, be self-limited.

An exception to the therapeutic failures is the relative success of ketogenic diet, which was efficacious in one of four patients treated in Paris (Mikaeloff et al., 2006). Based on these preliminary results, neurologists in Hôpital Necker-Enfants Malades in Paris further pursued this treatment modality in nine other patients and found it highly efficacious in six of them. The diet stopped seizure activity within 4-6 days (Nabbout et al., 2010). It should be emphasized, however, that all of the children continued to exhibit refractory epilepsy at follow-up. A positive response to ketogenic diet was described also by others (Ismail & Kossoff, 2012; Vaccarezza et al., 2012).

Positive response to treatment with immunomodulators such as IVIG or steroids is rare as the results of recent studies showed: IVIG – 3/44 and steroids 3/42 (Sakuma et al., 2010; Kramer et al., 2011; Illingworth et al., 2011). It might be reasonable, therefore, to pursue immunosuppressive therapy mainly in children with positive detection of autoantibodies; in theses specific cases, also plasma exchange, rituximab (Howell et al., 2012) and even cyclophosphamide might be tried.

A role for BSC therapy

The use of BSC is standard care in severe refractory status epilepticus (Rantala et al., 1999; Rossetti et al., 2005), even though its efficacy is questionable and the majority of the BSC-treated patients resume seizure activity following its cessation (Rantala et al., 1999). The Japanese retrospective survey, on the other hand, described a very good response in almost all patients treated with BSC, but at the same time they described an average treatment duration with BSC of 52 days, so the definition of good response is not clear (Sakuma et al., 2010). Pentobarbital may decrease cerebral blood flow in humans and animals (de Bray et al., 1993; Wada et al., 1996) and, although it may compensate for the cerebral edema that occurs during SE, these blood flow changes may induce insult to the vulnerable hippocampus (Nehling & Pereira de Vasconcelos, 1996). In addition, the use of barbiturates may paradoxically aggravate seizures (Nabbout et al., 2011). Sufficient information on the survivors' cognitive level at follow-up and on the duration of BSC was available for 32 of the survivors (Kramer et al., 2011). The statistical analysis clearly demonstrated that a BSC was not associated with an increased death rate. On the other hand, a longer period of therapeutically induced BSC was significantly associated with a poorer cognitive level at follow-up (p 0.005). This association should be considered cautiously, since induction of a longer BSC state is also the result of a longer disease process and thus likely to reflect a more severe condition.

In summary, there are increasing numbers of patients with FIRES described in the literature. The pathogenesis and the exact mechanism for this devastating encephalopathy are undefined. In addition, the efficacy of currently available treatments remains doubtful. The value of a ketogenic diet and immunomodulators as preferred treatments warrant further investigation.

References

- Baxter P, Clarke A, Cross H, et al. Idiopathic catastrophic epileptic encephalopathy presenting with acute onset intractable status. Seizure 2003; 12: 379-87.
- Carranza RD, Harvey S, Lona X, et al. Febrile infection-related epilepsy syndrome is not caused by SCN1A mutations. Epilepsy Res 2012; 100: 194-8.
- de Bray JM, Granry JC, Monrigal JP, Leftheriotis G, Saumet JL. Effects of thiopental on middle cerebral artery blood velocities: a transcranial Doppler study in children. Childs Nerv Syst 1993; 9: 220-3.
- Howell KB, Katanyuwong K, Mackay MT, et al. Long-term follow-up of febrile infection-related epilepsy syndrome. Epilepsia 2012; 53: 101-10.
- Illingworth MA, Hanrahan D, Anderson CE, et al. Elevated VGKC-complex antibodies ina boy with fever-induced refractory epileptic encephalopathy in school-age children (FIRES). Dev Med Child Neurol 2011; 53: 1053-7.
- Ismail F, Kossoff E. AERRPS, DESC, NORSE, FIRES: Multilabeling or distinct epileptic entities? Epilepsia 2011; 52: e185-9.
- Kramer U, Shorer Z, Ben-Zeev B, Lerman-Sagie T, Goldberg-Stern H, Lahat E. Severe refractory status epilepticus owing to presumed encephalitis. J Child Neurol 2005; 20: 184-7.
- Kramer U, Chi CS, Lin KL, et al. Febrile infection-related epilepsy syndrome (FIRES): pathogenesis, treatment and outcome. A multicenter study on 77 children. Epilepsia 2011; 52: 1956-65.
- Lin JJ, Lin KL, Wang HS, Hsia SH, Wu CT. Analysis of status epilepticus related presumed encephalitis in children. Eur J Paediatr Neurol 2008; 12: 32-7.
- Majoie HJ, de Baets M, Renier W, Lang B, Vincent A. Antibodies to voltage-gated potassium and calcium channels in epilepsy. Epilepsy Res 2006; 71: 135-41.
- Mikaeloff Y, Jambaque I, Hertz-Pannier L, et al. Devastating epileptic encephalopathy in school-aged children (DESC): a pseudo encephalitis. Epilepsy Res 2006; 69: 67-79.
- Nabbout R, Mazzuca M, Hubert P, et al. Efficacy of ketogenic diet in severe refractory status epilepticus initiating fever induced refractory epileptic encephalopathy in school age children (FIRES). Epilepsia 2010; 51: 2033-7.
- Nabbout R, Vezzani A, Dulac O, Chiron C. Acute encephalopathy with inflammation-mediated status epilepticus. Lancet Neurol 2011; 10: 99-108.
- Nehling A, Pereira de Vasconcelos A. The model of pentylenetetrazol-induced status epilepticus in the immature rat: short-and long-term effects. Epilepsy Res 1996; 26: 93-103.
- Rantala H, Saukkonen AL, Remes M, Uhari M. Efficacy of five days barbiturate anesthesia in the treatment of intractable epilepsies in children. Epilepsia 1999; 40: 1775-9.
- Rossetti AO, Logroscino G, Bromfield EB. Refractory status epilepticus: effects of treatment aggressiveness on prognosis. Arch Neurol 2005; 62: 1698-1702.
- Sahin M, Menache CC, Holmes GL, Riviello JJ. Outcome of severe refractory status epilepticus in children. Epilepsia 2001; 42: 1461-7.
- Sakuma H, Fukumizu M, Kohyama J. Efficacy of anticonvulsants on acute encephalitis with refractory, repetitive, partial seizures (AERRPS). No To Hattatsu 2001; 33: 385-90. (Japanese).

- Sakuma H, Awaya Y, Shiomi M, et al. Acute encephalitis with refractory, repetitive partial seizures (AERRPS): a peculiar form of childhood encephalitis. *Acta Neurol Scand* 2010; 121: 251-6.
- Shyu CS, Lee HF, Chi CS, Chen CH. Acute encephalitis with refractory, repetitive partial seizures. *Brain Dev* 2008; 30: 356-61.
- Specchio N, Fusco L, Claps D, Vigevano F. Epileptic encephalopathy in children possibly related to immune-mediated pathogenesis. *Brain Dev* 2010; 32: 51-6.
- Specchio N, Fusco L, Vigevano F. Acute-onset epilepsy triggered by fever mimicking FIRES (febrile infection-related epilepsy syndrome): the role of protocadherin 19 (PCDH19) gene mutation. *Epilepsia* 2011; 52: e172-5.
- Tian GF, Azmi H, Takano T, et al. An astrocytic basis of epilepsy. *Nat Med* 2005; 11: 973-81.
- Vaccarezza M, et al. Super-refractory status epilepticus: treatment with ketogenic diet in pediatrics. *Rev Neurol* 2012; 55: 20-5.
- van Baalen A, Hausler M, Boor R, et al. Febrile infection-related epilepsy syndrome (FIRES): a non-encephalitic encephalopathy in childhood. *Epilepsia* 2010; 51: 1323-8.
- van Baalen A, Hausler M, Piecko-Startinig B, et al. Febrile infection-related epilepsy syndrome without detectable autoantibodies and response to immunotherapy: a case series and discussion of epileptogenesis in FIRES. *Neuropediatrics* 2012; 43: 209-16.
- Vezzani A, Balosso S, Raizza T. The role of cytokines in the pathophysiology of epilepsy. *Brain Behav Immun* 2008; 72: 797-803.
- Wada DR, Harashima H, Ebling W, Osaki EW, Stanski DR. Effects of thiopental on regional blood flows in the rat. *Anesthesiology* 1996; 84: 596-604.
- Wiendi H, Bien CG, Bernasconi P, et al. GluR3 antibodies: prevalence in focal epilepsy but no specificity for Rasmussen's encephalitis. *Neurology* 2001; 57: 1511-4.
- Wilder-Smith EPV, Lim ECH, Teoh HL, et al. The NORSE (new-onset refractory status epilepticus) syndrome: defining a disease entity. *Ann Acad Med Singapore* 2005; 34: 417-20.

Are idiopathic epilepsy syndromes in neonates always "benign?"

Federico Vigevano[1], **Maria Roberta Cilio**[1,2], **Domenico Serino**[1], **Lucia Fusco**[1]

[1] *Neurology Unit, Bambino Gesù Children's Hospital, Rome, Italy*
[2] *Neonatal Brain Disorders Center, UCSF, San Francisco, USA*

■ Introduction

Seizures with onset during the neonatal period are mainly symptomatic in nature and secondary to acute or remote prenatal or perinatal pathologies. In 1964, Rett and Teubel reported, for the first time, the possible existence of seizures specifically related to a genetic predisposition with a benign evolution. Since then, other similar hereditary cases have been described, confirming its autosomal dominant nature. To date, two clinical entities with neonatal onset have been recognized among the *familial autosomal dominant* focal epilepsies group, which are the "benign familial neonatal seizure" syndrome (BFNS) and the "benign familial neonatal-infantile seizures" syndrome (BFNIS). These entities have many features in common with the infantile-onset "benign familial infantile seizures" (BFIS) syndrome, such as:

- autosomal dominant mode of inheritance;
- absence of other etiological factors;
- occurrence of seizures self-limited to a brief period of life;
- partial seizures in clusters, with variable site of onset;
- seizures with or without secondary generalization;
- absence of any typical interictal EEG traits;
- normal development;
- reported association with non-epileptic paroxysmal disorders.

Since autosomal dominant epileptic syndromes are rare, they have been object of many studies and today the genetic mutations which underlie them are known. For BFNS, the involved chromosomal loci are located on chromosomes 20 and 8 and the compromised genes are *KCNQ2* and *KCNQ3*, respectively, both encoding for potassium channels. The gene involved in BFNIS is *SCN2A*, located on chromosome 2 and encoding for a sodium channel subunit, while BFIS is related to mutations of the *PRRT2* gene located on chromosome 16, of the *ATP1A2* gene located on chromosome 1, and is also linked to a locus on chromosome 19. Such distinction is actually not so clear-cut, since mutations of the *KCNQ2* and *KCNQ3* genes may also be found in association with infantile-onset seizures.

The most commonly found mutation in BFNS is of the *KCNQ2* gene, which may be found in more than 90% of cases with onset during the neonatal period and in some cases with neonatal-infantile onset. Given the benign evolution of the patients presenting it, this gene mutation has been attributed with a positive prognostic value. Recently, however, several cases of neonatal-onset familial epilepsy with severe outcome have been described, for which mutations of the *KCNQ2* gene have surprisingly been found. Due to the severity of the relative clinical situation, the term "KCNQ2 encephalopathy" has been coined. To understand how the same genetic mutation may be responsible for two types of epilepsy with such a different prognosis, the clinical, EEG and genetic aspects of the two entities must be analyzed.

■ Benign familial neonatal seizures

Clinical and EEG features

Rett and Teubel (1964) reported on BFNS for the first time describing eight cases over three generations. On the third day of life the male proband developed a tonic seizure with cyanosis followed by bilateral clonic jerks also involving the face. He had 15-20 seizures on the following day. A brother born 16 months later had a similar clinical picture. Interictal EEG was reported as normal for these two newborns and for other affected relatives. The authors stressed the familial history, the normality of the interictal EEG and the benign outcome.

Since then, several similar families have been described, better defining the clinical characteristics of the syndrome (Plouin & Neubauer, 2012).

Seizure onset usually takes place between the second and the third day of life, but some newborns start having seizures later, during the first month of life or even up to the third month. Seizures are brief and frequent, lasting one to two minutes and often progressing towards status epilepticus. Mean cluster duration is of about 20 hours, varying from 2 hours to 3 days. With the help of video-EEG monitoring we now know that seizure semiology is characterized by a brief uni- or bilateral, asymmetrical, tonic component, with side dominance shifting between seizures, with brief apnea, followed by symmetrical or asymmetrical clonic jerks and autonomic oculo-facial features. The ictal EEG discloses a focal discharge, with variable site of onset, mainly in parieto-occipital areas, characterized by recruiting rhythm of increasing amplitude spreading over the hemisphere and involving then the entire brain. (Hirsch *et al.*, 1993; Ronen *et al.*, 1993; Bye, 1994).

Epileptic spasms and myoclonic jerks or purely tonic seizures are not reported.

Interictal EEG is described as normal, with mild abnormal patterns, rarely as "thèta pointu alternant", but never with patterns associated with a severe outcome, as generalized spike-wave bursts, multifocal spikes or suppression-burst patterns.

In contrast with the repetitive seizures, the neurological state of the babies remains normal in most cases; a mild hypotonia that may be transitory is noticed in some cases. None of these babies requires a neonatal intensive care unit.

Clinical evolution is characterized by disappearance of seizures within a few days and normal psychomotor development. Several patients have been treated with phenobarbital, valproic acid or phenytoin with similarly positive results. If treatment is initiated and diagnosis is correct, withdrawal seems reasonable between the third and the sixth month.

Febrile seizures have been reported in 5% of cases with the same incidence as for the general population. In relation to the subsequent development of epilepsy, the estimated risk is around 11%, mainly for benign forms; no case of severe epilepsy was noticed in BFNS.

Genetic aspects

BFNS is dominantly inherited with a penetrance as high as 85%. Gene mutations specifically involve *KCNQ2* in most of the reported families, but the syndrome exhibits genetic heterogeneity as it can be also caused by mutations of the *KCNQ3* gene. The KCNQ2 gene is located on chromosome 20q13.3 (Bievert *et al.*, 1998; Singh *et al.*, 1998; Lerche *et al.*, 1999; Miraglia *et al.*, 2000) whereas KCNQ3 is located on chromosome 8q24 (Charleir *et al.*, 1998; Hirose *et al.*, 2000). More than 10 mutations have been identified in *KCNQ2*, but only 2 in *KCNQ3*. In a recent paper (Zara *et al.*, 2013) in which genetic testing was performed in benign familial epilepsies of the first year of life, in 7 among 8 families with neonatal familial seizures, mutations specifically involved *KCNQ2* and were characterized by deletions whereas point mutations were characteristic of benign familial seizures with delayed onset.

■ KCNQ2 encephalopathy

The first recognized case of the clinical entity now known as "KCNQ2 encephalopathy" was described by one of us in 2003 (Dedek *et al.*, 2003) and had the following characteristics.

Case presentation

A.D. was the first child of non-consanguineous parents. After a full term uneventful pregnancy, he was born by cesarean section due to a prolonged delivery period and not better specified symptoms of fetal distress. The Apgar score was 6 (1 min) and 8 (5 min). Birth weight was 4 kg. While hospitalized in another institution, during his third day of life, A.D. developed multifocal seizures characterized by left or right head deviation and upper and lower limb involvement. The seizures were reported as being resistant to phenobarbitone, phenytoin, pyridoxine, phenobarbital and vigabatrin. Several neuroimaging exams were undertaken: computed tomography (CT) scans performed at days seven and 30 were reported as normal. Magnetic resonance imaging (MRI), performed at 18 days of life, was reported as normal. A.D. was first referred to our institute at 41 days of life. Neurological examination showed diffuse hypotonia. Biochemical screening (serum electrolytes, glucose level and ammonia), biotinidase screening, serum and cerebrospinal fluid (CSF) lactate and amino acids, serum ammonium, urine and CSF organic acids, urine guanidine-acetate-methyl-transferase (GAMT) and creatinine, CSF/serum glucose ratio) yielded no significant results. MRI imaging was normal and MR spectroscopy was within normal age parameters. At the age of 7 weeks the patient was treated with ACTH, resulting in a significant improvement in EEG activity and gradual reduction in seizure frequency, with cessation at age 13 weeks.

A.D.'s mother had a history of cyanotic spells and convulsions during the second post-natal day. The seizures, which occurred at a frequency of two to three per day, were characterized by right or left limb and facial jerks. After a temporary response to phenobarbital, ACTH therapy was started and she became seizure free within 1 month. Evidence of the aforesaid anamnestic data led to consequent genetic testing. PCR amplification and subsequent direct sequencing of KCQN2 exon 5 from both A.D.'s and his mother's DNA, revealed a heterozygous cytosine to guanine nucleotide exchange, leading to the substitution of serine by tryptophane in amino acid position 247 (S247W) of the predicted protein (data already published; Dedek et al., 2003).

At arrival to our institution, the patient was soporous and presented many seizures per day, alternating a state of apparent wakefulness with a state of apparent sleep. The interictal EEG showed a very discontinuous pattern which became a clear-cut burst-suppression during sleep. During wakefulness, the burst-suppression pattern was replaced by a multifocal random attenuation pattern in which bursts were asynchronous between the two hemispheres and attenuation randomly appeared after the paroxysms. Epileptiform abnormalities were mainly observed over the central, temporal and parietal regions.

Repetitive and prolonged video/EEG monitoring showed several focal seizures originating alternatively from both hemispheres, even more frequently from the left. Clinically seizures were characterized by unilateral eye and head deviation, upper limb hypertonia sometimes followed by asynchronous and asymmetrical clonic jerks, eyelid myoclonias and polypnea. Ictal EEG was characterized by focal low voltage fast activity, followed by recruiting theta rhythms and by bilateral focal spike-wave complexes alternatively localized to one hemisphere and subsequently diffusing to the other.

After one week from the beginning of ACTH therapy, EEG, while still pathological, improved and progressive reduction of abnormalities was recorded. Background activity became more continuous and the burst-suppression pattern disappeared. Interictal EEG pattern was characterized by frequent irregular spikes and polyspike – wave complexes over the right frontal and temporal regions associated with similar elements over the left parietal and temporal regions, with asynchronous trend.

During the following few weeks seizures were still recorded, while becoming more and more sporadic until finally disappearing after four weeks since the introduction of ACTH. Recorded seizures were tonic focal seizures, characterized by upper left limb contraction, right eye and head deviation, oral automatisms and hyperextension of head and trunk. Ictal EEG was still characterized by focal, right central, low voltage fast activity, followed by a recruiting alpha-like rhythm.

During a follow-up period of 4 years the patient was seizure-free. Psychomotor development was delayed and at the end of the first year a pyramidal paraparesis became evident. He was then referred to his local rehabilitation unit.

Clinical and genetic aspects

Since the first report of KCNQ2 encephalopathy (Dedek et al., 2003), a number of other cases with severe outcome including variable degrees of intellectual disability have been reported in families with KCNQ2 mutations (Borgatti et al., 2004; Steinlein et al., 2007). The clinical characteristics of these patients consisted of seizure persistence and psychomotor delay in association with normal neuroimaging.

In 2012, Weckhuysen et al. screened 80 cases of epilepsy of unknown etiology and onset during the neonatal period or the first months of life, for mutations of the KCNQ2 and KCNQ3 genes. In eight patients, representing 10% of all cases, seven different heterozygous mutations of the KCNQ2 gene and none of the KCNQ3 gene were found.

The clinical picture of the patients was characterized by onset of frequent, multiple daily, intractable seizures in the first week of life. The most frequent seizure semiology is a generalized tonic contraction, followed by myoclonic jerks. Seizures generally resolved by age 3 years, but all the children had profound or severe intellectual disability, with motor impairment. Interictal EEG at onset was characterized by multifocal spikes or burst suppression pattern. Early MRI of the brain showed characteristic hyperintensities in the basal ganglia and thalamus that later resolved.

The seizures were resistant to the majority of AEDs, but none of the Weckhuysen patients has been treated with ACTH. In relation to the eight KCNQ2 mutations, six arose *de novo*. One mutation was inherited from a less severely affected father who presented mosaicism for the mutation, which was found in around 30% of lymphocytes. The inheritance pattern of the remaining mutations was unknown. Interestingly, one of these mutations occurred twice de novo in 2 unrelated patients. None of the 7 different mutations were observed in 276 ethnically matched control individuals, or were previously published in association with BFNS. As has been already noted before (Steinlein et al., 2007), these mutations associated with an unfavorable outcome tend to be located within the functionally critical S5/S6 regions of the KCNQ2 gene.

■ Conclusions

The KCNQ2 gene family encodes for several subunits of voltage-gated potassium channels which are expressed in the central nervous system and which are responsible for the modulation of the M-current, a slowly activating, non-inactivating potassium conductance that inhibits neuronal excitability. Mutations of the KCNQ2 gene, which encodes for the channel Kv7.2 subunit, are closely associated with BNFS. However, previously quoted recently published data demonstrate that alterations of KCNQ2 may also be associated with an epileptic encephalopathy phenotype which differs from BNFS in both electroclinical presentation and evolution. In *Table I* we summarize the phenotype of the two syndromes.

It is easily noticed how the two syndromes differ not only in regard to prognosis, but mainly for seizure semiology and interictal EEG characteristics. Even if not in all cases of KCNQ2 encephalopathy, the MRI may also show transitional alterations never reported in relation to BFNS. Finally we have to highlight how the genetic similarities may only be apparent; mutations of the KCNQ2 gene found in "KCNQ2 encephalopathy" in fact, are not the same as those found in families with BFNS and are mostly localized in a restricted area around the S5/S6 segments. Further genetic investigations will allow a better understanding of the pathogenetic role of these mutations and furthermore of the possible role of other genetic and environmental factors, in the development of such a severe syndrome.

Table I. Electroclinical characteristics of the two syndromes

BFNS	KCNQ2 encephalopathy
Brief tonic seizures accompanied by motor and autonomic features	Similar type of seizures at onset, then predominantly tonic
Mutations in *KCNQ2* gene	Mutations in *KCNQ2* gene
Normal interictal EEG	EEG: burst-suppression pattern
Easy to treat seizures	Transient MRI abnormalities
Normal developmental outcome	Development of drug-resistant epilepsy
	Poor developmental outcome

In conclusion, because of their association with encephalopathy characterized by early onset suppression-burst EEG patterns, *KCNQ2* mutations must now accordingly be taken into consideration in the diagnostic work-up of neonatal encephalopathies when burst-suppression is the prevalent EEG pattern.

References

- Biervert C, Schroeder BC, Kubisch C, et al. A potassium channel mutation in neonatal human epilepsy. *Science* 1998; 279: 403-6.
- Borgatti R, Zucca C, Cavallini A, et al. A novel mutation in KCNQ2 associated with BFNC, drug resistant epilepsy, and mental retardation. *Neurology* 2004; 63: 57-65.
- Bye AM. Neonate with benign familial neonatal convulsions: recorded generalized and focal seizures. *Pediatr Neurol* 1994; 10: 164-5.
- Charlier C, Singh NA, Ryan SG. A pore mutation in a novel KQT-like channel gene in an idiopathic epilepsy family. *Nat Genet* 1998; 18: 53-5.
- Dedek K, Fusco L, Teloy N, Steinlein OK. Neonatal convulsions and epileptic encephalopathy in an Italian family with a missense mutation in the fifth transmembrane region of KCNQ2. *Epilepsy Res* 2003; 54: 21-7.
- Hirose S, Zenri F, Akiyoshi H, et al. A novel mutation of KCNQ3 (c.925T-->C) in a Japanese family with benign neonatal convulsions. *Ann Neurol* 2000; 47: 822-6.
- Hirsch E, Velez A, Sellal F, et al. Electroclinical signs of benign neonatal familial convulsions. *Ann Neurol* 1993; 134: 835-41.
- Lerche H, Biervert C, Alekov AK. A reduced K+ current due to a novel mutation in KCNQ2 causes neonatal convulsions. *Ann Neurol* 1999; 46: 305-12.
- Miraglia del Giudice E, Coppola G, Scuccimarra G, et al. Familial Neonatal Convulsions (BFNC) resulting from mutation of the KCNQ2 voltage sensor. *Eur J Med Genet* 2000; 8: 994-7.
- Plouin P, Neubauer BA. Benign familial and non-familial neonatal seizures. In: Bureau M, Genton P, Dravet C, Delgado-Escueta A, Tassinari CA, Thomas P, Wolf P (eds). *Epileptic Syndromes in Infancy, Childhood and Adolescence*, 5th ed. Montrouge: John Libbey, 2012, pp. 77-88.
- Rett AR, Teubel R. Neugeborenen Krampfe im Rahmen einer epileptisch belasten Familie. *Wiener Klinische Wochenschrift* 1964; 76: 609-13.
- Ronen GM, Rosales TO, Connolly M, et al. Seizure characteristics in chromosome 20 benign familial neonatal convulsions. *Neurology* 1993; 43: 1355-60.

- Singh NA, Charlier C, Stauffer D, *et al.* A novel potassium channel gene, KCNQ2, is mutated in an inherited epilepsy of newborns. *Nat Genet* 1998; 18: 25-9.
- Steinlein OK, Conrad C, Weidner B. Benign familial neonatal convulsions: always benign? *Epilepsy Res* 2007; 73: 245-9.
- Weckhuysen S, Mandelstam S, Suls A, *et al.* KCNQ2 encephalopathy: emerging phenotype of a neonatal epileptic encephalopathy. *Ann Neurol* 2012; 71: 15-25.
- Zara F, Specchio N, Striano P, *et al.* Genetic testing in benign familial epilepsies of the first year of life: Clinical and diagnostic significance. *Epilepsia* 2013; 54: 425-36.

Neonatal epilepsy and underlying aetiology (other than idiopathic): to what extent do the seizures and the EEG abnormalities influence outcome?

Georgia Ramantani

Epilepsy Centre, University Hospital Freiburg, Germany

■ Introduction

Seizure incidence is at its highest during the neonatal period compared to any other period of life (Volpe, 2008). The overall incidence is 1-3 in 1000 live births, with considerably higher rates in high-risk premature infants (Ronen *et al.*, 1999; Saliba *et al.*, 2001). Eighty percent of seizures occur in the first week of life, constituting the most common and distinctive sign of neurologic dysfunction (Volpe, 2008).

The recent technologic advances in obstetric and neonatal care have changed the spectrum of insults to which the immature brain is exposed and thus the etiologic profile of neonatal seizures (Arzimanoglou *et al.*, 2004; Mizrahi, 2005). Neonatal seizures are predominantly symptomatic, originating from acute perinatal events such as hypoxic-ischemic encephalopathy (HIE), metabolic disturbance, intracerebral haemorrhage, central nervous system (CNS) infection, stroke, or inborn errors of metabolism, in order of decreasing frequency (Mizrahi, 2005). Neonatal seizures constitute a grave condition that may lead to neonatal death or dire sequelae including neurologic impairment, developmental delay and postneonatal epilepsy. With mortality rates decreasing from 40% to 20% in the last decades, the prevalence of long-term neurodevelopmental sequelae in survivors remains unchanged at 30% (Volpe, 2008).

Several studies have sought to define predictors of long-term outcome in neonates with seizures, most focussing on the underlying aetiology or on specific seizure presentations and electroencephalography (EEG) abnormalities. However, no clear pattern has emerged so far, possibly due to the variable criteria of neonatal seizure identification and etiologic diagnosis through the years or among different institutions.

Identification of neonatal seizures

The detection and classification of neonatal seizures continues to be challenging, especially when based on clinical observation alone, as is often the case in clinical practice (Murray et al., 2008; Malone et al., 2009). The presentation of neonatal seizures is indeed highly variable and includes subtle, clonic, tonic, and myoclonic events of typically brief and focal nature (Scher, 2002). Seminal work postulated that clonic seizures are the most reliable and distinctive in terms of identification, followed by focal tonic seizures (Mizrahi & Kellaway, 1987). However, detection rate by clinical staff amounted to a mere 9% of electroclinical seizures in a recent study that included 70% clonic seizures (Murray et al., 2008). Similarly, in a study carried out among 137 health care professionals, participants correctly identified only half of clinical seizures in neonates, with identification rates of medical doctors similar to those of other health professionals (Malone et al., 2009).

Since neonatal seizures may present as clinical, electroclinical or electrographic events, their accurate identification and distinction from non-epileptic events is clearly not feasible when based on clinical evaluation alone (Scher, 2002). Encephalopathic neonates can exhibit abnormal motor behaviours not necessarily correlating with ictal EEG patterns and may correspond to "brainstem release" from functional decortication as a result of a severe neocortical dysfunction or damage (Mizrahi & Kellaway, 1987). On the other hand, healthy neonates can exhibit non-epileptic movements such as jitteriness, clonus, sleep myoclonus, sucking movements, and repetitive movements during rapid eye movement (REM) sleep that may further hamper detection (Scher, 2002). In addition, the clinical presentation of seizures in affected neonates may be suppressed despite persisting ictal EEG activity by the use of medications for ventilatory assistance or seizure control (Boylan et al., 2002).

Therefore, the diagnosis of neonatal seizures based on clinical observation alone is bound to include "false positives", consisting of neonates with either normal or non-epileptic pathologic behavioural patterns. Although amplitude integrated EEG (aEEG) can facilitate diagnosis and treatment monitoring of neonatal seizures to some extent, continuous multichannel simultaneous VIDEO-EEG recording remains the gold standard for their identification and classification. However, currently this remains largely inaccessible in most neonatal intensive care units (NICUs).

Pathophysiology of neonatal seizures and pharmacotherapy effects

The hyperexcitability of the newborn brain, a key feature for synaptogenesis and neuronal plasticity, ultimately predisposes the developing brain to seizures (Wirrell, 2005). G-Aminobutyric acid (GABA), the predominant inhibitory neurotransmitter in the brain, acts paradoxically as excitatory in neonates. This observation is crucial in understanding not only the pathophysiology of neonatal seizures but also the effect of anticonvulsant drugs. Widely used substances such as benzodiazepines and barbiturates accentuate the effect of GABA, thus suppressing clinical seizures through the inhibition exercised on spinal cord and brainstem, and at the same time may exacerbate ictal EEG abnormalities through the persistent excitation of cortical neurons (Dzhala et al., 2005). This may be one of the mechanisms that results in "uncoupling" or "electroclinical dissociation", with suppression of clinical seizures coexisting with ongoing ictal EEG patterns in affected neonates (Boylan et al., 2002).

■ Etiology and outcome of neonatal seizures

Neonatal seizures occur more often in premature infants, with seizure frequency and neonatal mortality increasing with the degree of prematurity (Bergman et al., 1983; Ronen et al., 2007). However, there is some controversy regarding the incidence of postneonatal epilepsy and neurodevelopmental disability in relation to gestational age, with recent studies highlighting an increased risk for impairment in preterm compared to term populations (Ronen et al., 2007; Yildiz et al., 2012), contrary to past reports (Garcias Da Silva et al., 2004). This discrepancy may correspond to a gradual shift from mortality to morbidity in premature neonates with seizures (Ronen et al., 2007). Innovations in neonatal care have facilitated the survival of premature neonates with their increased prevalence of intraventricular haemorrhage (IH) and have decreased the rate of transient metabolic disturbances with favourable prognosis, such as hypocalcaemia, that are associated with neonatal seizures (Tekgul et al., 2006). Furthermore, improved maternal and neonatal antimicrobial treatments have led to a marked decrease in seizures resulting from central nervous system infections compared to earlier cohorts (Bergman et al., 1983; Tekgul et al., 2006).

In a prospective study considering the entire population of live births in Newfoundland, Canada, in the years 1990-1994, 90 neonates with seizures identified by clinical observation alone were evaluated 10 years later (Ronen et al., 2007). In this population-based study, term neonates had increased chances of favourable outcomes compared to preterm neonates: 84% vs. 58% survived the neonatal period and 45% vs. 12% had normal outcomes, defined as the absence of neurodevelopmental impairment (Table I). Unfavourable prognosis was determined by aetiology including HIE and cortical malformations in term neonates as well as complicated IH and infections in premature neonates, EEG abnormalities, and poor response to anticonvulsants. It should be noted that HIE constituted the most prevalent seizure aetiology in this population-based study. Seizure semiology predicted long-term prognosis according to gestational ages, with clonic seizures in term neonates related to more favourable outcomes and generalised myoclonic seizures in premature neonates linked to increased mortality. Postneonatal epilepsy was established in 34% of infants; cerebral palsy and mental retardation developed in 35% and 32% of survivors respectively (Ronen et al., 2007). These observations are in line with a trend for increased rates of neurodevelopmental deficit and decreased mortality of extreme preterm or low-weight infants in developed countries.

In a prospective study considering all term neonates admitted to the NICUs of Children's Hospital and Brigham and Women's Hospital in Boston, USA, in 1997-2000, 100 infants with seizures diagnosed on the grounds of clinical observation alone were evaluated at least 12 months later (Tekgul et al., 2006). In this hospital-based study, mortality was 7% and morbidity, including postneonatal epilepsy, cerebral palsy and developmental delay, was 28% (Table 1). Unfavourable outcome was related to aetiology, especially to the presence of a structural lesion in neuroimaging, as well as to abnormal neurologic examination and EEG background activity (Table I). Contrary to previous reports (Brunquell et al., 2002), predominant seizure semiology did not relate to long-term outcome. Furthermore, seizure burden influenced developmental and neurologic deficit, but not the long-term risk of epilepsy. The authors underlined the role of aetiology, increasingly recognised due to novel diagnostic methodology, and of EEG background activity in determining long-term outcomes following neonatal seizures (Tekgul et al., 2006).

Table I. Outcome of neonatal seizures, as presented in selected studies published in the last decade. Normal outcome is defined as the absence of neurodevelopmental impairment

Authors & year	Period of recruitment	N at inclusion	N at last follow-up	Term neonates	Ictal EEG	Mortality	Normal outcome	Post-neonatal epilepsy	Cerebral palsy	Developmental delay	Predictors of poor outcome	Follow-up, m
Garcias Da Silva, 2004	1987-1997	158	127	65%	9%	15%	48%	34%	9%	7%	Etiology (CNS infection)	n.m.
Tekgul, 2006	1997-2000	100	89	100%	33%	7%	72%	20%	46%	48%	Etiology (HIE, CNS infection, MCD) Abnormal neurologic examination Structural lesion in neuroimaging Abnormal EEG background activity	12
Ronen, 2007	1990-1995	90	82	76%	n.m.	24%	35%	34%	35%	41%	Etiology (HIE, CNS infection, MCD) Abnormal EEG findings Drug resistant seizures Generalised myoclonic seizures	> 120

Table I. Outcome of neonatal seizures, as presented in selected studies published in the last decade. Normal outcome is defined as the absence of neurodevelopmental impairment (continued)

Authors & year	Period of recruitment	N at inclusion	N at last follow-up	Term neonates	Ictal EEG	Mortality	Normal outcome	Post-neonatal epilepsy	Cerebral palsy	Developmental delay	Predictors of poor outcome	Follow-up, m
Pisani, 2008	1999-2003	51	33	none	100%	34%	20%	18%	40%	36%	Apgar score at 1 min; Abnormal EEG background activity	58
Garfinkle, 2011	1991-2007	120	109	100%	n.m.	9%	49%	27%	28%	38%	Etiology (HIE, CNS infection, MCD); Abnormal EEG background activity; Seizure onset in the first 24h; Seizures other than focal clonic	> 24
Painter, 2012	1990-1995	59	52	n.m.	100%	8%	42%	48%	n.m.	58%	Structural lesion in neuroimaging	86
Yildiz, 2012	2007-2009	120	112	71%	n.m.	7%	37%	36%	28%	52%	Etiology (HIE, CNS infection, MCD); Myoclonic seizures	n.m.

n. m.: not mentioned; N: number of neonates; HIE: hypoxic ischemic encephalopathy; CNS: central nervous system; MCD: malformations of cortical development; EEG: electroencephalography; m: months

In a prospective study considering consecutively admitted preterm neonates in a tertiary NICU in Pisa, Italy, in the years 1999-2003, 51 infants with electroclinical seizures were included and assessed at age 30-91 months (mean 58) (Pisani et al., 2008). In this hospital-based study, mortality was 34% and only 20% of preterm neonates had a normal outcome. Postneonatal epilepsy was established in 18%, cerebral palsy in 40% and developmental delay in 36% of affected infants in long-term follow-up. Abnormal EEG background activity in the first days of life was related to increased mortality, while abnormal EEG background activity and Apgar score at 1 min predicted long-term outcome (Table I). Gestational age did not influence long-term outcome in this population of extremely premature neonates with 51% HIE and 29% IH. The development of postneonatal epilepsy was related to abnormal neuroimaging and EEG findings (Pisani et al., 2008).

Overall, current evidence regarding the relation of seizure types to long-term outcome is inconclusive (Brunquell et al., 2002; Pisani et al., 2009; Tekgul et al., 2006). In the largest study up to date, it has been postulated that neonates with predominantly focal clonic seizures were likely to have focal brain pathology and a more favourable short-term outcome than those presenting subtle seizures (Mizrahi and Kellaway, 1987). However, in other cohorts, generalised tonic seizures have been associated with unfavourable outcomes (Bergman et al., 1983; Brunquell et al., 2002). This discrepancy may be attributed to different underlying pathogenetic mechanisms giving rise to different seizure presentations at different time points during brain maturation and ultimately influencing outcome (Brunquell et al., 2002; Ronen et al., 2007). Generalised tonic seizures are indeed more common in preterm neonates in conjunction with structural lesions such as those resulting from severe IH and thus with unfavourable long-term outcomes.

■ Seizure-induced injury in the developing brain

The notion that recurrent seizures themselves, regardless of specific semiology, may cause irreversible injury to the developing brain beyond that of the underlying aetiology is crucial in terms of neonatal seizure management (Galanopoulou, 2007; Thibeault-Eybalin et al., 2009). However, the experimental evidence in neonatal animal models supporting this hypothesis is so far much stronger than the clinical evidence in human neonates (Thibeault-Eybalin et al., 2009). The effect of brain injury is linked to the specific stage in brain development at which the pathologic process occurs, with damage expected to be more severe in mid rather than late gestation. This effect may be accentuated by the metabolic stress and insult resulting from seizure activity, as in HIE (Wirell et al., 2001). In line with this observation, magnetic resonance spectroscopy studies in term neonates with HIE have shown that clinical seizures further compromise brain metabolism. Thus, the severity of neonatal seizures, rather than the severity of HIE, has been linked to outcome, although the critical seizure burden required to exacerbate brain damage remains unknown (Miller et al., 2002; Glass et al., 2009). Although the aetiology-specific and seizure-induced effects are still difficult to distinguish (Thibeault-Eybalin et al., 2009), recurrent or prolonged neonatal seizures can alter neuronal connectivity and thus lead to increased brain susceptibility to seizure induced brain injury later in life and to dire long-term consequences regarding learning and memory (Ben Ari & Holmes, 2006).

These observations add to the ongoing discussion as to whether all neonatal seizures, both clinical, identified solely by clinical observation, and electroclinical or electrograhic, diagnosed by ictal EEG recordings, justify antiepileptic drug (AED) treatment

(Thibeault-Eybalin et al., 2009). This is crucial, since current therapeutic options in the treatment of neonatal seizures are not only largely ineffective, but also contribute to the inaccurate estimation of seizure load and drug-induced injury to the developing brain (Ikonomidou and Turski, 2010).

■ EEG patterns as biomarkers in neonates with seizures

EEG abnormalities in neonates with seizures have been associated with a poor prognosis in numerous studies (Rowe et al., 1985; Holmes & Lombroso, 1993; Laroia et al., 1998; Tekgul et al., 2006; Pisani et al., 2009; Yildiz et al., 2012). Interictal EEG abnormalities remain the major disease severity indicator and outcome predictor, due to the limited availability of ictal EEG recordings. Identification of severe interictal EEG abnormalities, although not specific to particular aetiologies or to the timing of brain injury, may even predict seizure occurrence on subsequent EEG records (Laroia et al., 1998). Abnormal EEG background patterns were found to be more significant than interictal epileptic discharges (Laroia et al., 1998; Rowe et al., 1985; Tekgul et al., 2006; Pisani et al., 2008; Garfinkle et al., 2011). Furthermore, ictal epileptiform discharges regardless of their clinical correlates have been associated with an unfavourable outcome (Legido et al., 1991; Rowe et al., 1985).

The correlation of EEG findings during the neonatal period with long-term outcome was retrospectively studied in 118 term neonates assessed in the British Columbia Children's Hospital, Vancouver, British Columbia, Canada, in 1992-2009 with at least one EEG recording in the first month of life and at least one clinical evaluation 4-16 years later (Almubarak & Wong, 2011). The authors concluded that generalised EEG low-voltage background activity is highly correlated with unfavourable outcome, including postneonatal epilepsy and neurologic deficit at follow-up. The overall sensitivity was 94% and specificity was 42%. Interestingly, the underlying aetiology did not significantly correlate with outcome in this cohort.

Performing sequential EEG assessments in neonates was shown to enhance the prognostic value with persisting EEG abnormalities highly related to long-term outcome (Holmes & Lombroso, 1993; Khan et al., 2008). In particular, the persistence of EEG pathology beyond the first week of life has been linked to unfavourable outcomes, even if clinical abnormalities had resolved. In a recent study, two historical cohorts of newborns with seizures from 1987-1997 and 1999-2003 that were admitted to the NICU of University Hospital São Lucas, in Porto Alegre, Brazil, were combined and pairs of sequential EEGs of 58 newborns were classified into 4 groups: normal-normal, abnormal-normal, abnormal-abnormal and normal-abnormal. The presence of an abnormal background activity in both the first and second EEG increased the risk for epilepsy and developmental delay, while the abnormal background only in the second EEG increased the risk for developmental delay alone (Khan et al., 2008). Conversely, a recent study has postulated that there was no added value in considering sequential EEG studies in term neonates with seizures due to HIE (Tekgul et al., 2006).

Finally, paroxysmal fast activity in scalp EEGs of neonates with seizures has been recently assessed as a possible network marker and its correlation with long-term outcomes has been analyzed (Nagarajan et al., 2011). The EEG recordings of 42 neonates with seizures from the NICU of Princess Margaret Hospital for Children, Perth, Australia, were retrospectively studied. Ictal fast activity indeed correlated to the occurrence of clinical features during an EEG seizure, but not to neuroimaging abnormalities, neurodevelopmental impairment or postneonatal epilepsy.

■ Discussion

In spite of groundbreaking improvements in neonatal care in the past decade leading to a promising decrease in the mortality of neonates with seizures, the long-term neurodevelopmental morbidity in survivors remains substantial and unchanged compared to earlier studies (Arzimanoglou, 2004; Volpe, 2008).

Unresolved issues in seizure detection and classification, relations to underlying brain pathology, and to EEG abnormalities still impede clinical research in neonatal seizures. Past studies show some converging evidence towards EEG abnormalities and aetiology as predictors of unfavourable outcome. However, definite conclusions are not feasible due to the rapidly changing gestational ages and brain insults of neonates populating current NICUs, with hospital-based studies including high-risk deliveries and population-based studies reporting less affected neonates. Therefore, predictive factors of neonatal seizure outcome still remain to be validated on larger, representative contemporary cohorts.

Future approaches are bound to be enhanced by the use of amplitude integrated EEG and increased availability of continuous VIDEO-EEG and/or aEEG monitoring in the diagnosis and treatment evaluation of neonatal seizures. Furthermore, long established biomarkers such as seizure semiology and EEG findings are expected to play a new role in the context of genetic disease. Further than the resolution of diagnostic issues, novel therapies (Fürwentsches *et al.*, 2010; Ramantani *et al.*, 2011) deriving from lab research and aiming to minimize damage to the immature brain (Galanopoulou, 2007; Ikonomidou & Turski, 2010) may influence EEG findings and seizure presentations, as well as long-term outcomes. These challenges call for consensus in classification and treatment, close cooperation of clinicians and researchers, and ultimately for randomized, placebo-controlled, ethically acceptable trials of anticonvulsant efficacy and safety in the treatment of neonatal seizures.

References

- Almubarak S, Wong PK. Long-term clinical outcome of neonatal EEG findings. *J Clin Neurophysiol* 2011; 28: 185-9.
- Arzimanoglou A, Guerrini R, Aicardi J. *Neonatal Seizures: Aicardi's Epilepsy in Children*, 3rd ed. Philadelphia: Lippincott Williams &Wilkins; 2004, pp. 188-209.
- Ben-Ari Y, Holmes GL. Effects of seizures on developmental processes in the immature brain. *Lancet Neurol* 2006; 5: 1055-63.
- Bergman I, Painter MJ, Hirsch RP, Crumrine PK, David R. Outcome in neonates with convulsions treated in an intensive care unit. *Ann Neurol* 1983; 14: 642-7.
- Boylan GB, Rennie JM, Pressler RM, Wilson G, Morton M, Binnie CD. Phenobarbitone, neonatal seizures, and video-EEG. *Arch Dis Child Fetal Neonatal Ed* 2002; 86: 165-70.
- Brunquell PJ, Glennon CM, DiMario FJ Jr, Lerer T, Eisenfeld L. Prediction of outcome based on clinical seizure type in newborn infants. *J Pediatr* 2002; 140: 707-12.
- Dzhala VI, Talos DM, Sdrulla DA, *et al.* NKCC1 transporter facilitates seizures in the developing brain. *Nat Med* 2005; 11: 1205-13.

- Fürwentsches A, Bussmann C, Ramantani G, *et al*. Levetiracetam in the treatment of neonatal seizures: a pilot study. *Seizure* 2010; 19: 185-9.
- Galanopoulou AS. Developmental patterns in the regulation of chloride homeostasis and GABA(A) receptor signaling by seizures. *Epilepsia* 2007; 48 (Suppl 5): 14-8.
- Garcias Da Silva LF, Nunes ML, Da Costa JC. Risk factors for developing epilepsy after neonatal seizures. *Pediatr Neurol* 2004; 30: 271-7.
- Garfinkle J, Shevell MI. Prognostic factors and development of a scoring system for outcome of neonatal seizures in term infants. *Eur J Paediatr Neurol* 2011; 15: 222-9.
- Glass HC, Glidden D, Jeremy RJ, Barkovich AJ, Ferriero DM, Miller SP. Clinical neonatal seizures are independently associated with outcome in infants at risk for hypoxic-ischemic brain injury. *J Pediatr* 2009; 155: 318-23.
- Holmes GL, Lombroso CT. Prognostic value of background patterns in the neonatal EEG. *J Clin Neurophysiol* 1993; 10: 323-52.
- Ikonomidou C, Turski L. Antiepileptic drugs and brain development. *Epilepsy Res* 2010; 88: 11-22.
- Khan RL, Nunes ML, Garcias da Silva LF, da Costa JC. Predictive value of sequential electroencephalogram (EEG) in neonates with seizures and its relation to neurological outcome. *J Child Neurol* 2008; 23: 144-50.
- Laroia N, Guillet R, Burchfiel J, McBride MC. EEG background as predictor of electrographic seizures in high-risk neonates. *Epilepsia* 1998; 39: 545-51.
- Legido A, Clancy RR, Berman PH. Neurologic outcome after electroencephalographically proven neonatal seizures. *Pediatrics* 1991; 88: 583-96.
- Malone A, Ryan CA, Fitzgerald A, Burgoyne L, Connolly S, Boylan GB. Interobserver agreement in neonatal seizure identification. *Epilepsia* 2009; 50: 2097-101.
- Miller SP, Weiss J, Barnwell A, *et al*. Seizure-associated brain injury in term newborns with perinatal asphyxia. *Neurology* 2002; 58: 542-8.
- Mizrahi EM, Kellaway P. Characterization and classification of neonatal seizures. *Neurology* 1987; 37: 1837-44.
- Mizrahi EM, Watanabe K. Symptomatic neonatal seizures. In: Roger J, Bureau M, Dravet C, Genton P, Tassinari CA, Wolf P, (eds). *Epileptic Syndromes in Infancy, Childhood and Adolescence*, 4th ed. Montrouge: John Libbey Eurotext, 2005, pp. 17-38.
- Murray DM, Boylan GB, Ali I, Ryan CA, Murphy BP, Connolly S. Defining the gap between electrographic seizure burden, clinical expression and staff recognition of neonatal seizures. *Arch Dis Child Fetal Neonatal Ed* 2008; 93: 187-91.
- Nagarajan L, Ghosh S, Palumbo L, Akiyama T, Otsubo H. Fast activity during EEG seizures in neonates. *Epilepsy Res* 2011; 97: 162-9.
- Pisani F, Barilli AL, Sisti L, Bevilacqua G, Seri S. Preterm infants with video-EEG confirmed seizures: outcome at 30 months of age. *Brain Dev* 2008; 30: 20-30.
- Ramantani G, Ikonomidou C, Walter B, Rating D, Dinger J. Levetiracetam: safety and efficacy in neonatal seizures. *Eur J Paediatr Neurol* 2011; 15: 1-7.
- Ronen GM, Penney S, Andrews W. The epidemiology of clinical neonatal seizures in Newfoundland: a population-based study. *J Pediatr* 1999; 134: 71-5.
- Ronen GM, Buckley D, Penney S, Streiner DL. Long-term prognosis in children with neonatal seizures: a population-based study. *Neurology* 2007; 69: 1816-22.
- Rowe JC, Holmes GL, Hafford J, *et al*. Prognostic value of the electroencephalogram in term and preterm infants following neonatal seizures. *Electroencephalogr Clin Neurophysiol* 1985; 60: 183-96.
- Saliba RM, Annegers FJ, Waller DK, Tyson JE, Mizrahi EM. Risk factors for neonatal seizures: a population-based study, Harris County, Texas, 1992-1994. *Am J Epidemiol* 2001; 154: 14-20.

- Scher MS. Controversies regarding neonatal seizure recognition. *Epileptic Disord* 2002; 4: 139-58.
- Tekgul H, Gauvreau K, Soul J, *et al.* The current etiologic profile and neurodevelopmental outcome of seizures in term newborn infants. *Pediatrics* 2006; 117: 1270-80.
- Thibeault-Eybalin MP, Lortie A, Carmant L. Neonatal seizures: do they damage the brain? *Pediatr Neurol* 2009; 40: 175-80.
- Volpe JJ. Neonatal seizures. In: Neurology of the Newborn. Philadelphia, PA: WB Saunders; 2008, pp. 203-244.
- Wirrell EC, Armstrong EA, Osman LD, Yager JY. Prolonged seizures exacerbate perinatal hypoxic-ischemic brain damage. *Pediatr Res* 2001; 50: 445-54.
- Wirrell EC. Neonatal seizures: to treat or not to treat? *Semin Pediatr Neurol* 2005; 12: 97-105.
- Yildiz EP, Tatli B, Ekici B, *et al.* Evaluation of etiologic and prognostic factors in neonatal convulsions. *Pediatr Neurol* 2012; 47: 186-92.

Infantile spasms: what matters more? Seizures, EEG, underlying aetiology, or treatment?

Andrew L. Lux

Paediatric Neurology, Bristol Royal Hospital for Children, Bristol, United Kingdom

---

Infantile spasms constitute the commonest epilepsy syndrome with onset in infancy. There is tremendous interest in identifying factors that might predict prognosis, and in particular to determine which of four different factors – the seizures, the EEG features, the underlying aetiology, and existing treatments – might be most influential or most amenable to effective interventions to improve long-term outcomes.

■ Which outcomes matter most?

Although seizures and spasms are important in their own right as causes of stress and concern to families and carers, most clinicians and investigators would argue that their main importance rests on an observed or assumed increase in risk for other morbidity or mortality, and in particular the increased risk for subsequent epilepsy and for a poor neurodevelopmental outcome. The neurodevelopmental spectrum includes autism, which is strongly associated with a history of infantile spasms.

Infantile spasms can be associated with developmental regression at onset. Indeed, developmental regression was considered to be one element of a triad of features that defined West syndrome until a consensus statement suggested that early-onset developmental regression is too difficult to identify and time with sufficient reliability to constitute a suitable definitional criterion (Lux & Osborne, 2004). The preservation of developmental function at onset of spasms, and in particular preserved visual function, is considered to be a favourable prognostic factor for longer-term neurodevelopment (Dulac et al., 1993).

Early studies of natural history and prognosis suggested that infantile spasms tend to resolve over time, but also to develop into other seizure types. A study of 150 children with infantile spasms, not all of whom had been treated with adrenocorticotropin (ACTH) or steroids, reported that 34 (23%) died during follow-up, and that of the remaining 116 infants, cumulatively reported cessation of spasms was 28% by age 1 year, 49% by age 2 years, 57% by age 3 years, 74% by age 4 years and 85% by age 5 years (Jeavons & Bower,

1973). A study of 214 cases of infantile spasms who were followed for at least 20 years reported that 11% died by age 3 years, 19% by 10 years, and 28% by 20 years (Riikonen, 1996; Riikonen, 2001); and that there was a normal developmental outcome (IQ above 85) in 25 cases (12%), with normal or near-normal development (IQ above 68) in 36 cases (17%).

Over time, there has been a shift in emphasis away from descriptive cohort studies and towards interventional studies in which the primary outcome measures have tended to be combinations of cessation of spasms, electrographic resolution of hypsarrhythmia, and developmental assessments that, if done at all, have tended to be performed at a young age. This shift in emphasis makes it difficult to find valid and fully generalizable information about longer-term developmental and survival outcomes for infantile spasms. However, available data permit some exploration of which factors are likely to help most with predicting or modifying outcomes.

■ Seizures

Do the seizures matter, and if so, which aspects of the seizures matter most? The evidence we might draw on to answer this question relates to whether the clinical semiology of the seizure has features that independently predict outcome; and also whether the type or duration of seizure activity can be proven to have any specific effect. It is known that younger age at onset of spasms is associated with poorer neurodevelopmental outcomes, and data from one randomised-controlled clinical trial using outcomes based on Vineland Adaptive Behavior Scale (VABS) at age 4 years showed that scores were on average 3.1 points lower for each month of earlier onset of witnessed spasms (O'Callaghan et al., 2011). The question of duration of spasms will be considered in more detail later, in the section on treatment.

Epileptic spasms have many features, including flexor or extensor movements of limbs and/or trunk, synchrony, symmetry, frequency, and duration of the ictus; and whether there are such features as onset occurring during sleep or wakefulness, a crescendo-decrescendo pattern in the prominence of spasms within a cluster, and other seizure types occurring around the time of the epileptic spasms. Since epileptic spasms are biological events that are categorised and distinguished from myoclonic seizures and tonic seizures mainly by their duration, they exist within a spectrum that might overlap with these other seizure types, leading to potential ambiguity or misclassification. For example, it is challenging to distinguish the briefest of epileptic spasms from the longest of myoclonic seizures, or the shortest tonic seizure from the longest epileptic spasm.

There remains debate about what constitutes the true ictal event with infantile spasms, but most clinicians and clinical investigators would probably agree that the cluster of periodic spasms forms a unitary event that is more worthy of study and record than the single spasm occurring within a cluster (Lux & Osborne, 2004). This propensity for clustering with a degree of predictable periodicity seems to be characteristic of epileptic spasms and rare with other epilepsies. We do not understand the pathophysiological reasons for this characteristic semiological feature, and neither do we know whether it independently predicts better or worse outcome. It has been suggested that reappearance of hypsarrhythmia between the electrographic ictal patterns within a cluster of epileptic spasms is associated with the "idiopathic" aetiological category, and therefore with a better prognosis for neurodevelopment (Dulac et al., 1993; Fusco & Vigevano, 1993).

There is evidence that preceding and coexisting epileptic seizures of other types increase the risk of poorer neurodevelopmental outcomes (Jeavons & Bower, 1973; Koo et al., 1993). And there is also evidence that coexisting seizures can modify the clinical semiology of the epileptic spasms. For example, there might be isolated myoclonic seizures independently of any epileptic spasms, or there might be focal seizures, which have been described to have variable temporal relationships with epileptic spasms (Fusco & Vigevano, 1993). However, it is not so clear that these associations are due to effects that are independent of the underlying aetiology.

Although there have been many papers describing the clinical features associated with infantile spasms, there has not been a systematic review or study of these features in the context of specifically predicting neurodevelopmental outcomes. Phenotyping on the basis of clinical semiology is probably most helpful in the context of identifying underlying etiologic categories. Consistently asymmetric spasms, for example, are likely to be associated with a structural aetiology (Fusco & Vigevano, 1993).

There is much interest in the prognosis for evolution into other seizure types and epilepsy syndromes, and in particular the well recognised evolution into Lennox-Gastaut syndrome. A study in Japan described 116 children with Lennox-Gastaut syndrome, 42 of whom (36%) had preceding infantile spasms, which was considered a poor prognostic factor for remission of seizures and for developmental outcomes (Ohtahara et al., 1976). A cohort study in Canada reported that 11/17 children (65%) with Lennox-Gastaut syndrome had preceding infantile spasms (Camfield & Camfield, 2007). A study of infants presenting with infantile spasms after the age of one year described many of the clustered spasms to have tonic features, and electroclinical events reminiscent of "atypical absences", suggesting a possible intermediate state between West and Lennox-Gastaut syndromes (Eisermann et al., 2006).

EEG

Considering the EEG in infantile spasms, it is possible to focus on the prognostic value of ictal or interictal patterns. The interictal pattern, hypsarrhythmia, is the most characteristic electrographic feature, and in combination with the epileptic spasms constitutes West syndrome (Lux & Osborne, 2004). The essential elements of hypsarrhythmia are asynchronous and chaotic high-amplitude slow waves, and multifocal epileptiform discharges, generally spikes. Gibbs and Gibbs described them as occasionally becoming more generalised, but never rhythmically repetitive or highly organised (Gibbs & Gibbs, 1952). They stated that hypsarrhythmia is an "almost continuous" abnormality, although it is not clear that, in clinical practice, the near-continuity and other features are categorised as hypsarrhythmia with high interrater reliability.

Should the interictal pattern of hypsarrhythmia be considered to constitute a form of non-convulsive status epilepticus (NCSE)? Given that NCSE is an electroclinical, rather than solely electrographic, construct a strict response to this question would be that hypsarrhythmia cannot in itself constitute NCSE. However, it is well recognised that both cognitive impairment – manifest as developmental delay or regression – and hypsarrhythmia can precede the onset of any witnessed infantile spasms, and that this scenario does provide the core elements of NCSE. This is reflected in NCSE schemes of classification (Kaplan, 2002; Shorvon, 2005; Lux, 2007; Sutter & Kaplan, 2012).

Investigators in several German centres retrospectively examined pre-hypsarrhythmic EEGs and demonstrated good interrater agreement in the categorisation by frequency of non-REM sleep (NREM) interictal epileptiform discharges, which were associated with the subsequent development of infantile spasms, and with a small subgroup appearing to have a modified clinical course when exposed to presymptomatic treatment (Philippi et al., 2008).

There have been a number of scoring systems for hypsarrhythmia, none of which have developed broad use in clinical practice or recognition as a standard in clinical studies (Jeavons & Bower, 1961; Rating et al., 1987; Kramer et al., 1997). The system developed and evaluated by Kramer et al. scores degrees of "disorganization" (a composite of interhemispheric synchrony and gradient), the amount of diffuse delta activity, voltage amplitude, the frequency of epileptiform discharges, episodes of electrodecrement or relative normalisation, absence of normal sleep patterns, and burst-suppression patterns in sleep. Any scoring system has to deal with issues of sampling and potential selection bias. Hypsarrhythmia is detected more sensitively in NREM sleep than in wakefulness, consistently disappears in REM sleep, and is less likely to be found at older ages (Watanabe et al., 1993).

Factors that are regarded as "modifying" hypsarrhythmia also vary with behavioural state and age, and a classical pattern of hypsarrhythmia pattern is unlikely when spasms have onset after one year of age (Eisermann et al., 2006). Interhemispheric synchrony, for example, becomes commoner with increasing age but reduces in progressively deeper stages of sleep. Hypsarrhythmia with significant interhemispheric asymmetry is associated with "symptomatic" and structural causes (Watanabe et al., 1993; Kramer et al., 1997). In one case series, asymmetric infantile spasms were consistently associated with asymmetric hypsarrhythmia, although asymmetric hypsarrhythmia did not consistently manifest as asymmetric spasms (Donat & Lo, 1994). One study described asymmetric and asynchronous spasms to be associated with ipsilateral focal seizures and underlying pathology in the contralateral cerebral hemisphere (Gaily et al., 1995).

In infants with perinatal brain insults, paroxysms of abnormal electrographic fast activity have been shown to precede onset of infantile spasms and to have topographical similarities to ictal EEG features after onset of infantile spasms (Endoh et al., 2007; Endoh et al., 2011). One clinical observation is that the timing of hypoxic-ischaemic brain injury can influence the prognosis for control of infantile spasms and subsequent epileptic seizures, which tend to be better where there has been a preterm delivery than when the brain insult occurs with a term delivery, possibly due to the differential predilections for involvement of cerebral subcortical white matter and cortical grey matter, respectively (Cusmai et al., 1993; Dulac et al., 2010).

There are several ictal patterns associated with epileptic spasms. These include electrodecrement (diffuse flattening), sharp-and-slow-wave complexes, a generalised slow-wave with or without fast activity, and medium-amplitude spindle-like activity (Kellaway et al., 1979; Fusco & Vigevano, 1993). It is not clear that any of these patterns or combinations of electrographic ictus is associated with a better or worse prognosis.

■ Aetiology

There are many underlying aetiologies for infantile spasms, and one of the great challenges is to define a scheme of categorisation that captures the essence of similarities and difference that are likely to be of clinical and prognostic significance. Most specific causes of infantile spasms are uncommon, although collectively they constitute a large proportion of all cases. For example, in the United Kingdom Infantile Spasms Study (UKISS), there was an identified aetiology in 127 (61%) of 207 enrolled cases, but none of the commonest identified causes – hypoxic-ischemic encephalopathy, chromosomal abnormalities (themselves heterogeneous), cerebral malformations, perinatal stroke, tuberous sclerosis complex, or periventricular leukomalacia or haemorrhage – constituted more than 10% of the total (Osborne et al., 2010).

There has been an established but inconsistently applied classification of underlying aetiology into idiopathic, symptomatic, and cryptogenic groups. The Commission on Classification and Terminology of the International League Against Epilepsy has recently suggested that these aetiological categories are broadly congruent with the preferred terms terms "genetic", "structural-metabolic", and "unknown", respectively, and that these new terms represent modified aetiological concepts (Berg et al., 2010). In this context, the terms "genetic" and "idiopathic" are congruent where the genetic cause is a channelopathy or monogenic mutation without associated structural or neurodevelopmental features. There have been various approaches to sub-categorising symptomatic causes, mainly with the intention of defining subgroups to determine modified expectations for outcome or identifying preferred first-line treatments; for example, into the categories "clastic", "degenerative", and "malformative" (Dalla Bernardina & Dulac, 1994).

Certain patterns of clinical semiology combined with EEG and neuroimaging findings are considered characteristic of specific underlying aetiologies and to have a moderate degree of predictive value. For example, the combination of dystonia and epileptic spasms in a male infant suggests a mutation in the ARX gene, and onset of epileptic spasms after 12 months of age in combination with spastic diplegia is said to suggest diagnoses of duplications of the MECP2 gene (in a male infant) or periventricular leukomalacia (Dulac et al., 2010). Aetiologies with structural or functional involvement of the temporal lobes are considered to have associations with behavioural outcomes that include autism (Chugani et al., 1996).

Paciorkowski et al., have suggested an aetiological classification drawing on the links between clinical presentations, gene ontology and molecular function, and identified genes that are known to be associated with infantile spasms (Table I) (Paciorkowski et al., 2011).

For a specific underlying aetiology, the occurrence of infantile spasms may be associated with a poorer prognosis for neurodevelopment. A study of tuberous sclerosis complex reported that mean IQ was 70.7 in 11/41 cases (27%) who had a history of infantile spasms compared with a mean IQ of 97.3 in the 30 spasm-free cases (Mann-Whitney U test, $p < 0.001$); and that the history of infantile spasms predicted a lower IQ independently of other factors, such as number of tubers on MRI head scan (O'Callaghan et al., 2004). An entry criterion for this study was that patients would tolerate MRI head scan without sedation, which biases the sample of study participants towards higher IQs on both groups and limits the generalizability of these findings.

Table I. Phenotypic characteristics associated with known genetic causes of infantile spasms according to the classification scheme suggested by Paciorkowski *et al.*, 2011

Clinical phenotype	Gene ontology & molecular function	Identified genes
Group A Features of autism Movement disorders Severe cognitive impairment	Transcription factors	*ARX* *FOXG1* *MEF2C*
Group B1 Severe brain malformation Severe cognitive impairment Intractable epilepsy	Binding	*DCX* *PAFAH1B1/LIS1* *TUBA1A*
Group B2 Brain malformation of TSC Severe cognitive impairment Autism Intractable epilepsy	Signal transduction	*TSC1* *TSC2*
Group C1 Metabolic disease Variable cognitive impairment Variable subsequent epilepsy	Binding Catalytic activity	*GLDC* *PAH*
Group C2 Metabolic disease Intractable epilepsy	Transporter Catalytic activity	*ATP7A* *KCNJ11*
Group D Intractable epilepsy Severe cognitive impairment	Binding	*GRIN1* *GRIN2A* *MAGI2* *SPTAN1* *STXBP1*
Group E Intractable epilepsy Retinitis	Transporter	*SLC25A22*

It would be naive to conclude, on the basis of this evidence alone, that infantile spasms are the cause of the lower IQs because there might be underlying pathophysiological mechanisms that predispose both to the poorer neurodevelopmental outcomes and to the epileptic spasms, with the spasms being a confounding factor. However, the causal argument finds support in an open-label study of prophylactic vigabatrin treatment based on finding presymptomatic epileptiform abnormalities in infants with tuberous sclerosis (Jóźwiak et al., 2011). And there is other evidence supporting the hypothesis that infantile spasms, or at least a factor that coexists with infantile spasms, directly affect neurodevelopmental outcomes, by virtue of the spasms exhibiting a "dose-response effect" on neurodevelopment when assessed in terms of lead-time to treatment.

■ Treatment

Lead-time to treatment is a measure of the infant's exposure to infantile spasms and, it is reasonable to assume, also a measure of exposure to an hypsarrhythmic or otherwise abnormal EEG. It has long been suggested that longer lead-time to diagnosis and treatment is associated with poorer neurodevelopmental outcome, particularly in cases where no underlying aetiology is identified and in whom earlier intervention might be expected to modify outcome more substantially (Matsumoto *et al.*, 1981).

Two informative retrospective studies have investigated the potential effects of longer lead-time to treatment intervention in cohorts with relatively homogeneous underlying causes (Eisermann *et al.*, 2003; Kivity *et al.*, 2004). Eisermann and colleagues described outcomes in 18 children with infantile spasms in whom the underlying aetiology was Down syndrome. They found that a longer lead-time to treatment intervention was associated with a longer time to treatment response, lower intelligence quotient (IQ) and higher scores on measures of autism-spectrum behaviours. Kivity and colleagues described outcomes in 37 children who had been treated with adrenocorticotropic hormone (ACTH) for infantile spasms and in whom no underlying aetiology had been identified. Of these cases, 22 had been treated within a month of the first witnessed spasms and 15 had been treated after the spasms had been present for longer than a month. Subsequent neurodevelopment was described as normal in all 22 cases treated within a month but in only 6/15 cases (40%) treated after a longer duration of spasms. Subsequent epileptic seizures were described in only 1/22 in the first group but in almost half (7/15) of cases in the second group, with five of those seven cases being described as having Lennox-Gastaut syndrome.

Even though there is a long history of clinical trials and descriptive studies of treatments for infantile spasms, the usual primary outcome measures have been cessation of spasms or some form of electroclinical outcome rather than a direct measure of neurodevelopment, and information relating to longer-term neurodevelopmental outcomes suggests that they have not improved substantially over several decades (Jobst, 2011). The most recent Cochrane Database Systematic Review of treatment for infantile spasms summarised 14 randomised controlled trials, of which only two had more than 100 enrolled participants (Hancock *et al.*, 2008). Only one of these larger trials reported neurodevelopmental and subsequent epilepsy outcomes (Elterman *et al.*, 2010; Lux *et al.*, 2005). Both classes of outcome were reported in a trial that enrolled only nine participants, and two other trials reported one or other of these outcomes (Askalan *et al.*, 2003; Vigevano & Cilio, 1997; Yanagaki *et al.*, 1999).

The United Kingdom Infantile Spasms Study (UKISS) assessed neurodevelopmental outcomes using Vineland Adaptive Behavior Scales at the ages of 14 months and 4 years (Lux *et al.*, 2004; Lux *et al.*, 2005; Darke *et al.*, 2010). Cases whose aetiology was tuberous sclerosis complex (TSC) were excluded from the trial because most clinicians consider the appropriate first-line treatment to be vigabatrin and because there is some evidence that corticosteroids, and in particular hydrocortisone, is a less effective treatment of infantile spasms in this circumstance (Chiron *et al.*, 1997). The primary outcome measure, cessation of spasms on days 13 and 14 of the study, showed a better response to the hormonal treatments (prednisolone or tetracosactide depot) (40/55; 73%) than to vigabatrin (28/52; 54%). However, relapse-free response at 14 months of age was similar in both groups (22/55; 40% and 19/52; 37% respectively).

Analysis of neurodevelopmental outcomes was made in two aetiological groups: one with identified and proven aetiology, and the other with no identified aetiology. The rationale for this subgroup analysis was the assumption that underlying aetiology would be a very strong influence on neurodevelopmental outcomes, and that the effects of treatment intervention or other factors upon neurodevelopment would be detected most sensitively and reliably in cases with no proven underlying aetiology, a subgroup that tends on average to have better neurodevelopmental outcomes.

With developmental assessments at age 14 months, there was found to be a better neurodevelopmental outcome in cases where there was no identified aetiology (the groups formerly described as "idiopathic" and "cryptogenic") and a statistically significant test for interaction between treatment intervention and the dichotomised aetiological categories. In the group with no identified aetiology, there was a better neurodevelopmental outcome in infants who had been randomly allocated hormonal treatments rather than vigabatrin, a difference that was of borderline statistical significance but replicable with a repeated developmental assessment at age 4 years (Darke et al., 2010).

One important factor relating to neurodevelopment is visual function. Given the efficacy of vigabatrin in controlling epileptic spasms and focal seizures, a combination that seems to be particularly challenging to treat, it is important to monitor the risks and prevalence of vigabatrin-associated visual field losses. A recent initiative is a registry that enrols all infants who are treated with vigabatrin in the United States, and an open question is whether monitoring and supplementation of taurine levels would help to mitigate the risks of vigabatrin-related retinal toxicity in humans (Pellock et al., 2011; Heim & Gidal, 2012).

Although there remains much debate about the relative effectiveness of treatment interventions, the most recent report from the guideline development and practice committees of the American Academy of Neurology and the Child Neurology Society considers there to be sufficient evidence that, "short lag time to treatment leads to better long-term developmental outcome," and that, "successful short-term treatment of cryptogenic infantile spasms with ACTH or prednisolone leads to better long-term developmental outcome than treatment with vigabatrin," (Go et al., 2012).

■ Summary and conclusions

Given the advances that have occurred in all areas of medicine, it would be surprising if we were not able, over time, to demonstrate clear improvements in neurodevelopmental outcomes with infantile spasms. As we gather a better understanding of infantile spasms, its underlying causes, and pathophysiological mechanisms that are potentially amenable to treatment, we should bear in mind the biases that might be introduced by period effects and changes in outcome measures. For example, better survival rates associated with generally improved supportive care for infants with serious and severe medical conditions might produce a bias that makes average neurodevelopmental scores appear poorer even if there has in reality been an improvement in neurodevelopmental outcomes for individuals with like conditions. And in future clinical studies, applying the more rigorous primary clinical outcome measure suggested by the West Delphi consensus will bias future studies such that they will appear to have poorer outcomes unless this is qualified by appropriate discussion.

Intuitively and evidentially, the strongest influence on neurodevelopmental prognosis is underlying aetiology, and many factors that might appear to independently predict outcome probably do so via strong links with aetiology. Such adverse prognostic factors would include: other seizures prior to onset of the epileptic spasms; atypical clinical features or focal seizures during the clinical attacks; EEG asymmetry; and onset of spasms before 4 months of age (Riikonen, 2010). However, some other prognostic factors are potentially independent of aetiology and therefore more amenable to treatment interventions. Such factors include shorter duration of spasms prior to treatment intervention, which would be influenced by greater diagnostic awareness and more rapid referral practices; early and sustained response to treatment, measured as relapse-free cessation of spasms, which would be informed by appropriately designed and robust randomised controlled trials that also systematically collect neurodevelopmental outcomes; and shorter duration of hypsarrhythmia.

The EEG with infantile spasms remains a fascinating biomarker that is likely to yield further valuable information as there is increasing insight into its association with underlying aetiology, clinical semiology, and neurodevelopmental status. It is very likely that there will be further ideas and debate about how the interictal EEG relates to evolving concepts such as epileptic encephalopathy and nonconvulsive status epilepticus, and innovative approaches to investigating its diagnostic and prognostic value using techniques that co-register neurophysiological techniques and functional neuroimaging.

References

- Askalan R, Mackay M, Brian J, *et al*. Prospective preliminary analysis of the development of autism and epilepsy in children with infantile spasms. *J Child Neurol* 2003; 18: 165-70.
- Berg AT, Berkovic SF, Brodie MJ, *et al*. Revised terminology and concepts for organization of seizures and epilepsies: Report of the ILAE Commission on Classification and Terminology, 2005-2009. *Epilepsia* 2010; 51: 676-85.
- Camfield P, Camfield C. Long-term prognosis for symptomatic (secondarily) generalized epilepsies: A population-based study. *Epilepsia* 2007; 48: 1128-32.
- Chiron C, Dumas C, Jambaqué I, Mumford J, Dulac O. Randomized trial comparing vigabatrin and hydrocortisone in infantile spasms due to tuberous sclerosis. *Epilepsy Res* 1997; 26: 389-95.
- Chugani HT, Da Silva E, Chugani DC. Infantile spasms: III. Prognostic implications of bitemporal hypometabolism on positron emission tomography. *Ann Neurol* 1996; 39: 643-9.
- Cusmai R, Ricci S, Pinard JM, Plouin P, Fariello G, Dulac O. West syndrome due to perinatal insults. *Epilepsia* 1993; 34: 738-42.
- Dalla Bernardina B, Dulac O. Introduction to etiology. In: Dulac O, Chugani HT, Dalla Bernardina B (eds). *Infantile Spasms and West Syndrome*. London: WB Saunders, 1994, pp. 166-71.
- Darke K, Edwards SW, Hancock E, *et al*. Developmental and epilepsy outcomes at age 4 years in the UKISS trial comparing hormonal treatments to vigabatrin for infantile spasms: A multicentre randomised trial. *Arch Dis Child* 2010; 95: 382-6.
- Donat JF, Lo WD. Asymmetric hypsarrhythmia and infantile spasms in West syndrome. *J Child Neurol* 1994; 9: 290-6.
- Dulac O, Bast T, Dalla Bernardina B, Gaily E, Neville B. Infantile spasms: Toward a selective diagnostic and therapeutic approach. *Epilepsia* 2010; 51: 2218-9; author reply 2221.
- Dulac O, Plouin P, Jambaqué I. Predicting favorable outcome in idiopathic West syndrome. *Epilepsia* 1993; 34: 747-56.
- Eisermann MM, DeLaRaillère A, Dellatolas G, *et al*. Infantile spasms in Down syndrome – effects of delayed anticonvulsive treatment. *Epilepsy Res* 2003; 55: 21-7.
- Eisermann MM, Ville D, Soufflet C, *et al*. Cryptogenic late-onset epileptic spasms: An overlooked syndrome of early childhood? *Epilepsia* 2006; 47: 1035-42.

- Elterman RD, Shields WD, Bittman RM, Torri SA, Sagar SM, Collins SD. Vigabatrin for the treatment of infantile spasms: Final report of a randomized trial. *J Child Neurol* 2010; 25: 1340-7.
- Endoh F, Yoshinaga H, Ishizaki Y, Oka M, Kobayashi K, Ohtsuka Y. Abnormal fast activity before the onset of West syndrome. *Neuropediatrics* 2011; 42: 51-4.
- Endoh F, Yoshinaga H, Kobayashi K, Ohtsuka Y. Electroencephalographic changes before the onset of symptomatic West syndrome. *Brain Dev* 2007; 29: 630-8.
- Fusco L, Vigevano F. Ictal clinical electroencephalographic findings of spasms in West syndrome. *Epilepsia* 1993; 34: 671-8.
- Gaily EK, Shewmon DA, Chugani HT, Curran JG. Asymmetric and asynchronous infantile spasms. *Epilepsia* 1995; 36: 873-82.
- Gibbs FA, Gibbs EL. Infantile spasms. In: *Atlas of Electroencephalography: Epilepsy*. Cambridge, Mass.: Addison-Wesley, 1952, pp. 24-30.
- Go CY, Mackay MT, Weiss SK, *et al*. Evidence-based guideline update: Medical treatment of infantile spasms. Report of the Guideline Development Subcommittee of the American Academy of Neurology and the Practice Committee of the Child Neurology Society. *Neurology* 2012; 78: 1974-80.
- Hancock EC, Osborne JP, Edwards SW. Treatment of infantile spasms. *Cochrane Database Syst Rev* 2008: CD001770.
- Heim MK, Gidal BE. Vigabatrin-associated retinal damage: Potential biochemical mechanisms. *Acta Neurol Scand* 2012; 126: 219-28.
- Jeavons PM, Bower BD. The natural history of infantile spasms. *Arch Dis Child* 1961; 36: 17-22.
- Jeavons PM, Bower BD. Long-term prognosis of 150 cases of "West syndrome". *Epilepsia* 1973; 14: 153-64.
- Jobst BC. Infantile spasms: The devil is in the details, but do we see the forest for the trees? *Epilepsy Curr* 2011; 11: 151-2.
- Jóźwiak S, Kotulska K, Domańska-Pakieła D, *et al*. Antiepileptic treatment before the onset of seizures reduces epilepsy severity and risk of mental retardation in infants with tuberous sclerosis complex. *Eur J Paediatr Neurol* 2011; 15: 424-31.
- Kaplan PW. Behavioral manifestations of nonconvulsive status epilepticus. *Epilepsy Behav* 2002; 3: 122-39.
- Kellaway P, Hrachovy RA, Frost JD, Zion T. Precise characterization and quantification of infantile spasms. *Ann Neurol* 1979; 6: 214-8.
- Kivity S, Lerman P, Ariel R, Danziger Y, Mimouni M, Shinnar S. Long-term cognitive outcomes of a cohort of children with cryptogenic infantile spasms treated with high-dose adrenocorticotropic hormone. *Epilepsia* 2004; 45: 255-62.
- Koo B, Hwang PA, Logan WJ. Infantile spasms: Outcome and prognostic factors of cryptogenic and symptomatic groups. *Neurology* 1993; 43: 2322-7.
- Kramer U, Sue WC, Mikati MA. Hypsarrhythmia: Frequency of variant patterns and correlation with etiology and outcome. *Neurology* 1997; 48: 197-203.
- Lux AL. Is hypsarrhythmia a form of non-convulsive status epilepticus in infants? *Acta Neurol Scand* 2007 (Suppl); 186: 37-44.
- Lux AL, Osborne JP. A proposal for case definitions and outcome measures in studies of infantile spasms and West syndrome: Consensus statement of the West delphi group. *Epilepsia* 2004; 45: 1416-28.
- Lux AL, Edwards SW, Hancock E, *et al*. The United Kingdom Infantile Spasms Study comparing vigabatrin with prednisolone or tetracosactide at 14 days: A multicentre, randomised controlled trial. *Lancet* 2004; 364: 1773-8.
- Lux AL, Edwards SW, Hancock E, *et al*. The United Kingdom Infantile Spasms Study (UKISS) comparing hormone treatment with vigabatrin on developmental and epilepsy outcomes to age 14 months: A multicentre randomised trial. *Lancet Neurol* 2005; 4: 712-7.

- Matsumoto A, Watanabe K, Negoro T, *et al*. Infantile spasms: Etiological factors, clinical aspects, and long term prognosis in 200 cases. *Eur J Pediatr* 1981; 135: 239-44.
- O'Callaghan FJ, Harris T, Joinson C, *et al*. The relation of infantile spasms, tubers, and intelligence in tuberous sclerosis complex. *Arch Dis Child* 2004; 89: 530-3.
- O'Callaghan FJ, Lux AL, Darke K, *et al*. The effect of lead time to treatment and of age of onset on developmental outcome at 4 years in infantile spasms: Evidence from the United Kingdom Infantile Spasms Study. *Epilepsia* 2011; 52: 1359-64.
- Ohtahara S, Yamatogi Y, Ohtsuka Y. Prognosis of the Lennox syndrome – Long-term clinical and electroencephalographic follow-up study, especially with special reference to relationship with the West syndrome. *Folia Psychiatr Neurol Jpn* 1976; 30: 275-87.
- Osborne JP, Lux AL, Edwards SW, *et al*. The underlying etiology of infantile spasms (West syndrome): Information from the United Kingdom Infantile Spasms Study (UKISS) on contemporary causes and their classification. *Epilepsia* 2010; 51: 2168-74.
- Paciorkowski AR, Thio LL, Dobyns WB. Genetic and biologic classification of infantile spasms. *Pediatr Neurol* 2011; 45: 355-67.
- Pellock JM, Faught E, Sergott RC, *et al*. Registry initiated to characterize vision loss associated with vigabatrin therapy. *Epilepsy Behav* 2011; 22: 710-7.
- Philippi H, Wohlrab G, Bettendorf U, *et al*. Electroencephalographic evolution of hypsarrhythmia: Toward an early treatment option. *Epilepsia* 2008; 49: 1859-64.
- Rating D, Seidel U, Grimm B, Hanefeld F. The prognostic value of EEG patterns in epilepsies with infantile spasms. *Brain Dev* 1987; 9: 361-4.
- Riikonen R. Long-term outcome of West syndrome: A study of adults with a history of infantile spasms. *Epilepsia* 1996; 37: 367-72.
- Riikonen R. Long-term outcome of patients with West syndrome. *Brain Dev* 2001; 23: 683-7.
- Riikonen RS. Favourable prognostic factors with infantile spasms. *Eur J Paediatr Neurol* 2010; 14: 13-8.
- Shorvon S. The definition, classification and frequency of NCSE. *Epileptic Disord* 2005; 7: 253-96.
- Sutter R, Kaplan PW. Electroencephalographic criteria for nonconvulsive status epilepticus: Synopsis and comprehensive survey. *Epilepsia* 2012; 53 (Suppl 3): 1-51.
- Vigevano F, Cilio MR. Vigabatrin versus ACTH as first-line treatment for infantile spasms: A randomized, prospective study. *Epilepsia* 1997; 38: 1270-4.
- Watanabe K, Negoro T, Aso K, Matsumoto A. Reappraisal of interictal electroencephalograms in infantile spasms. *Epilepsia* 1993; 34: 679-85.
- Yanagaki S, Oguni H, Hayashi K, *et al*. A comparative study of high-dose and low-dose ACTH therapy for West syndrome. *Brain Dev* 1999; 21: 461-7.

Lennox-Gastaut syndrome: nosographic limits and long term outcome

Giuseppe Capovilla[1], Alberto Verrotti[2]

[1] Child Neuropsychiatry Department, Epilepsy Center "C. Poma Hospital", Mantova, Italy
[2] Alberto Verrotti, Department of Pediatrics, University of Chieti, Italy

---

The Lennox-Gastaut Syndrome (LGS) is a severe form of epileptic encephalopathy starting in childhood with polymorphic seizures and mental deterioration. The presence of the EEG slow spike and wave complexes completes the classical triad of symptoms. The first descriptions of the syndrome date back to the sixties when Gastaut and collaborators (Gastaut et al., 1963, Gastaut et al., 1966) as well as Sorel (Sorel, 1964), recognized the syndrome and wrote the first papers about it. Gastaut and co-workers suggested generously naming it "Lennox syndrome" because earlier cases had been reported by Lennox and Davis in 1950 (Lennox & Davis, 1950). The term "Lennox-Gastaut syndrome" was introduced later and the final definition of LGS was proposed by Beaumanoir (Beaumanoir & Blume, 2005) and adopted by the ILAE Classification Commission in 1989 (Commission on Classification and Terminology of the International League Against Epilepsy, 1989). Despite this long lifespan, clinical descriptions of the syndrome are scarce as are reports of series of patients. The overwhelming majority of the papers focuses on the treatment of the syndrome and, in particular, LGS has been and is used as a useful tool to test the efficacy of new antiepileptic drugs. The etiology is extensive and diverse, varying from congenital to acquired lesions. About one-third of LGS cases occur without antecedent history or evidence of brain pathology (Panayiotopoulos, 2005) and it is unclear whether they should be considered cryptogenic or idiopathic (Kaminska et al., 1999). The long-term prognosis is generally considered very poor, with persistence of seizures in more than 75% of patients and severe mental retardation in more than 50% of patients (Dulac & Engel, 2003). Despite the relatively high frequency of LGS (see below), there are very few papers that have reported the long-term prognosis of the syndrome.

Nosographic limits

The frequency of LGS has been estimated to account for 1-10% of childhood epilepsies. As stressed by Camfield in 2011, this wide range must be attributed to the tendency to label as LGS all patients presenting with intellectual disability, seizure polymorphism with generalized tonic-atonic-myoclonic fits and multifocal and/or diffuse EEG abnormalities (Camfield, 2011). So, in the past, many patients presenting with some electroclinical signs common to LGS have been so classified without having the true and complete electroclinical phenotype. For example, some authors published about the myoclonic variant of LGS (Chevrie & Aicardi, 1972), others about the so called atypical benign partial epilepsy or pseudo-Lennox syndrome (Aicardi, 1982; Doose et al., 2001; Hahn et al., 2001; Hahn, 2002), and others again reported patients with an incomplete electroclinical picture and used the eponym Lennox-like for their cases (Cukiert et al., 2006). So, LGS has become a spectrum of conditions with clear electroclinical, prognostic and nosographic differences. Consequently, follow-up studies yielded conflicting results about the severity of its prognosis. To avoid this nosographic confusion, we think that strict inclusion criteria should be adopted for the diagnosis of LGS. The presence of the interictal slow spike and wave activity has always been considered as a prerequisite for the diagnosis and must remain mandatory. Moreover, agreeing with Arzimanoglou and Resnick (2011), and remembering that Gastaut himself described this clinical seizure type as a typical feature, we consider also the presence of tonic seizures as mandatory for the diagnosis. The last feature necessary for the diagnosis of LGS, according to Beaumanoir (Beaumanoir & Blume, 2005), are the fast rhythms. To make sure that a patient complies with the electroencephalographic criteria, it may be necessary to perform multiple EEG registrations, as both signs may not be continuously present in an individual patient.

In our chapter, we will present the long-term evolution of a group of patients presenting with all the electroclinical features that we consider mandatory for the diagnosis.

Personal series of patients

The study included 33 children who were admitted to the Department of Child Neuropsychiatry of Mantova and to the Department of Pediatrics, University of Chieti, tertiary hospital epilepsy centers, between 1990 and 2000. The medical records collected from these departments were retrospectively reviewed to select patients with LGS according to the classical symptomatic triad of epileptic seizures, retardation or decline of intellectual level and/or personality features and slow spike and wave complexes (Beaumanoir & Blume, 2005; Arzimanoglou et al., 2009). Moreover, to be included in our series, the cases should present tonic seizures and show fast rhythms in their EEG records. Finally, a follow-up period of more than 10 years was required.

Children's data were collected by searching a database of all patients with a diagnosis of LGS. Not all the cases have been followed up from the first seizure but EEG documentations of the first period of their illness was always available for the included cases. All patients had personal seizure diaries and these diaries included documentation of (a) description of the seizures; (b) school performance and neuropsychological assessment; (c) seizure frequency; (d) anticonvulsant regimens prior and during our follow-up.

All patients underwent MRI at the onset of the epilepsy or during the follow-up and the neuroimaging studies were abnormal in 25 children. The different etiologies of LSG are listed in *Table I*. Biochemical, endocrinological, haematological and metabolic evaluations were performed in all patients and showed normal results. Genetic tests were not available in some of the older cases or were omitted if they were not considered clinically relevant, for example if a clear anoxic-ischemic etiology was present. Conversely, all the cryptogenic/idiopathic cases have been studied with genetic tests often including CGH and *SCN1A* gene or other specific genetic tests depending on the clinical picture.

Neuropsychological assessment was performed in all patients using the routine neuropsychological tests according to the different ages of the patients.

Table I. Different etiologies of the patients

Etiologies	Number of patients	Number of patients (%)
Dysmorphic syndromes	6	18.2
Tuberous Sclerosis Complex	3	9.1
Non Syndromic MCD	2	6.1
Leucodystrophy	2	6.1
Post-Infectious or acquired lesions	4	12.1
Anoxic-ischemic	8	24.2
Idiopathic	8	24.2

Electroclinical data

Onset of epilepsy

Age at onset ranged from 2.5 to 5.1 (mean 3.5) years. Overall, male (23/33) patients significantly predominated. Family history of epilepsy was positive in 9 of 33 (27.3%) cases and a history of febrile seizures was seen in 5 of 33 children (15.1%). Twenty-six subjects suffered from previous types of epilepsy (16 West syndrome and 10 focal epilepsy) while 7 patients showed *de novo* LGS. Cryptogenic/idiopathic patients always showed normal cognitive development before the seizure onset.

Seizure scenario

All patients showed tonic seizures: they were usually symmetrical, brief (2-10 sec.) and of variable degree of severity. Three different types of tonic seizures were reported by the parents: 1) axial seizures that affected the facial, nuchal, trunk and, rarely, abdominal muscles; 2) axo-rhizomelic seizures which were axial seizures but also involved the proximal muscles of all limbs; 3) global seizures that were axo-rhizomelic with the involvement of the distal part of all limbs also. Often, global seizures caused sudden falls of the patients. Sometimes, tonic seizures were subtle and could manifest, clinically, with eye opening, so being recognized by the parents. Atypical absences (sometimes associated with myoclonic jerks) occurred in all patients. They occurred many times per day and always had gradual onset and gradual termination. Their length ranged between few and several seconds and in about half of the patients (17/33), one or more absence status with a prolonged important confusional state occurred. In the large majority of our patients epileptic falls caused severe injuries. These episodes were determined by an atonic seizure with sudden loss of postural tone or by one type of the typical tonic seizures that characterize LGS. Often, a mixed combination of these types of seizures was present (demonstrated by video-EEG documentation). Other not infrequently associated seizure types were focal seizures with or without secondary generalization.

Ictal EEG

Two types of seizures equally present in all cases characterize the EEG recordings of our patients:

- tonic seizures with variable length and degree of severity *(Figures 1 and 2)*. They could be subtle, go unnoticed clinically and be detected only by using surface EMG electrodes or video-EEG *(Figure 3)*;
- atypical absences with a sequence of slow spike and wave complexes *(Figure 4)*, also present in all patients. Atypical absence status *(Figure 5)* was also video-EEG recorded in some patients.

Interictal EEG

Background activity was variably altered depending on the etiology and timing of the EEG recording. In the cryptogenic/idiopathic cases, for example, it could be normal in the early first stages of the disease and returned to normality at the end of follow-up in the patients showing a favorable outcome. However, the lack of a clear alpha rhythm was almost invariably present at some stage of the evolution. Paroxysms of frequent diffuse slow spike and wave discharges less than 2.5 Hz in frequency, often with a frontal predominance and more evident during slow sleep, were invariably present. With disease evolution, EEG changed and multifocal spikes appeared in various areas of both hemispheres. Fast rhythms at 10-20 Hz were the other characteristic EEG marker in all our patients *(Figure 6)*. Also fast rhythms showed an anterior predominance and were markedly prevalent during drowsiness or slow sleep stages.

Therapy

All our patients have been treated with variously combined antiepileptic drugs. Polytherapy, even if not at onset, was invariably present for long periods of the evolution. In some cases, ketogenic diet, vagus nerve stimulation and callosotomy were also used as therapeutic options.

Neuropsychological profile

After seizure onset, slowing of cognitive development with behavioral problems including hyperactivity and autistic traits occurred in about two thirds of the patients. The degree of developmental delay was variable and in some cases a (partial) recovery of neuropsychological competences was present, as explained in the next subhead at the end of follow-up. In the remaining, mental and neurological retardation was, prior to the onset, so severe as to make a precise evaluation impossible.

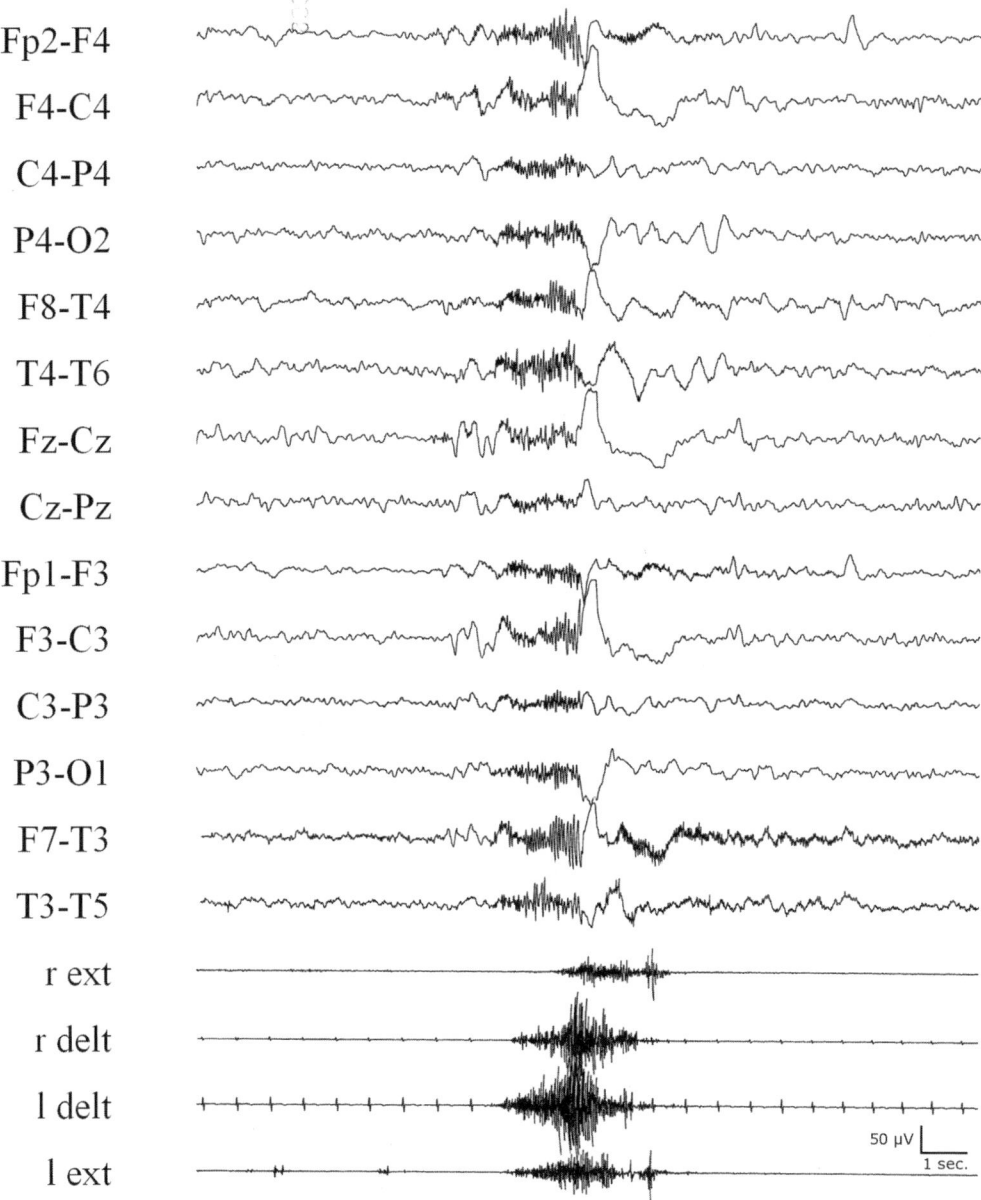

Figure 1. Polygraphic recording of a brief tonic seizure.

End of follow-up

The main data of the long-term follow-up of the patients (subdivided according to three main groups of etiologies) are reported in *Table II*. Seven out of 33 patients were seizure-free at the end of follow-up: the etiologies of these patients were: cryptogenic-idiopathic in 4 cases, acquired lesions in 2 and congenital lesion in the last. All these patients showed normal background EEG activity without spikes or polyspikes at the end of follow-up.

Table II. Long term evolution of patients divided in three main groups

	Number of patients	M/F	Seizure free	Persistence of seizures	Normal EEG at end of follow-up	Normal or borderline cognitive development
Congenital lesions	11	5/6	1	10	1	1
Acquired lesions	14	7/7	2	12	2	2
Cryptogenic-idiopathic	8	4/4	4	4	4	4
Total	33	33	7	26	7	7

Five of them had their therapy discontinued, parent's decision was to continue the AED treatment in the other two. Discontinuation of anticonvulsant therapy was decided after at least 3 years from the last seizure. The other children showed a persistence of seizures with a combination of tonic axial seizures, atypical absences and focal seizures with or without secondary generalization. Persistence of seizures was associated with persistence of multifocal EEG abnormalities and diffuse slow spike and wave complexes, even if attenuated compared with the more active phases of the illness.

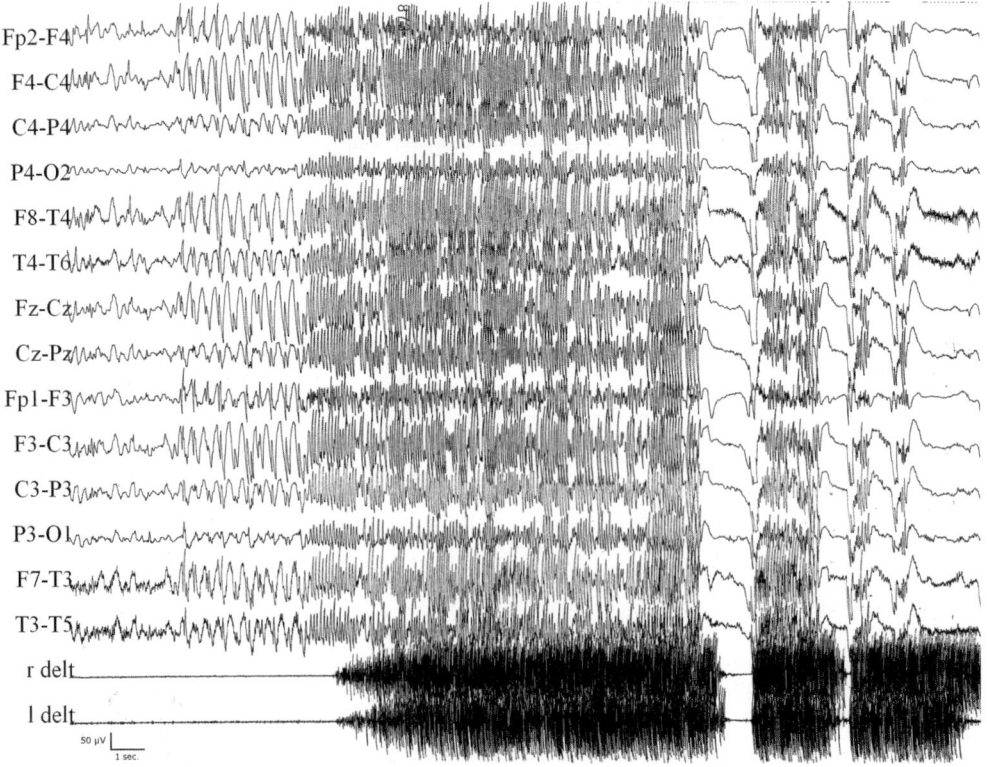

Figure 2. Polygraphic recording of a longer tonic seizure.

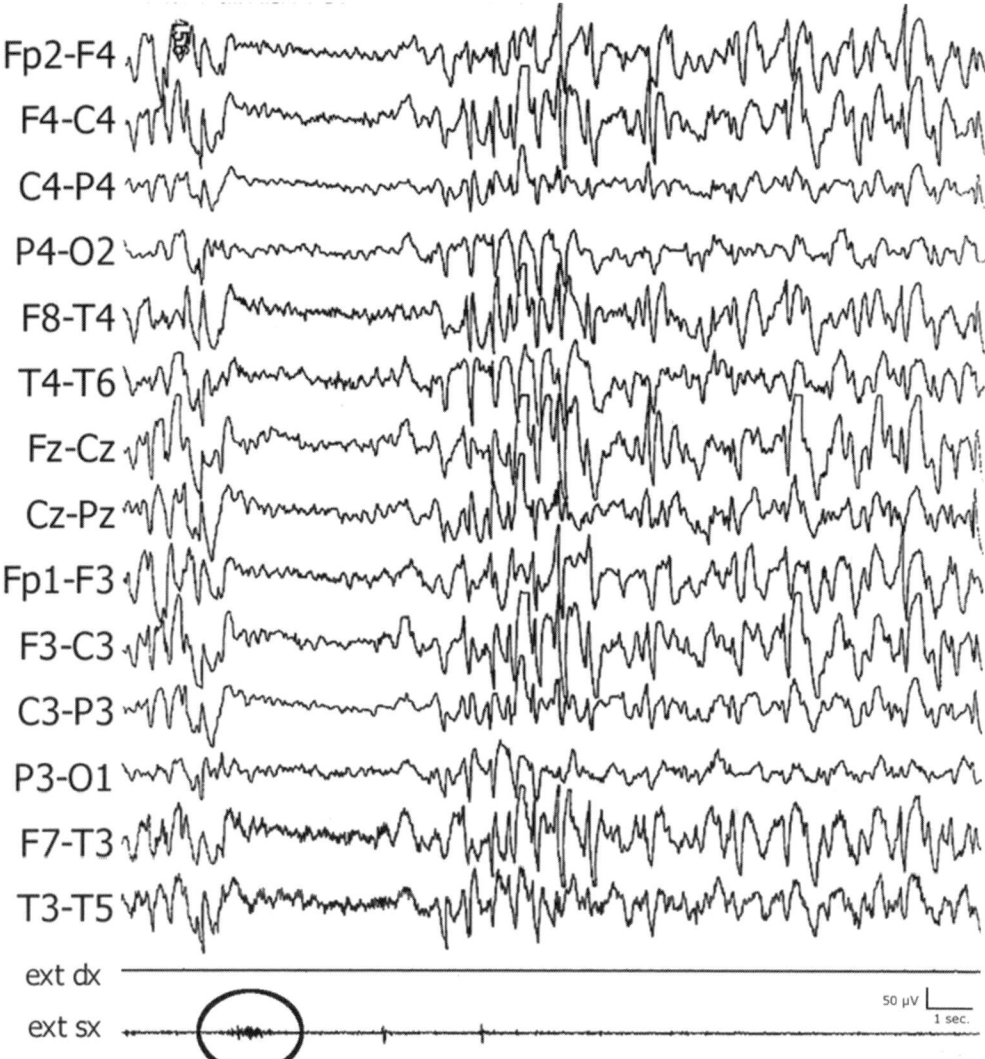

Figure 3. Slight tonic contraction of the left arm (ellipsis) is detected using surface EMG electrodes. Eye opening was documented by video-EEG.

Seven out of 33 (21%) children showed normal or borderline IQ without important behavioral problems and the majority of them (4 cases) had cryptogenic/idiopathic etiology. Half of the patients with cryptogenic/idiopathic etiology showed a good cognitive evolution. Among the other 26 patients, 14 had profound or severe and 12 moderate or mild mental retardation combined with autistic or other types of personality disorders.

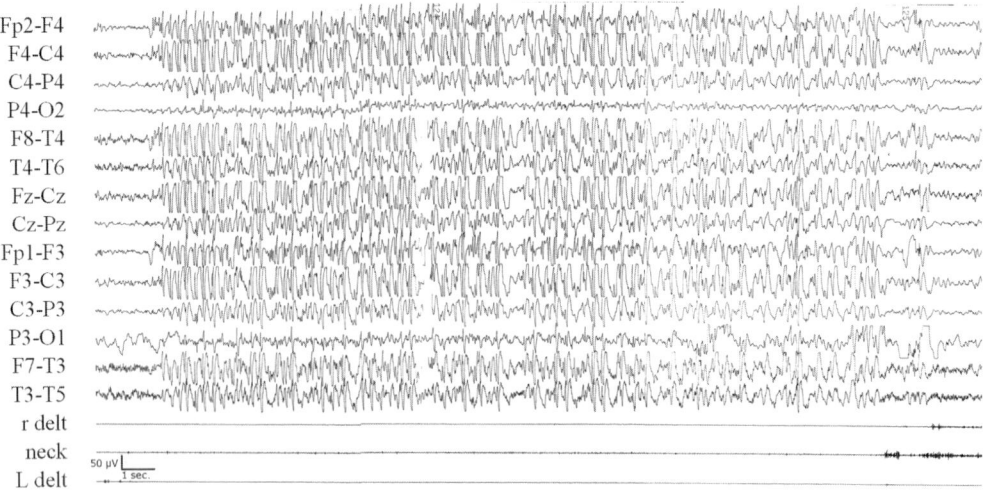

Figure 4. Atypical absence.

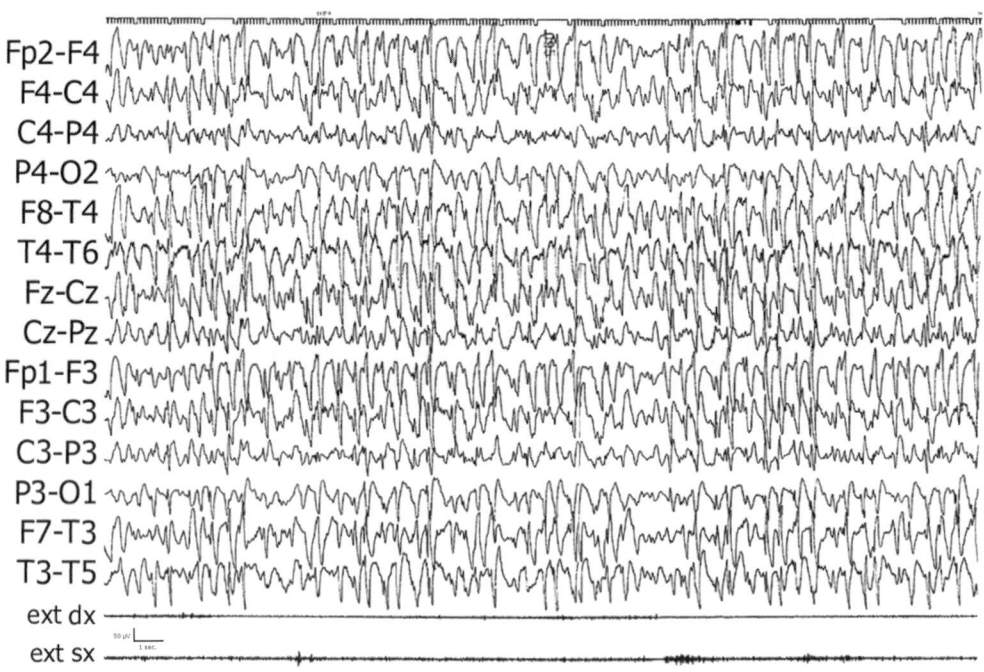

Figure 5. Atypical absence status of slow and wave complexes.

■ Discussion

The overwhelming majority of clinical reports about LGS are focused, in particular, on the therapeutic response to a more or less novel antiepileptic drug or to the differential diagnosis of drop attacks. Very few papers discuss the nosological boundaries and, consequently, semiological aspects are not strictly delineated with no well-defined clinical and

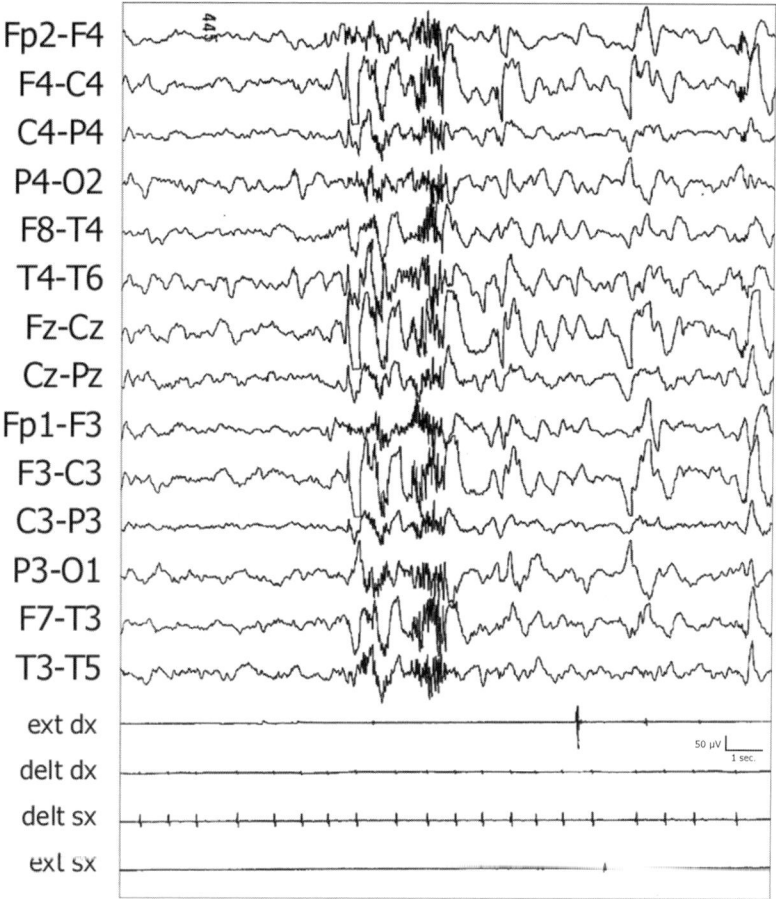

Figure 6. Fast rhythms during slow sleep in a 2 years and 8 months old child.

EEG limits. So, a precise definition remains elusive (Arzimanoglou & Resnick, 2011) with obvious consequences for the prognostic aspect. The overlap with other types of generalized and focal epilepsies can occur at different levels. A first typical example is myoclonic-astatic epilepsy (MAE) or Doose syndrome where the distinction with LGS can be difficult if a dramatic psychomotor deterioration with tonic seizures is present (Beaumanoir & Blume, 2005). Again, some authors included among their LGS patients cases without tonic seizures, others included in their MAE series cases with tonic seizures. It is not so clear how the inclusion criteria are used and the choice to include similar patients in one or another category seems to have been arbitrary. Both LGS and MAE are associated with multiple seizure types, but tonic seizures are the rule in LGS (Dulac, 2001; Beaumanoir & Blume, 2005) and rarely present in MAE (Tang & Pal, 2012), and eventually develop during its evolution (Oguni et al., 2002; Trivisano et al., 2011). Focal seizures are virtually absent in MAE (Trivisano et al., 2011; Tang & Pal, 2012) but not infrequently present in LGS (Dulac, 2001; Arzimanoglou & Resnick, 2011). EEG findings also differ in the two epilepsy syndromes. LGS is characterized by slow spike and wave complexes enhanced during slow-wave sleep and altered background EEG activity, whereas normal background activity with generalized spike and wave discharges are more likely in Doose syndrome.

Furthermore, fast rhythms have not been described in MAE. LGS is almost regularly highly resistant to anti-epileptic medication with an overall poor prognosis (in spite of new therapeutic strategies), often requiring some rational polytherapy that is rarely successful (Van Straten & Ng, 2012). The pharmacoresistance is often enduring and sometimes can persist during the entire life. On the other hand, Doose syndrome has a more variable outcome with cases presenting a favorable outcome after a first period of pharmacoresistance (Oguni et al., 2002; Kelley & Kossoff, 2010; Trivisano et al., 2011; Tang & Pal, 2012). Myoclonic seizures in LGS are considered rare (Furune et al., 1988; Oguni et al., 1996) and we have also rarely observed this type of seizure in our patients, whereas they are almost the rule in MAE (Oguni et al., 2002; Trivisano et al., 2011; Tang & Pal, 2012). Focal epilepsies are another example of possible nosographic confusion: if aggravation of the EEG picture with mental deterioration occurs, some authors (Aicardi, 1982; Doose et al., 2001; Hahn et al., 2001; Hahn, 2002; Cukiert et al., 2006) include these cases in the LGS spectrum, either classical or one of its variants (pseudo-Lennox, Lennox-like). The same phenomenon occurred in the past to Doose syndrome, when (benign) myoclonic epilepsy in infancy, severe myoclonic epilepsy or Dravet syndrome and atypical benign partial epilepsy of childhood have been included by Doose himself in the first published series of MAE patients (Doose, 1970; Doose & Baier, 1987).

The pathophysiology of LGS has long been debated. Recently, some authors (Capovilla et al., 2009; Avanzini et al., 2012) proposed the hypothesis of so-called "system epilepsies". Epileptic encephalopathies, in general, have the ideal profile to be considered as system epilepsies and LGS is one of the best prototypes. The hypothesis postulates that system epilepsies are the result of the enduring propensity to generate seizures in different brain areas that, alone, are unable to create a specific electroclinical phenotype. This goes beyond the classical dichotomy between focal and generalized epilepsy. Apart from the conventional neurophysiologic methods for studying brain activities and the pathophysiological mechanisms underlying epileptic syndromes, other new methods support this hypothesis. For example, EEG-functional MRI (fMRI) combines MRI spatial resolution with EEG time resolution, and can be used to study the structure and function of neural systems involved in LGS. As suggested for West syndrome (Lado & Moshe, 2002; Avanzini et al., 2012), the electroclinical phenotype could originate from the abnormal interaction of cortical and subcortical circuits rather than in a specific region alone. Blume (2001), to explain the pathophysiological mechanisms at the basis of LGS, hypothesized that "the occurrence of factors enhancing excitability during a vulnerable period of cortical and thalamic development may permanently imprint a bilateral, diffuse epileptogenic system upon the mammalian brain". "Thus, enduring synaptic and non-synaptic epileptic systems would form" and could be at the basis of the mechanisms underlying LGS. The elegant paper of Siniatchkin et al. (2011), who studied, with fMRI, LGS patients, evidenced how both cortical and subcortical structures (thalamus, brainstem, reticular formation and cerebellum) are activated in LGS cases, both with symptomatic and cryptogenic etiology. In contrast to children with LGS, there were no consistent positive BOLD signal changes in subcortical structures in children with multifocal partial epilepsy. Because LGS is an epileptic syndrome with variable aetiology, we suggest that multiple causes may activate a syndrome-specific neuronal network.

Concluding remarks

LGS continues to lack exact criteria for its definition and series of published patients studying the long-term prognosis are scarce. It is important to underline that the strict inclusion criteria comprising not only the classical triad but also tonic attacks and fast EEG rhythms, restrict the nosographic boundaries of the LGS, making us return to the original cases described by Gastaut *et al.* and Sorel. To prevent the inclusion of atypical, incomplete or, possibly, different cases, the exact description of the initial electroclinical documentation was available for all our patients. With the increasing level of clinical epileptology and considering that tonic seizures are a prerequisite to the diagnosis, a prospective multicenter study with video-EEG confirmation of seizures would certainly yield a more accurate picture of the prognosis, also taking in mind the at times subtle nature of seizures in LGS.

References

- Aicardi J, Chevrie JJ. Atypical benign partial epilepsy of childhood. *Dev Med Child Neurol* 1982; 24: 281-92.
- Arzimanoglou A, French J, Blume W, *et al.* Lennox-Gastaut syndrome: a consensus approach on diagnosis, assessment, management, and trial methodology. *Lancet Neurol* 2009; 8: 82-93.
- Arzimanoglou A, Resnick T. All children who experience epileptic falls do not necessarily have Lennox-Gastaut syndrome... but many do. *Epileptic Disord* 2011; 13 (Suppl 1): 3-13.
- Avanzini G, Manganotti P, Meletti S, *et al.* The system epilepsies: A pathophysiological hypothesis. *Epilepsia* 2012; 53: 771-8.
- Beaumanoir A, Blume W. The Lennox-Gastaut syndrome. In: Roger J, Bureau M, Dravet C, Genton P, Tassinari CA, Wolf P (eds). *Epileptic Syndromes in Infancy, Childhood and Adolescence,* 4th edition. Montrouge: John Libbey Eurotext, 2005, pp. 125-48.
- Blume WT. Pathogenesis of Lennox-Gastaut syndrome: considerations and hypotheses. Epileptic Disord. 2001; 4: 183-96.
- Camfield P. Definition and natural history of Lennox-Gastaut syndrome. *Epilepsia* 2011; 52: 3-9.
- Capovilla G, Berg AT, Cross JH, Moshe SL, Vigevano F, Wolf P, Avanzini G. Conceptual dichotomies in classifying epilepsies: Partial versus generalized and idiopathic *versus* symptomatic (April 18-20, 2008, Monreale, Italy). *Epilepsia* 2009; 50: 1645-9.
- Chevrie JJ, Aicardi J. Childhood epileptic encephalopathy with slow spike-wave. A statistical study of 80 cases. *Epilepsia* 1972; 13: 259-71.
- Commission on Classification and Terminology of the International League Against Epilepsy. Proposal for revised classification of epilepsies and epileptic syndromes. *Epilepsia* 1989; 30: 389-99.
- Cukiert A, Burattini JA, Mariani PP, *et al.* Extended, one-stage callosal section for treatment of refractory secondarily generalized epilepsy in patients with Lennox-Gastaut and Lennox-like syndromes. *Epilepsia* 2006; 47: 371-4.
- Doose H, Gerken H, Leonhardt R, Völzke E, Völz C. Centrencephalic myoclonic-astatic petit mal. Clinical and genetic investigation. *Neuropaediatrie* 1970; 2: 59-78.
- Doose H, Baier WK. Epilepsy with primarily generalized myoclonic-astatic seizures: a genetically determined disease. *Eur J Pediatr* 1987; 146: 550-4.
- Doose H, Hahn A, Neubauer BA, Pistohl J, Stephani U. Atypical "benign" partial epilepsy of childhood or pseudo-lennox syndrome. Part II: family study. *Neuropediatrics* 2001; 32: 9-13.

- Doose H, Hahn A, Neubauer BA, Pistohl J, Stephani U. Atypical "benign" partial epilepsy of childhood or pseudo-lennox syndrome. Part II: family study. *Neuropediatrics* 2001; 32: 9-13.
- Dulac O. Epileptic encephalopaty. *Epilepsia* 2001; 42: 23-6.
- Dulac O, Engel J. Report of the International League against Epilepsy. 2003, http://www.ilae-epilepsy.org/ctf/lennox_gastaut.html
- Furune S, Watanabe K, Negoro T. Long-term prognosis and clinico-electroencephalographic evolution of Lennox-Gastaut syndrome. *Brain Dysfunct* 1988; 1: 146-53.
- Gastaut H, Roger J, Ouahchi S, Timsit M, Broughton R. An electroclinical study of generalized epileptic seizures of tonicexpression. *Epilepsia* 1963; 4: 15-44.
- Gastaut H, Roger J, Soulayrol R, *et al*. Childhood epileptic encephalopathy with diff use slow spike-waves (otherwise known as "petit mal variant") or Lennox syndrome. *Epilepsia* 1966; 7: 139-79.
- Hahn A. Atypical benign partial epilepsy/pseudo-Lennox syndrome. *Epileptic Disord* 2000; 2: S11-17.
- Hahn A, Pistohl J, Neubauer BA, Stephani U. Atypical "benign" partial epilepsy or pseudo-Lennox syndrome. Part I: symptomatology and long-term prognosis. *Neuropediatrics* 2001; 32: 1-8.
- Kaminska A, Ickowicz A, Plouin P, Brum M, Dellatolas G, Dulac O. Delineation of cryptogenic Lennox-Gastaut syndrome and myoclonic astatic epilepsy using multiple correspondence analysis. *Epilepsy Res* 1999; 36: 15-29.
- Kelley SA, Kossof E. Doose syndrome (myoclonic-astatic epilepsy): 40 years of progress. *Dev Med Child Neurol* 2010; 52: 988-93.
- Lado FA, Moshe SL. Role of subcortical structures in the pathogenesis of infantile spasms: what are possible subcortical mediators? *Int Rev Neurobiol* 2002; 49: 115-40.
- Lennox WG, Davis JP. Clinical correlates of the fast and slow spikewave electroencephalogram. *Pediatrics* 1950; 5: 626-44.
- Ng YT, Conry J, Paolicchi J, *et al*.; on behalf of the OV-1004 study investigators (see Appendix A). Long-term safety and efficacy of clobazam for Lennox-Gastaut syndrome: Interim results of an open-label extension study. *Epilepsy Behav* 2012; 25: 687-94.
- Oguni H, Hayashi K, Osawa M. Long term prognosis of Lennox-Gastaut syndrome. *Epilepsia* 1996; 37: 44-7.
- Oguni H, Tanaka T, Hayashi K, *et al*. Treatment and long-term prognosis of myoclonic-astatic epilepsy of early childhood. *Neuropediatrics* 2002; 33: 122-32.
- Panayiotopoulos C. *The Epilepsies. Seizures, Syndromes and Management*. Chipping Norton: Blandon Medical Publishing, 2005, pp. 159-76.
- Siniatchkin M, Coropceanu D, Moeller F, Boor R, Stephani U. EEG-fMRI reveals activation of brainstem and thalamus in patients with Lennox-Gastaut syndrome. *Epilepsia* 2011; 52: 766-74.
- Sorel L. L'épilepsie myokinétique grave de la première enfance avec pointe-onde lente (petit mal variant) et son traitement. *Rev Neurol* 1964; 116: 110-5.
- Stephani U. The Natural History of Myoclonic Astatic Epilepsy (Doose Syndrome) and Lennox-Gastaut Syndrome. *Epilepsia* 2006; 47: 53-5.
- Tang S, Pal DK. Dissecting the genetic basis of myoclonic-astatic epilepsy. *Epilepsia* 2012; 53: 1303-13.
- Trivisano M, Specchio N, Cappelletti S, *et al*. Myoclonic astatic epilepsy: An age-dependent epileptic syndrome with favorable seizure outcome but variable cognitive evolution. *Epilepsy Res* 2011; 97: 133-41.
- Van Rijckevorsel K. Treatment of Lennox-Gastaut syndrome: overview and recent findings. *Neuropsychiatr Dis Treat* 2008; 4: 1001-19.
- Van Straten AF, Ng YT. Update on the management of Lennox-Gastaut Syndrome. *Pediatr Neurol* 2012; 47: 153-61.

Dravet syndrome
What matters more: seizures or the underlying aetiology?

Ingrid E. Scheffer

Florey Institute and Department of Medicine, University of Melbourne, Austin Health; Department of Paediatrics, University of Melbourne, Royal Children's Hospital, Melbourne, Australia

In many ways, Dravet syndrome can be regarded as the archetypal genetic epileptic encephalopathy. The epileptic encephalopathies are a group of disorders typically associated with refractory epilepsy in which frequent epileptic activity is thought to contribute to the cognitive and behavioural deterioration beyond that which would be expected from the underlying pathology alone (Berg *et al.*, 2010). Dravet syndrome was the first epileptic encephalopathy in which a genetic cause was found and now more than 70% of patients have sodium channel gene mutations (Claes *et al.*, 2001; Harkin *et al.*, 2007; Depienne *et al.*, 2009a). Dravet syndrome served to illustrate that epileptic encephalopathies could have a genetic rather than an acquired aetiology as previously surmised.

Dravet syndrome

Charlotte Dravet described severe myoclonic epilepsy of infancy, as it was originally known, in 1978 in French and in 1982 in English (Dravet *et al.*, 1982). Dravet syndrome is a distinctive electroclinical syndrome with seizure onset at about 6 months of age in a previously normal and typically developing infant. The infant presents with febrile status epilepticus which is often hemiclonic but may be generalized. The infant returns over the next six to twelve months with further episodes of febrile status; a clinical clue is that the hemiclonic attacks may have different lateralization in different seizures suggesting that a structural lesion is less likely. Between one to five years of age, the child develops other seizure types including focal dyscognitive seizures, absence and myoclonic seizures. Episodes of non-convulsive status epilepticus, also known as obtundation status, are common.

Although seizures may be frequent between 6 and 12 months of age, the infant's development continues normally until one year. It then starts to slow. Regression may occur particularly with episodes of convulsive status epilepticus. The mean age of walking is slightly late at 17 months and physiological ataxia may be more protracted than usual (Rodda et al., 2012). Most individuals ultimately have intellectual disability.

Despite this complex clinical picture, children may present with atypical features such as never experiencing episodes of status, no predilection for seizures with fever and normal developmental outcome. There is a group of patients who only experience convulsive seizures without absence, myoclonic or focal dyscognitive seizures, but show similar developmental decline. These patients were recognised by German groups as severe idiopathic generalized epilepsy of infancy with generalized tonic-clonic seizures (Doose et al., 1998) and Japanese authors as one of the borderline variants of severe myoclonic epilepsy of infancy called intractable childhood epilepsy with generalized tonic-clonic seizures (Oguni et al., 1994).

Despite frequent seizures, the EEG is usually normal in the first two years of life. Irregular generalized spike wave and multifocal discharges emerge and photosensitivity may be seen. Imaging is usually normal although non-specific changes such as diffuse atrophy may be observed. Up to one third of children develop hippocampal sclerosis, yet it is somewhat surprising that not all have mesial temporal lobe changes as the majority experience febrile status epilepticus, which is a known predisposing factor for hippocampal sclerosis (Falconer et al., 1964).

The aetiology of Dravet syndrome is genetic with about 75% of patients having mutations of the sodium channel alpha 1 subunit gene, *SCN1A* (Claes et al., 2001; Harkin et al., 2007; Depienne et al., 2009a). About 70% have sequencing mutations of *SCN1A* and most patients have novel, rather than recurrent, mutations. A further 3-5% have copy number variants (CNVs) of *SCN1A*, including exonic deletions or duplications and may involve one or more exons or the entire gene and even contiguous genes. CNV analysis requires specific testing using methods such as multiplex ligation-dependent probe amplification or multiplex amplicon quantification (Mulley et al., 2006; Suls et al., 2006). Ninety percent of *SCN1A* mutations arise *de novo* in the patient. Ten percent are inherited and family members tend to have mild phenotypes within the GEFS+ (genetic epilepsy with febrile seizures plus) spectrum (Singh et al., 2001). Parental testing is essential to inform recurrence risks.

What is the aetiology in the remaining 25% of *SCN1A*-negative Dravet syndrome patients? Firstly some have *SCN1A* mutations that have been missed by sequencing and CNV studies. Our recent study of 13 cases with whole exome sequencing revealed three patients with *SCN1A* mutations that had been missed by techniques employed over the last ten years. Other mutations in splice sites or intronic regions may be missed. It may therefore be worth repeating mutational analysis if *SCN1A* sequencing was performed with older technologies.

A proportion of girls with a Dravet-like picture have mutations of *PCDH19*, encoding protocadherin 19. These girls resemble Dravet syndrome with a predilection to seizures with fever and a slightly later mean onset of seizures at 9 months (Depienne et al., 2009b). The seizure pattern differs, however, with clusters of brief focal or convulsive seizures with fever rather than status epilepticus (Scheffer et al., 2008). Their seizures cluster with many per day for a few days, often persisting after the fever has abated. Rare cases present with febrile status epilepticus and resemble Dravet syndrome more closely. Girls with *PCDH19* female-limited epilepsies are less likely to have absence and myoclonic seizures and have a better prognosis than children with Dravet syndrome (Depienne *et al.*, 2009b). The inheritance pattern for *PCDH19* mutations is unusual as it follows X-linked inheritance with male sparing (Dibbens *et al.*, 2008, Scheffer *et al.*, 2008). This means that all daughters of normal transmitting fathers will be affected and half of the daughters of affected mothers. Therefore the parents of affected girls should be tested for the *PCDH19* mutation to determine if it is a *de novo* or inherited mutation and referred for genetic counseling.

■ Outcome of Dravet syndrome

The outcome of Dravet syndrome is poor from the point of view of cognition, motor skills, psychosocial outcome and mortality. There are, however, rare patients who do well and have normal outcome. It is not clear why these patients have a much better outcome. Perhaps they would previously have escaped diagnosis because with better recognition of Dravet syndrome, increasing numbers of cases at the milder end of the spectrum are being identified. An alternative and more likely explanation is that there are genetic modifiers or epigenetic factors that are protective in individuals of normal intellect. A key question is whether these rare normal patients reach their intellectual potential. An extraordinary pair of monozygotic twins shed light on this question. The twin with Dravet syndrome was discordant for a *SCN1A* nonsense mutation with her unaffected monozygotic twin. The affected twin was of low average intellect while her co-twin was of average intellect suggesting that Dravet syndrome had impacted on her cognition but to a far lesser extent than usually observed (Vadlamudi *et al.*, 2010).

The vast majority of patients with Dravet syndrome have intellectual disability which is evident by the end of the first decade (Brunklaus *et al.*, 2012). There may be two groups with a different trajectory of intellectual decline; most show a rapid decline between 12 and 60 months of age and a smaller group show mild decline (Ragona *et al.*, 2011). By adult life, 69% (50/72) have severe intellectual disability, 19% (14/72) moderate and 8% (6/72) mild intellectual impairment (Jansen *et al.*, 2006; Akiyama *et al.*, 2010; Catarino *et al.*, 2011). In adult life, cognitive decline may parallel seizure activity with more preservation of intellect in those with better seizure control (Akiyama *et al.*, 2010). In addition, a recent study of 241 cases with *SCN1A* mutations found that a worse developmental outcome was associated with the occurrence of status epilepticus, EEG abnormalities in the first year of life, and motor disorder (Brunklaus *et al.*, 2012).

The evolution of seizures with age in Dravet syndrome follows a distinctive but not universal pattern. The episodes of convulsive status epilepticus, with or without fever, settle by about 5 years of age although they can still occur out of the blue or if the patient develops a fever or illness. Brief convulsive seizures become the predominant pattern initially both awake and asleep but with age, they occur predominantly during sleep. The patients often develop two types of episodic loss of awareness comprising focal dyscognitive seizures and absence seizures. The focal dyscognitive seizures typically have temporal lobe semiology with prominent pallor and longer duration compared with absence seizures which are sometimes accompanied by eyelid fluttering. Myoclonic seizures are not always present and may fluctuate markedly with time. Atonic seizures rarely occur.

Seizures persist into adult life with most patients having refractory seizures despite multiple anti-epileptic therapies (Catarino et al., 2011). Overall seizure frequency tends to reduce with age. The most frequent semiology comprises brief nocturnal tonic-clonic seizures, often occurring weekly although this varies from daily to yearly in different individuals (Jansen et al., 2006; Akiyama et al., 2010). Focal features were frequently observed in video-EEG studies often with frontal onset although multifocal and generalized patterns were also observed (Akiyama et al., 2010). Focal dyscognitive, myoclonic and absence seizures continue in a small proportion of patients (Jansen et al., 2006; Akiyama et al., 2010). Ongoing non-convulsive status epilepticus occurs in a minority of adult patients (Akiyama et al., 2010). Triggers in adult life continue to include fever, elevated environmental temperature and illness (Akiyama et al., 2010; Catarino et al., 2011). Seizure-freedom can occur as reported in 5/48 (16%) Japanese adults (Akiyama et al., 2010). Seizure freedom correlated with a milder early course: fewer than three episodes of convulsive status epilepticus and the disappearance of epileptiform activity on follow up EEG studies.

Behavioural problems and autistic features are common and persist into adult life (Catarino et al., 2011). By the end of the first decade, 50% or more of 241 children had autistic features, behavioural problems and motor disorder (Brunklaus et al., 2012). Motor features include ataxia, spasticity, dyskinesia and hypotonia (Brunklaus et al., 2012). The behavioural issues often pose greater difficulties for families than the seizures and place the child at risk of injury.

With age, motor difficulties become more prominent with the evolution of an abnormal gait in adolescence in the majority of patients. This crouch gait has a pattern of increased hip and knee flexion and ankle dorsiflexion (Rodda et al., 2012). It is associated with bony malalignment with medial femoral torsion, lateral tibial torsion and planoabductovalgus of the feet together with weakness in the antigravity muscles. The crouch gait is associated with mild pyramidal, cerebellar and extrapyramidal signs (Jansen et al., 2006; Catarino et al., 2011; Rilstone et al., 2012). Despite quite an abnormal appearance to their gait, patients are relatively stable and can run, albeit awkwardly. The gait produces functional impairment with aid increasingly required for walking long distances by adult life (Rodda et al., 2012). The aetiology of the gait is not known but is likely to relate to the underlying *SCN1A* mutation and does not appear related to seizures per se.

The recent study by Catarino and co-authors (2011) found ongoing cognitive and motor deterioration in 22 adults with Dravet syndrome aged up to 60 years. They identified progressive features including kyphoscoliosis (6/22), dysphagia (5/22), from the fourth decade requiring percutaneous endoscopic gastrostomy, recurrent chest infections (6/22) and non-ictal urinary incontinence. They made the important observation that there was still evidence of reversibility of the encephalopathic state with optimization of anti-epileptic therapy for Dravet syndrome and removal of aggravating drugs in adult life.

Dravet syndrome is associated with a significant mortality of 15% by early adult life. Although death can occur at any age, it occurs most frequently in childhood (Dravet et al., 2012). Death can be in the setting of sudden unexpected death in epilepsy (SUDEP), convulsive status epilepticus with multi-organ failure, chest infection and accidental causes.

■ Do known genetic or environmental factors predict outcome?

Intuitively one would predict that a more severe type of SCN1A mutation may be more likely to cause a more severe Dravet phenotype. There are now more than 800 SCN1A mutations described (more still on the online Belgian and US databases) and the vast majority is associated with Dravet syndrome. Mutations include missense mutations in about 50% of cases and truncation mutations in around 50%; the latter comprise nonsense, frameshift and splice site mutations, small intragenic insertions and duplications, and larger CNVs (Zuberi et al., 2011). While the majority of truncation mutations are associated with Dravet syndrome, missense mutations occur in both Dravet syndrome and mild GEFS+ phenotypes. Zuberi and colleagues (2011) performed an elegant analysis of 833 mutations and found that truncation mutations were associated with an earlier mean onset of prolonged seizures (7 compared with 9 months), myoclonic seizures (16 *versus* 19 months) and atypical absence seizures (19 *versus* 30 months). There was a predilection for missense mutations in Dravet syndrome to occur in the voltage sensor and pore-forming regions of the protein, confirming earlier Japanese work (Kanai et al., 2004). Zuberi and co-workers also scrutinized the degree of change in the physico-chemical properties of the mutated protein using the Grantham score which incorporates polarity, molecular volume and composition of the amino acid substitution. A higher Grantham score correlated with earlier seizure onset. Overall these findings are not particularly practical in predicting outcome in a patient with Dravet syndrome.

We do not understand why many individuals with Dravet syndrome have severe intellectual disability and few have mild impairment. It is likely that the genetic background affects the impact of a SCN1A mutation with specific genes potentially rescuing the detrimental effects of a mutation. Support for this hypothesis comes from murine studies of SCN1A mutants. The SCN1A knockout mouse recapitulates the Dravet phenotype and shows strain-dependent penetrance. The 129SvJ background *Scn1a* heterozygote mouse shows improved survival and no seizures compared with the C57BL/6 background animal which has frequent seizures and 80% of heterozygotes die by thirteen weeks of age (Yu et al., 2006). They also found upregulation of another sodium channel subunit, Nav1.3, in hippocampal interneurons suggesting that this may be compensatory for Nav1.1 haploinsufficiency (Yu et al., 2006).

In human studies, only two genetic modifiers have been studied to date. These include the sodium channel alpha 9 subunit gene, SCN9A, and very recently, the calcium channel subunit gene, CACNA1A (Singh et al., 2009; Ohmori et al., 2012). Confirmation of these studies is required before conclusions can be drawn to assist with clinical utility. Another hypothesis would be that variations in the remaining SCN1A allele may influence outcome. It is likely that many factors contribute to the outcome.

Little is known about the effects of environmental factors on outcome. One particularly contentious area is the effect of vaccination in Dravet syndrome. Many families and clinicians have observed that seizure onset in Dravet syndrome occurs within a day or two of vaccination (Berkovic et al., 2006). This temporal association has led to large medico-legal payouts and vocal claims by the anti-vaccination lobby (Perez-Pena 2003). Our study of 37 patients with Dravet syndrome and SCN1A mutations found that one-third had onset within 72 hours of vaccination. Careful analysis of the phenotypes between those associated with vaccination and those without a temporal association revealed no differences apart from onset seven weeks earlier in those triggered by vaccination

(McIntosh et al., 2010). There was no difference in degree of intellectual impairment, seizures or any other parameter studied. Thus vaccination was a trigger for a disorder that these infants were destined to have. The timing of onset presumably relates to when the SCN1A protein becomes functionally relevant and the next fever or illness would have triggered the first seizure if immunization had not occurred. The mouse model supports this contention by providing evidence for age-dependent expression of the Scn1a protein (Ogiwara et al., 2007).

■ Outcome is more dependent on the underlying genetic basis than seizures

Dravet syndrome is an epileptic encephalopathy where ongoing seizures and epileptic activity impact on developmental outcome. There is no doubt, however, that factors other than seizures also influence outcome. As seizures settle with age, there is the emergence of an abnormal gait and ongoing evidence of cognitive decline. Further evidence for the pathogenicity of *SCN1A* lesions can be drawn from the autism literature where rare cases with autism spectrum disorders without seizures have *SCN1A* mutations (Weiss et al., 2003; O'Roak et al., 2011, 2012). These observations suggest that the underlying aetiology may be more important than seizures but it is more likely that both contribute to long term outcome.

Some solace can be sought from evidence that optimization of anti-epileptic therapy to improve seizure control, especially episodes of status, is likely to benefit developmental outcome. By selecting medications that work in Dravet syndrome (such as topiramate, stiripentol, valproate, clobazam as well as levetiracetam and the ketogenic diet), and avoiding those that aggravate seizures (such as carbamazepine and vigabatrin), seizures may be less frequent and debilitating (Catarino et al., 2011; Brunklaus et al., 2012). Lamotrigine has been reported to exacerbate seizures in young children with Dravet syndrome but this may not be universal and it may be beneficial in some patients particularly older ones (Guerrini et al., 1998). This raises the spectre of age-specific treatments where drugs have different beneficial and adverse effects at different ages.

References

- Akiyama M, Kobayashi K, Yoshinaga H, Ohtsuka Y. A long-term follow-up study of Dravet syndrome up to adulthood. *Epilepsia* 2010; 51: 1043-52.
- Berg AT, Berkovic SF, Brodie MJ, et al. Revised terminology and concepts for organization of seizures and epilepsies: report of the ILAE Commission on Classification and Terminology, 2005-2009. *Epilepsia* 2010; 51: 676-85.
- Berkovic SF, Harkin L, McMahon JM, et al. De-novo mutations of the sodium channel gene SCN1A in alleged vaccine encephalopathy: a retrospective study. *Lancet Neurol* 2006; 5: 488-92.
- Brunklaus A, Ellis R, Reavey E, Forbes GH, Zuberi SM. Prognostic, clinical and demographic features in SCN1A mutation-positive Dravet syndrome. *Brain* 2012; 135: 2329-36.
- Catarino CB, Liu JY, Liagkouras I, et al. Dravet syndrome as epileptic encephalopathy: evidence from long-term course and neuropathology. *Brain* 2011; 134: 2982-3010.
- Claes L, Del-Favero J, Ceulemans B, Lagae L, Van Broeckhoven C, De Jonghe P. De novo mutations in the sodium-channel gene SCN1A cause severe myoclonic epilepsy of infancy. *Am J Hum Genet* 2001; 68: 1327-32.

- Depienne C, Trouillard O, Saint-Martin C, *et al.* Spectrum of SCN1A gene mutations associated with Dravet syndrome: analysis of 333 patients. *J Med Genet* 2009a; 46: 183-91.
- Depienne C, Bouteiller D, Keren B, *et al.* Sporadic infantile epileptic encephalopathy caused by mutations in PCDH19 resembles Dravet syndrome but mainly affects females. *PLoS Genet* 2009b; 5: e1000381.
- Dibbens LM, Tarpey PS, Hynes K, *et al.* X-linked protocadherin 19 mutations cause female-limited epilepsy and cognitive impairment. *Nat Genet* 2008; 40: 776-81.
- Doose H, Lunau H, Castiglione E, Waltz S. Severe idiopathic generalised epilepsy of infancy with generalised tonic-clonic seizures. *Neuropediatrics* 1998; 29: 229-38.
- Dravet C, Roger J, Bureau M, Dalla Bernardina M. Myoclonic pilepsies in childhood. In: Akimoto H, Kazamatsuri H, Seino M, Ward A (eds). *Advances in Epileptology, XIIIth Epilepsy International Symposium.* New York: Raven Press; 1982, pp. 135-41.
- Dravet C, Bureau M, Oguni H, Cokar O, Guerrini R. Dravet syndrome (Severe Myoclonic Epilepsy in Infancy). In: Bureau M, Genton P, Dravet C, *et al.* (eds). *Epileptic Syndromes in Infancy, Childhood and Adolescence, 5th ed.* Paris: John Libbey Eurotext; 2012, pp. 125-56.
- Falconer MA, Serafetinides EA, Corsellis JA. Etiology and pathogenesis of temporal lobe epilepsy. *Arch Neurol* 1964; 10: 233-48.
- Guerrini R, Dravet C, Genton P, Belmonte A, Kaminska A, Dulac O. Lamotrigine and seizure aggravation in severe myoclonic epilepsy. *Epilepsia* 1998; 39s: 508-12.
- Harkin LA, McMahon JM, Iona X, *et al.* The spectrum of SCN1A-related infantile epileptic encephalopathies. *Brain* 2007; 130: 843-52.
- Jansen FE, Sadleir LG, Harkin LA, *et al.* Severe myoclonic epilepsy of infancy (Dravet syndrome): recognition and diagnosis in adults. *Neurology* 2006; 67: 2224-6.
- Kanai K, Hirose S, Oguni H, *et al.* Effect of localization of missense mutations in SCN1A on epilepsy phenotype severity. *Neurology* 2004; 63: 329-34.
- McIntosh AM, McMahon J, Dibbens LM, *et al.* Effects of vaccination on onset and outcome of Dravet syndrome: a retrospective study. *Lancet Neurol* 2010; 9: 592-8.
- Mulley JC, Nelson P, Guerrero S, *et al.* A new molecular mechanism for severe myoclonic epilepsy of infancy: exonic deletions in SCN1A. *Neurology* 2006; 67: 1094-5.
- O'Roak BJ, Deriziotis P, Lee C, *et al.* Exome sequencing in sporadic autism spectrum disorders identifies severe de novo mutations. *Nat Genet* 2011; 43: 585-9.
- O'Roak BJ, Vives L, Girirajan S, *et al.* Sporadic autism exomes reveal a highly interconnected protein network of de novo mutations. *Nature* 2012; 485: 246-50.
- Ogiwara I, Miyamoto H, Morita N, *et al.* Nav1.1 localizes to axons of parvalbumin-positive inhibitory interneurons: a circuit basis for epileptic seizures in mice carrying an *SCN1A* gene mutation. *J Neurosci* 2007; 27: 5903-14.
- Oguni H, Hayashi K, Oguni M, *et al.* Treatment of severe myoclonic epilepsy in infants with bromide and its borderline variant. *Epilepsia* 1994; 35: 1140-5.
- Ohmori I, Ouchida M, Kobayashi K, *et al.* CACNA1A variants may modify the epileptic phenotype of Dravet syndrome. *Neurobiol Dis* 2013; 50: 209-17.
- Perez-Pena R. Vaccine refusal is cited in whooping cough cases. *The New York Times* 2003; (7 October): sect. 1 (col. 2).
- Ragona F, Granata T, Dalla Bernardina B, *et al.* Cognitive development in Dravet syndrome: a retrospective, multicenter study of 26 patients. *Epilepsia* 2011; 52: 386-92.
- Rilstone JJ, Coelho FM, Minassian BA, Andrade DM. Dravet syndrome: seizure control and gait in adults with different SCN1A mutations. *Epilepsia* 2012; 53: 1421-8.
- Rodda JM, Scheffer IE, McMahon JM, Berkovic SF, Graham HK. Progressive gait deterioration in adolescents with Dravet syndrome. *Arch Neurol* 2012; 69: 873-8.

- Scheffer IE, Turner SJ, Dibbens LM, et al. Epilepsy and mental retardation limited to females: an under-recognized disorder. Brain 2008; 131: 918-27.
- Singh NA, Pappas C, Dahle EJ, et al. A role of SCN9A in human epilepsies, as a cause of febrile seizures and as a potential modifier of Dravet syndrome. PLoS Genet 2009; 5: e1000649.
- Singh R, Andermann E, Whitehouse WPA, et al. Severe myoclonic epilepsy of infancy: Extended spectrum of GEFS+? Epilepsia 2001; 42: 837-44.
- Suls A, Claeys KG, Goossens D, et al. Microdeletions involving the SCN1A gene may be common in SCN1A-mutation-negative SMEI patients. Hum Mutat 2006; 27: 914-20.
- Vadlamudi L, Dibbens LM, Lawrence KM, et al. Timing of de novo mutagenesis--a twin study of sodium-channel mutations. N Engl J Med 2010; 363: 1335-40.
- Weiss LA, Escayg A, Kearney JA, et al. Sodium channels SCN1A, SCN2A and SCN3A in familial autism. Mol Psychiatry 2003; 8: 186-94.
- Yu FH, Mantegazza M, Westenbroek RE, et al. Reduced sodium current in GABAergic interneurons in a mouse model of severe myoclonic epilepsy in infancy. Nat Neurosci 2006; 9: 1142-9.
- Zuberi SM, Brunklaus A, Birch R, Reavey E, Duncan J, Forbes GH. Genotype-phenotype associations in SCN1A-related epilepsies. Neurology 2011; 76: 594-600.

Epileptic encephalopathy with continuous spike-waves during slow-wave sleep including Landau-Kleffner syndrome: what determines the outcome?

Patrick Van Bogaert

Université Libre de Bruxelles (ULB), Department of Pediatric Neurology, Hôpital Erasme, Brussels, Belgium

■ What is epileptic encephalopathy with CSWS including LKS?

Landau-Kleffner syndrome (LKS) is a childhood disorder in which an acquired aphasia and interictal epileptiform discharges (IED) are associated (Commission, 1989). First described by Landau and Kleffner in six children with normal early language development who became aphasic after the onset of subtle seizures (Landau & Kleffner, 1957), the aphasia was characterized as auditory verbal agnosia, *i.e.*, the inability to decode phonemes despite intact peripheral hearing mechanisms, leading to a severe receptive and expressive verbal deficit (Rapin *et al.*, 1977). Further observations showed that language regression may occur without clinical seizures (Deonna, 1991; Paquier *et al.*, 1992; Soprano *et al.*, 1994; Tassinari *et al.*, 2002). Patients have IED that are generally multifocal, bilateral, often with a predominance over temporal and parietal regions, and activated during non rapid eye movement (NREM) sleep (Aicardi, 1986; Deonna & Roulet-Perez, 2010; Galanopoulou *et al.*, 2000; Tassinari *et al.*, 2002). A pattern of continuous spike-waves during slow-wave sleep (CSWS), *i.e.*, diffuse spike-waves occurring during at least 85% of slow sleep (Tassinari *et al.*, 2002), was found in the course of the disease in all patients reported in some series (Dulac *et al.*, 1983; Hirsch *et al.*, 1990; Massa *et al.*, 2000; Paquier *et al.*, 1992; Robinson *et al.*, 2001), but only in a minority of patients in another series (McVicar *et al.*, 2005).

CSWS is synonymous with electrical status epilepticus during slow sleep (ESES). ESES was described in children having the CSWS pattern combined with different types of seizures (partial or generalized seizures during sleep or atypical absences when awake), and with cognitive regression that was either global, leading to severe mental retardation, or more selective for language (Patry *et al.*, 1971). LKS and ESES are thus overlapping conditions and are no more considered as separate syndromes. The term "epileptic encephalopathy with CSWS including LKS" is now proposed for this particular childhood epileptic syndrome (Engel 2006). This terminology also encompasses children presenting types of acquired cognitive impairment other than aphasia or dementia in association with CSWS, i.e., frontal lobe dysfunction, apraxia and hemineglect, pseudo-bulbar palsy, visual agnosia, and learning arrest (Roulet Perez et al., 1993; Van Bogaert et al., 2006). It encompasses also atypical rolandic epilepsy, i.e., an epileptic syndrome resembling benign epilepsy with central temporal spikes (BECTS) but with atypical features like frequent brief seizures (atypical absences, focal positive or negative myoclonia), cognitive impairment, and CSWS (Aicardi & Chevrie, 1982; Fejerman, 2009; Fujii et al., 2010).

Observations of classical BECTS cases evolving to an epileptic encephalopathy with CSWS, sometimes precipitated by the use of certain anti-epileptic drugs (AED), like carbamazepine (Saltik et al., 2005; Tassinari et al., 2000), and of CSWS and BECTS cases coexisting within the same family (De Tiege et al., 2006), led to the assumption that some cases of CSWS have to be classified among the idiopathic (genetic) focal epileptic syndromes. On the other hand, CSWS was also reported in children with cerebral palsy showing brain lesions like porencephalic cysts, polymicrogyria, congenital hydrocephalus or thalamic perinatal ischemic lesions (Guerrini et al., 1998; Guzzetta et al., 2005), demonstrating that some cases of CSWS belong to the group of symptomatic (structural/metabolic) focal epilepsies.

In summary, epileptic encephalopathy with CSWS is a spectrum of epileptic conditions best defined by the association of cognitive or behavioral impairment acquired during childhood and not related to another factor than the presence of abundant IED during sleep, which tend to diffuse over the whole scalp. It is part of the childhood focal epileptic syndromes, some cases being idiopathic (genetic) and overlapping with BECTS, others being structural/metabolic, and others being of unknown etiology. LKS is a particular presentation where acquired aphasia is the core symptom.

■ What causes cognitive regression in this epileptic syndrome?

Epileptic encephalopathy with CSWS is one of the best illustrations of the concept of epileptic encephalopathy, i.e., conditions in which epileptiform abnormalities may contribute to progressive cognitive dysfunction, so that early effective intervention may improve developmental outcome (Berg et al., 2010; Engel 2006). Indeed, clinical improvement is evident and sometimes impressive when EEG normalization is obtained using drugs (Aeby et al., 2005; Buzatu et al., 2009). A recent study showed impaired consolidation of a declarative memory task during sleep in two children with epileptic encephalopathy with CSWS, and normalization of overnight memory performance after successful treatment of CSWS with hydrocortisone in one of them, suggesting that CSWS could impair the mechanisms of sleep related brain plasticity (Urbain et al., 2011).

The initial hypothesis of a "functional ablation" of eloquent cortical areas by the "persistent convulsive discharge" to explain the neuropsychological impairment, as proposed half a century ago by Landau and Kleffner (Landau & Kleffner, 1957), remains the most largely accepted hypothesis. However, some observations are not fully explained with this theory. Firstly, the temporal association between CSWS on EEG and neurological regression is not always strict (Hirsch et al., 1990; Rapin et al., 1977). Secondly, while some authors found a strict association between the pattern of neuropsychological derangement and the location of the interictal focus, others did not. Patients showing clinical frontal dysfunction and parietal epileptic focus have been reported (De Tiege et al., 2004). A tentative physiopathological hypothesis which has the advantage to reconcile these apparent discrepancies emerged from connectivity studies obtained from FDG-PET data in children investigated at the active phase of the disease as well as at remission (De Tiege et al., 2008; De Tiege et al., 2004). This hypothesis is based on the concept of surrounding and remote inhibition, which has been demonstrated in animal models of epilepsy (Bruehl & Witte, 1995; Schwartz & Bonhoeffer, 2001). It proposes that the foci of increased glucose metabolism are the epileptic foci (which may in some patients not be intense enough to be imaged by PET), and that these foci inhibit other cortical areas which become hypometabolic and may be located either at the border of the hypermetabolic area (surrounding inhibition) or distant from it (remote inhibition). Therefore, it is not only the location of the epileptic focus but also the location of the inhibited cortical area which determine the type of neuropsychological profile. Arguments favoring this hypothesis are that, at remission, regression of both focal hypermetabolism and hypometabolism is observed and functional connectivity between regions showing increased and decreased regional metabolism for glucose during the active phase of CSWS returns to normal (De Tiege et al., 2008). This theory is also supported by EEG-fMRI investigations performed in children with CSWS having shown increases in perfusion at the site of the epileptic focus that were associated to decreases in perfusion in distinct connected brain areas, including structures of the default mode network (De Tiege et al., 2007; Siniatchkin et al., 2010).

■ Which factors determine long-term outcome?

In epilepsy, outcome commonly refers to seizure freedom. In epileptic encephalopathy with CSWS, seizure freedom is a secondary objective, as some patients do not present any clinical seizures or only rare seizures. Moreover, the literature agrees that long-term outcome for seizures is good, with seizures persisting in adulthood only in a small minority of patients. Therefore, the primary end-point in epileptic encephalopathy with CSWS is the cognitive outcome. This section will focus only on long-term cognitive outcome.

Several factors might theoretically affect long-term cognitive outcome in epileptic encephalopathy with CSWS. The first one is the underlying aetiology. The outcome could be better in genetic cases than in structural/metabolic cases. The second one is age at onset of epilepsy. Younger age at onset could be associated with worse outcome considering that the impact of epileptic activity on brain plasticity should be greater at earlier stages of brain development. The third factor is the duration of CSWS. Considering the hypothesis of a direct impact of CSWS on cognition, shorter duration of CSWS should be associated with better outcome. The fourth is the severity of the cognitive deficit during the acute phase of the disease. A severe auditory agnosia is expected to be associated with more severe long-term deficits than an isolated attention deficit disorder. The fifth is the type of anti-epileptic drugs (AED) used. The influence of AED on cognitive functions, particularly in polytherapy at high doses, is well known in children. This factor is not specific for epileptic encephalopathy with CSWS and will not be discussed here.

Studies on long-term cognitive outcome in epileptic encephalopathy with CSWS are few, retrospective, and do not address systematically the above cited risk factors. However, despite these important limitations, some conclusions may be drawn from the available literature.

Impact of underlying aetiology

Concerning the impact of underlying aetiology on outcome, it may be difficult to correctly classify a patient with normal structural MRI between the idiopathic (genetic) subgroup and the subgroup of unknown aetiology. Indeed, while patients with atypical rolandic epilepsy clearly belong to the idiopathic subgroup, there is no consensus as to the classification of patients who present either EEG abnormalities non suggestive of BECTS (for instances focal IED in areas other than the centro-temporal regions, or only secondary generalized discharges even at the awake state), or pre-existing psychomotor delay. Therefore, in most studies, the idiopathic and unknown aetiology subgroups are considered as one group. In two papers, the cognitive outcome of atypical rolandic epilepsy with CSWS was specifically assessed. The first study showed that epileptic encephalopathy with CSWS is rare in BECTS (less than 5% of all BECTS cases in this retrospective study), and that full cognitive recovery occurred only in 2 of the 5 patients who were successfully treated with AED (Tovia et al., 2011). The second study followed 12 patients until ages 6 to 14 years, and showed that long duration of the period with negative motor seizures was later associated with low IQ, 4 patients having IQ less than 70 (Fujii et al., 2010).

Another difficulty when trying to correlate aetiology with outcome is that a great heterogeneity exists within the structural/metabolic subgroup. Indeed, structural MRI may show highly variable lesions in terms of extension and location, going from thalamic infarcts to bilateral polymicrogyria. Studies have shown that the long-term outcome for seizures is also good in this subgroup, and disappearance of CSWS using AED is accompanied by cognitive improvement (Guerrini et al., 1998; Guzzetta et al., 2005). This suggests that the underlying lesion is not the only determinant of long-term cognitive outcome. Cognitive improvement of lesion-related cases after corticosteroids (Buzatu et al., 2009) or after epilepsy surgery (Peltola et al., 2011) also supports this hypothesis.

Impact of age at onset and duration of CSWS/cognitive regression

Young age at onset of CSWS as well as long duration of CSWS are both risk factors for long-term cognitive sequels that are difficult to assess for several reasons. Firstly, sleep EEG data at onset of cognitive regression are often missing. Secondly, EEG abnormalities may fluctuate within short periods of time without any drug intervention (Fernandez et al., 2012), and sleep EEG may even be normal in the active phase of LKS (Van Bogaert et al., 2012). Thirdly, there is no consensus for a neurophysiological definition of CSWS, and some questions are still unanswered. Is the threshold of 85% of epileptic activity during NREM sleep as defined by Tassinari valid, considering that LKS was described in patients having a spike-wave index (SWI) inferior to 85% during sleep (McVicar et al., 2005; Van Bogaert et al., 2012)? What is the best way to calculate the SWI? Is it necessary or not to calculate the SWI on a full night recording? Is it relevant to take into account the secondary generalized discharges only, considering that unilateral CSWS may be associated with cognitive impairment (Paquier et al., 2009)? For all these reasons, the age at onset of cognitive regression is a more reliable parameter than the age at appearance of the CSWS pattern, but it should be kept in mind that these two parameters do not necessarily overlap.

Young age at onset of CSWS was considered as a factor of a poor prognosis by some investigators but without statistical assessment (Scholtes *et al.*, 2005; Veggiotti *et al.*, 2002). On the contrary, authors who searched for statistical association between age at onset and cognitive outcome did not find it (Robinson *et al.*, 2001; Seegmuller *et al.*, 2012).

Long duration of CSWS (or regression) was found to be predictive of a poor cognitive outcome in many studies (Kramer *et al.*, 2009; Paquier *et al.*, 1992; Robinson *et al.*, 2001; Scholtes *et al.*, 2005; Seegmuller *et al.*, 2012; Veggiotti *et al.*, 2002). In some studies, this factor reached statistical significance. In a series of 18 LKS patients followed for a mean of 67 months, long duration of CSWS was associated with outcome, no child with CSWS of more than 36 months duration having normal outcome (Robinson *et al.*, 2001). In a series of 30 patients with epileptic encephalopathies with CSWS of various aetiologies (lesion-related, idiopathic and cryptogenic cases) followed for a mean of 6.6 years, the duration of CSWS correlated significantly with residual intellectual deficit (Kramer *et al.*, 2009). Long duration of CSWS was statistically associated with poor cognitive outcome in a recent series of 10 patients with different types of cognitive regression and normal MRI followed at long term (Seegmuller *et al.*, 2012).

Short duration of CSWS was, on the contrary, found to be significantly associated with positive response in terms of cognitive improvement after hydrocortisone in one series (Buzatu *et al.*, 2009).

■ Impact of type and severity of initial regression

The type and severity of cognitive regression in the acute phase of the disease also have a major impact on long-term outcome. Several studies showed persistence of neuropsychological dysfunctions particular to each syndrome at long-term, so that patients with prolonged global intellectual regression had the worst outcome, whereas those with more specific deficits recovered best (Debiais *et al.*, 2007; Praline *et al.*, 2003; Seegmuller *et al.*, 2012). Concerning more specifically LKS, patients usually have language difficulties in adulthood, but the disability is highly variable, depending on response to treatment (Deonna *et al.*, 2009; Paquier *et al.*, 1992; Praline *et al.*, 2003; Van Bogaert *et al.*, 2012). Persistent dysfunction of the brain areas affected during the acute phase of auditory agnosia is suggested by a functional imaging study performed in LKS patients years after remission of epilepsy (Majerus *et al.*, 2003).

■ Conclusion

Severity and duration of initial regression are the most important risk factors of cognitive impairment at the long term. Therefore, efforts should be made to make a diagnosis of this condition a soon as possible in order to start appropriate treatment without delay. First line treatment remains a subject of debate. Treatment should be more aggressive, *i.e.*, a trial with corticosteroids is warranted early in the course of the disease, especially if the initial cognitive regression is severe.

References

- Aeby A, Poznanski N, Verheulpen D, Wetzburger C, Van Bogaert P. Levetiracetam efficacy in epileptic syndromes with continuous spikes and waves during slow sleep: experience in 12 cases. *Epilepsia* 2005; 46: 1937-42.
- Aicardi J. *Epilepsy in Children*. New York: Raven Press, 1986.
- Aicardi J, Chevrie JJ. Atypical benign partial epilepsy of childhood. *Dev Med Child Neurol* 1982; 24: 281-92.
- Berg AT, Berkovic SF, Brodie MJ, et al. Revised terminology and concepts for organization of seizures and epilepsies: report of the ILAE Commission on Classification and Terminology, 2005-2009. *Epilepsia* 2010; 51: 676-85.
- Bruehl C, Witte OW. Cellular activity underlying altered brain metabolism during focal epileptic activity. *Ann Neurol* 1995; 38: 414-20.
- Buzatu M, Bulteau C, Altuzarra C, Dulac O, Van Bogaert P. Corticosteroids as treatment of epileptic syndromes with continuous spike-waves during slow-wave sleep. *Epilepsia* 2009; 50 (Suppl 7): 68-72.
- Commission on Classification and Terminology of the International League Against Epilepsy. Proposal for revised classification of epilepsies and epileptic syndromes. *Epilepsia* 1989; 30: 389-99.
- De Tiege X, Goldman S, Verheulpen D, Aeby A, Poznanski N, Van Bogaert P. Coexistence of idiopathic rolandic epilepsy and CSWS in two families. *Epilepsia* 2006; 47: 1723-7.
- De Tiege X, Ligot N, Goldman S, Poznanski N, de Saint Martin A, Van Bogaert P. Metabolic evidence for remote inhibition in epilepsies with continuous spike-waves during sleep. *Neuroimage* 2008; 40: 802-10.
- De Tiege X, Harrison S, Laufs H, et al. Impact of interictal epileptic activity on normal brain function in epileptic encephalopathy: an electroencephalography-functional magnetic resonance imaging study. *Epilepsy Behav* 2007; 11: 460-5.
- De Tiege X, Goldman S, Laureys S, et al. Regional cerebral glucose metabolism in epilepsies with continuous spikes and waves during sleep. *Neurology* 2004; 63: 853-7.
- Debiais S, Tuller L, Barthez MA, et al. Epilepsy and language development: the continuous spike-waves during slow sleep syndrome. *Epilepsia* 2007; 48: 1104-10.
- Deonna T, Roulet-Perez E. Early-onset acquired epileptic aphasia (Landau-Kleffner syndrome, LKS) and regressive autistic disorders with epileptic EEG abnormalities: the continuing debate. *Brain Dev* 2010; 32: 746-52.
- Deonna T, Prelaz-Girod AC, Mayor-Dubois C, Roulet-Perez E. Sign language in Landau-Kleffner syndrome. *Epilepsia* 2009; 50 (Suppl 7): 77-82.
- Deonna TW. Acquired epileptiform aphasia in children (Landau-Kleffner syndrome). *J Clin Neurophysiol* 1991; 8: 288-98.
- Dulac O, Billard C, Arthuis M. [Electroclinical and developmental aspects of epilepsy in the aphasia-epilepsy syndrome]. *Arch Fr Pediatr* 1983; 40: 299-308.
- Engel J, Jr. Report of the ILAE classification core group. *Epilepsia* 2006; 47: 1558-68.
- Fejerman N. Atypical rolandic epilepsy. *Epilepsia* 2009; 50 (Suppl 7): 9-12.
- Fernandez IS, Peters JM, Hadjiloizou S, et al. Clinical staging and electroencephalographic evolution of continuous spikes and waves during sleep. *Epilepsia* 2012; 53: 1185-95.
- Fujii A, Oguni H, Hirano Y, Osawa M. Atypical benign partial epilepsy: recognition can prevent pseudocatastrophe. *Pediatr Neurol* 2010; 43: 411-9.
- Galanopoulou AS, Bojko A, Lado F, Moshe SL. The spectrum of neuropsychiatric abnormalities associated with electrical status epilepticus in sleep. *Brain Dev* 2000; 22: 279-95.
- Guerrini R, Genton P, Bureau M, et al. Multilobar polymicrogyria, intractable drop attack seizures, and sleep-related electrical status epilepticus. *Neurology* 1998; 51: 504-12.

- Guzzetta F, Battaglia D, Veredice C, *et al*. Early thalamic injury associated with epilepsy and continuous spike-wave during slow sleep. *Epilepsia* 2005; 46: 889-900.
- Hirsch E, Marescaux C, Maquet P, *et al*. Landau-Kleffner syndrome: a clinical and EEG study of five cases. *Epilepsia* 1990; 31: 756-67.
- Kramer U, Sagi L, Goldberg-Stern H, Zelnik N, Nissenkorn A, Ben-Zeev B. Clinical spectrum and medical treatment of children with electrical status epilepticus in sleep (ESES). *Epilepsia* 2009; 50: 1517-24.
- Landau WM, Kleffner FR. Syndrome of acquired aphasia with convulsive disorder in children. *Neurology* 1957; 7: 523-30.
- Majerus S, Laureys S, Collette F, *et al*. Phonological short-term memory networks following recovery from Landau and Kleffner syndrome. *Hum Brain Mapp* 2003; 19: 133-44.
- Massa R, de Saint-Martin A, Hirsch E, *et al*. Landau-Kleffner syndrome: sleep EEG characteristics at onset. *Neurophysiol Clin* 2000; 111 (Suppl 2): S87-93.
- McVicar KA, Ballaban-Gil K, Rapin I, Moshe SL, Shinnar S. Epileptiform EEG abnormalities in children with language regression. *Neurology* 2005; 65: 129-31.
- Paquier PF, Van Dongen HR, Loonen CB. The Landau-Kleffner syndrome or'acquired aphasia with convulsive disorder'. Long-term follow-up of six children and a review of the recent literature. *Arch Neurol* 1992; 49: 354-9.
- Paquier PF, Verheulpen D, De Tiege X, Van Bogaert P. Acquired cognitive dysfunction with focal sleep spiking activity. *Epilepsia* 2009; 50 (Suppl 7): 29-32.
- Patry G, Lyagoubi S, Tassinari CA. Subclinical "electrical status epilepticus" induced by sleep in children. A clinical and electroencephalographic study of six cases. *Arch Neurol* 1971; 24: 242-52.
- Peltola ME, Liukkonen E, Granstrom ML, *et al*. The effect of surgery in encephalopathy with electrical status epilepticus during sleep. *Epilepsia* 2011; 52: 602-9.
- Praline J, Hommet C, Barthez MA, *et al*. Outcome at adulthood of the continuous spike-waves during slow sleep and Landau-Kleffner syndromes. *Epilepsia* 2003; 44: 1434-40.
- Rapin I, Mattis S, Rowan AJ, Golden GG. Verbal auditory agnosia in children. *Dev Med Child Neurol* 1977; 19: 197-207.
- Robinson RO, Baird G, Robinson G, Simonoff E. Landau-Kleffner syndrome: course and correlates with outcome. *Dev Med Child Neurol* 2001; 43: 243-7.
- Roulet Perez E, Davidoff V, Despland PA, Deonna T. Mental and behavioural deterioration of children with epilepsy and CSWS: acquired epileptic frontal syndrome. *Dev Med Child Neurol* 1993; 35: 661-74.
- Saltik S, Uluduz D, Cokar O, Demirbilek V, Dervent A. A clinical and EEG study on idiopathic partial epilepsies with evolution into ESES spectrum disorders. *Epilepsia* 2005; 46: 524-33.
- Scholtes FB, Hendriks MP, Renier WO. Cognitive deterioration and electrical status epilepticus during slow sleep. *Epilepsy Behav* 2005; 6: 167-73.
- Schwartz TH, Bonhoeffer T. In vivo optical mapping of epileptic foci and surround inhibition in ferret cerebral cortex. *Nat Med* 2001; 7: 1063-7.
- Seegmuller C, Deonna T, Dubois CM, *et al*. Long-term outcome after cognitive and behavioral regression in nonlesional epilepsy with continuous spike-waves during slow-wave sleep. *Epilepsia* 2012; 53: 1067-76.
- Siniatchkin M, Groening K, Moehring J, *et al*. Neuronal networks in children with continuous spikes and waves during slow sleep. *Brain* 2010; 133: 2798-813.
- Soprano AM, Garcia EF, Caraballo R, Fejerman N. Acquired epileptic aphasia: neuropsychologic follow-up of 12 patients. *Pediatr Neurol* 1994; 11: 230-5.

- Tassinari CA, Rubboli G, Volpi L, Billard C, Bureau M. État de mal électrique épileptique pendant le sommeil lent (ESES ou POCS) incluant l'aphasie épileptique acquise (syndrome de Landau-Kleffner). In: Roger J, Bureau M, Dravet C, Genton P, Tassinari CA, Wolf P, eds. *Les syndromes épileptiques de l'enfant et de l'adolescent*. Eastleigh: John Libbey, 2002: 265-83.
- Tassinari CA, Rubboli G, Volpi L, *et al*. Encephalopathy with electrical status epilepticus during slow sleep or ESES syndrome including the acquired aphasia. *Clin Neurophysiol* 2000; 111 (Suppl 2): S94-S102.
- Tovia E, Goldberg-Stern H, Ben Zeev B, *et al*. The prevalence of atypical presentations and comorbidities of benign childhood epilepsy with centrotemporal spikes. *Epilepsia* 2011; 52: 1483-8.
- Urbain C, Di Vincenzo T, Peigneux P, Van Bogaert P. Is sleep-related consolidation impaired in focal idiopathic epilepsies of childhood? A pilot study. *Epilepsy Behav* 2011; 22: 380-4.
- Van Bogaert P, King MD, Paquier P, *et al*. Acquired auditory agnosia in childhood and normal sleep EEG subsequently diagnosed as Landau-Kleffner syndrome: report of 3 cases. *Dev Med Child Neurol* 2012 [Epub ahead of print].
- Van Bogaert P, Aeby A, De Borchgrave V, *et al*. The epileptic syndromes with continuous spikes and waves during slow sleep: definition and management guidelines. *Acta Neurol Belg* 2006; 106: 52-60.
- Veggiotti P, Termine C, Granocchio E, Bova S, Papalia G, Lanzi G. Long-term neuropsychological follow-up and nosological considerations in five patients with continuous spikes and waves during slow sleep. *Epileptic Disord* 2002; 4: 243-9.

Outcome of idiopathic generalized epilepsy and the role of EEG discharges

Elaine C. Wirrell
Mayo Clinic, Rochester MN, USA

Idiopathic generalized epilepsy accounts for approximately 15-20% of all new-onset pediatric epilepsy (Camfield *et al.*, 1996; Wirrell *et al.*, 2011) and is presumed to have a genetic etiology. A number of well-defined electroclinical syndromes comprise the idiopathic generalized epilepsies. This paper will review long-term prognosis of these syndromes, focusing on both seizure outcome as well as intellectual and psychosocial functioning.

■ Electroclinical syndromes of idiopathic generalized epilepsy

Table I outlines the clinical and electrographic characteristics of the specific electroclinical syndromes which comprise idiopathic generalized epilepsy. The four most common syndromes include childhood absence epilepsy (CAE), comprising 32-58%, juvenile absence epilepsy (JAE), comprising 9-20%, juvenile myoclonic epilepsy (JME) comprising 10-20% and epilepsy with generalized tonic clonic seizures alone (IGE-GMA), comprising 11% of idiopathic generalized epilepsy (Camfield *et al.*, 1996, Wirrell *et al.*, 2011).

■ Long-term prognosis of seizures

While many idiopathic generalized epilepsies that begin in childhood are both pharmacoresponsive and self-limited, identification of the specific electroclinical syndrome is essential to more clearly define the natural history. Several, less common forms of absence epilepsy exist with unique semiological features and greater rates of pharmacoresistance, and these must be distinguished from the more common CAE or JAE.

Childhood absence epilepsy

Several studies have examined long-term seizure outcome in CAE and shown that the majority of children will ultimately achieve remission of their epilepsy. In a population-based study of 72 children with CAE followed for a mean of 14 years, 65% of children were seizure-free and off antiepileptic drugs, and the mean age of remission was 12 years (range 4-24) (Wirrell *et al.*, 1996). Factors predicting against remission on multivariate

Table I. Electroclinical syndromes of idiopathic generalized epilepsy

Syndrome	Age at onset	Seizure type(s)	Self-limited	Pharmaco-responsive	EEG features
Myoclonic epilepsy in infancy	4 mos-3 years	Myoclonic jerks only. GTCS may occur later in life	Yes	Yes	GSW in brief bursts, usually with clinical accompaniment
Myoclonic-atonic epilepsy	Early childhood	Myoclonic-atonic, absence, myoclonic, GTCS	Often	Usually not early in course, but ultimate seizure control often obtained	2-3 Hz GSW, some PSW, parietal theta rhythms, slow background
Childhood absence epilepsy	Early-mid childhood	Absences 20-50x/d	Often	Usually	3 Hz GSW, act by HV
Juvenile absence epilepsy	Young-mid adolescence	Absences (<1-2/d) and GTCS in 80%	Rarely	Usually	3-4 Hz GSW
Juvenile myoclonic epilepsy	Adolescence/ young adult	GTCS, myoclonus, absence rare	Rarely	Usually	Generalized 3.5-6 Hz polyspike and spike-wave, 40% PS
IGE with grand mal alone	Adolescence/ young adult	GTCS	Rarely	Usually	GSW
Epilepsy with myoclonic absences	Early-mid childhood	Myoclonic absences, absence, GTCS	Rarely	Rarely	3 Hz SW
Perioral myoclonia with absence	2-13 yrs	Absences with perioral myoclonia, GTCS, absence SE common	Rarely	Rarely	4-7 Hz spike-wave and PSW
Phantom absences with generalized tonic clonic seizure	Early adulthood	GTCS, preceding inconspicuous absences, absence SE common	Rarely	Often	3-4 Hz GSW and PSW and fragments
Eyelid myoclonia with absence "Jeavons"	Childhood	Eyelid myoclonia with brief absences	No	Rarely	3-6 Hz GSW and PSW triggered by E/C and photic
Early onset absence epilepsy	< 3 yrs	Absences, rare GTCS	Often	Often	3-4 Hz GSW

analysis were myoclonic seizures occurring while on antiepileptic medication, absence status epilepticus, family history of generalized seizures and EEG background slowing. Of those who failed to remit, 44% had progressed to JME.

In a study of 47 children with new-onset CAE recruited from several centers in the Netherlands and followed for 12-17 years, only 7% had ongoing seizures at final follow-up, and only 13% had developed generalized tonic-clonic seizures over the course of their epilepsy (Callenbach et al., 2009). The mean age at remission was 9.5 years. While children who did not achieve seizure control within six months of treatment onset had higher remission rates and longer epilepsy duration, most did well in the long-term.

Several epilepsy clinic cohorts of CAE have also been reported. However, these cohorts may select more refractory patients, and thus give a more pessimistic long-term outcome. In a hospital-based prevalence cohort of 64 patients with CAE followed for a mean of 30 years, 56% had been seizure-free for at least two years at final follow-up (Trinka et al., 2004). Over the course of their epilepsy, over two thirds developed generalized tonic-clonic seizures, and 5% developed myoclonic seizures, however only 5% had progressed to JME. The development of other seizure types predicted against final remission. In another study following 53 children treated in a single epilepsy clinic in France for a mean of 3 years, Bartolomei noted that 40% continued to have persisting seizures, and predictors for this outcome were polyspike and wave on EEG, and occurrence of generalized tonic-clonic seizures (Bartolomei et al., 1997).

Juvenile absence epilepsy

JAE is less well-studied than CAE, however is felt to be rarely self-limited. Most cases require life-long antiepileptic drug therapy. Loiseau et al. followed 62 patients to a mean age of 30 years (Loiseau et al., 1995). Seventy-nine percent had generalized tonic- clonic seizures, which began at a mean age of 17 years, or, on average, 5 years after onset of absences. All subjects were treated with valproic acid, with or without other antiepileptic drugs, and only 47% achieved complete control of absences. While "most" cases were said to have remission of their generalized tonic-clonic seizures, the actual number is not reported. A somewhat improved outcome was reported in a single-center study of 64 cases of JAE followed for a mean of 22 years (Trinka et al., 2004). Nearly two thirds were seizure-free for at least two years at final follow-up and 19% had evolved to JME. Two smaller studies with shorter follow-up report similar results – 56-60% were seizure-free with valproate with or without other antiepileptic agents (Bartolomei et al., 1997; Obeid, 1994). Overall, generalized tonic-clonic seizures were more likely to be controlled than absences. Both higher generalized tonic-clonic seizure frequency at onset and the presence of polyspike and wave on EEG tended to predict poorer outcome.

Juvenile myoclonic epilepsy

Similar to JAE, JME is felt to be frequently pharmacoresponsive but rarely self-limited, and as such, life-long antiepileptic therapy is usually required. Several long-term follow-up studies have now been reported, which confirm these findings, but somewhat surprisingly, note that a significant minority of patients were able to successfully discontinue antiepileptic medications. In the largest study of 48 patients followed for a mean of 20 years, 67% were shown to have a benign course (defined as no generalized tonic-clonic seizures and less than two myoclonic seizures per month at final follow-up), 17% were resistant (defined as more than one generalized tonic-clonic seizure per year despite adequate medications), and 17% had pseudoresistance (defined as ongoing seizures due to lifestyle issues, lack of compliance or inappropriate medication treatment) (Baykan et al., 2008). Only 8.3% had been able to successfully stop antiepileptic medication and remain seizure-free.

A small, population-based cohort, followed for a mean of 26 years, showed a similar proportion with intractable epilepsy (13%) (Camfield & Camfield, 2009). One quarter of this cohort had remission of their epilepsy, meaning they were seizure-free off medication.

A slightly larger cohort identified through a single hospital center noted that 68% of subjects with JME were seizure-free after a mean follow-up of 39 years (Geithner et al., 2012). Forty three percent of those who were seizure-free had attempted to discontinue antiepileptic medication, and two thirds of these were successful. Factors which predicted against seizure freedom at follow-up included generalized tonic-clonic seizures preceded by bilateral myoclonic jerks, longer duration of epilepsy with unsuccessful treatment and polytherapy.

Idiopathic generalized epilepsy with grand mal alone

Only a single, small, population-based study has reported on long-term seizure outcome in IGE-GMA with a mean age at onset of 6.7 years and showed that 75% were in complete terminal remission after a mean follow-up of 22 years (Camfield & Camfield, 2010).

Other idiopathic generalized epilepsies

Myoclonic epilepsy in infancy is a rare syndrome that presents with myoclonic seizures beginning between 4 months to three years of age in otherwise healthy infants (Dravet et al., 1992). Myoclonus is often more subtle at initial presentation but increases in intensity and frequency early in the course. A family history of generalized epilepsy is present in nearly one third of cases, suggesting a possible genetic etiology. Nearly one third may have preceding febrile convulsions and a small proportion progress to generalized tonic-clonic seizures. The EEG shows generalized spike-wave and polyspike discharges with the myoclonic jerks, but the background is normal. Valproate is often the first drug used, but other medication including ethosuximide, benzodiazepine and phenobarbital may be effective. Epilepsy is usually self-limited and most infants can discontinue medication early in the toddler years.

Myoclonic atonic epilepsy often presents with very frequent generalized seizures which are both nonconvulsive and convulsive. Seizures often initially respond suboptimally to medication, and nonconvulsive status epilepticus is seen in a significant minority (Trivisano et al., 2011). While long-term seizure outcome is variable, many patients ultimately experience resolution of seizures, although may be left with some degree of intellectual disability.

The outcome for early onset absence epilepsy, presenting before 3 years of age is heterogenous. While Chaix et al. reported persisting absences in half of their cohort (Chaix et al., 2003), Giordano et al. reported excellent response to therapy in 85% of their cases (Giordano et al., 2011). Glucose transporter (GLUT1) deficiency is an important cause of early-onset absence epilepsy, accounting for approximately 12% of cases (Suls et al., 2009) and should be screened for in this population, particularly in the setting of intellectual disability or pharmacoresistance. Factors predicting poorer seizure outcome include abnormal neurological status (Chaix et al., 2003) and associated generalized tonic-clonic seizures (Grosso et al., 2005).

Epilepsy with myoclonic absences (Tassinari syndrome) is characterized by absence seizures with associated prominent jerking of the upper limbs and head. Myoclonic absence seizures begin at a mean age of 7 years and generalized tonic-clonic seizures develop in nearly two thirds of patients but are usually infrequent. Compared to CAE, pharmacoresistance is more common and this syndrome is less likely to remit. Approximately 18% of cases may evolve to a more severe epilepsy similar to Lennox-Gastaut syndrome (Bureau & Tassinari, 2005).

Perioral myoclonia with absence has a relatively broad range of onset from 2 to 13 years (Rubboli et al., 2009). Absences vary in frequency but are typically brief (< 4-8 s) and associated with rhythmic contractions of the orbicularis oris, depressor anguli oris, or muscles of mastication, resulting in twitching of the mouth, protrusion of the lips, and jerking of the jaw. Generalized tonic-clonic seizures occur in nearly all patients but are infrequent. Over half will develop one or more episodes of absence status epilepticus, which may end with a generalized tonic-clonic seizure. The interictal EEG shows brief bursts or fragments of spike wave. Ictally, irregular, generalized polyspike-wave discharge at 3 to 4 Hz without photosensitivity is seen. This syndrome also persists into adulthood and tends to be more resistant to antiepileptic therapy.

Eyelid myoclonia with absence (Jeavon's syndrome) presents at a peak age of 6-8 years with frequent but brief absences associated with myoclonia of the eyelids, upward deviation of the eyes and retropulsion of the head. Seizures are frequently triggered by eye closure and photosensitivity is usual. Generalized tonic-clonic seizures commonly also occur, and although these may respond to antiepileptic medications, the absences with eyelid myoclonia are usually pharmacoresistant. Again, remission is rare and this is usually a lifelong condition (Striano et al., 2009).

The entity of phantom absences with generalized tonic-clonic seizures was reported by Panayiotopoulos et al. in 13 adults, representing 9.6% of all adults with idiopathic generalized epilepsy (Panayiotopoulos et al., 1997). Absences were very mild, usually lasting 2 to 4 seconds, and associated with inconspicuous impairment of cognition. Generalized tonic-clonic seizures occurred without consistent circadian distribution or specific provoking factors, and appeared later (mean age 32 years) than in most other idiopathic generalized epilepsies. Patients were not photosensitive and did not have associated myoclonic jerks. One or more bouts of absence status epilepticus occurred in half of all patients (Panayiotopoulos et al., 1997, Rubboli et al., 2009).

■ Long-term intellectual and psychosocial outcome

Cognitive delays and psychosocial comorbidities are common in pediatric epilepsy and frequently present at the time of diagnosis (Camfield & Camfield, 2007). Several studies have surprisingly shown that these comorbidities are for the most part unrelated to biological or epilepsy-related factors.

It has been previously assumed that the idiopathic generalized epilepsies were "more benign" and that children with these disorders had favorable long-term social outcomes, particularly if their epilepsy is self-limited. However, careful studies have raised significant concerns, suggesting that long-term outcome is often poor.

Intellectual outcomes

Caplan et al., compared cognitive and linguistic function in 69 children with CAE (all with IQ ≥ 70) identified from community and tertiary care centers to 103 controls without epilepsy (Caplan et al., 2008). All children with CAE had at least one seizure in the preceding year. Cognition was evaluated using the Wechsler Intelligence Scale for Children-Revised (from 1994-98) and the Wechsler Intelligence Scale for Children – 3rd edition (from 1999-2005). Language was evaluated using the Test of Language Development. The CAE cohort scored significantly lower than controls on full scale IQ ($p < 0.0001$), verbal IQ ($p < 0.0001$), performance IQ ($p = 0.001$) and spoken language quotient ($p < 0.0001$). One fourth had subtle cognitive difficulties and just under half had linguistic deficits. Increased duration of epilepsy predicted both lower verbal IQ ($p < 0.02$) and lower spoken language quotient ($p < 0.0008$), and antiepileptic drug treatment was also associated with lower IQ ($p < 0.005$) and spoken language quotient ($p < 0.002$) scores.

Attention deficit hyperactivity disorder

Attentional problems are very common amongst children with epilepsy. Using the cohort described above, Caplan et al. found that 37% of children with CAE had comorbid ADHD compared to only 8% of controls (Caplan et al., 2008). ADHD was significantly more prevalent with longer duration of epilepsy ($p < 0.008$) and higher seizure frequency ($p < 0.05$). Similarly, when controlled for age and IQ, Vega et al. found that children with CAE scored significantly higher than healthy controls on the Attention Problems subscale, but not the Hyperactivity subscale of the Behavior Assessment System for Children (Vega et al., 2010). Unlike Caplan's study however, they found no significant relationship between Attention subscale score and seizure control, duration of illness or age at onset.

Affective disorders

Anxiety and depression are significant comorbidities of idiopathic generalized epilepsy. These conditions are poorly recognized but frequently impair quality of life. Caplan et al., compared 171 children with epilepsy (100 – complex partial seizures, 71 – CAE) to 93 healthy controls (Caplan et al., 2005). All children underwent a structured psychiatric interview (K-SADs) and completed mood self-report scales (Child Depression Inventory and Multidimensional Anxiety Scale for Children). Additionally, parents completed the Child Behavior Checklist and provided behavioral information through a structured interview. Rates of affective and anxiety disorders were significantly higher in children with epilepsy compared to controls (33% vs. 6%, $p < 0.0008$). While no patient had attempted suicide, 20% of those with epilepsy admitted to suicidal ideation. Compared to children with complex partial seizures, those with CAE had much higher rates of anxiety but lower rates of depression and comorbid depression/anxiety ($p < 0.02$). Lower verbal IQ and greater school problems reported on the Child Behavior Checklist were predictive of higher risk of affective disorders. Another study by Vega et al. compared the Anxiety and

Depression subscales of the parent-completed Behavior Assessment System for Children, in children with CAE to healthy controls (Vega *et al.*, 2011). A greater proportion of children with CAE had scores in the clinically significant range on both the Anxiety (11% *vs.*2%) and Depression (24% *vs.* 2%) subscales. Neither disease duration, medical intractability nor medication effects predicted higher risk of affective problems.

Similarly, psychiatric disorders also appear common in JME. In 48 patients followed for a mean of 20 years, Baykan *et al.*, noted psychiatric disorders in 31% (Baykan *et al.*, 2008). Depression was the most common diagnosis, in 21% of patients, while 4% each had been diagnosed with either anxiety or psychosis. Psychiatric disorders were most common amongst the pharmacoresistant group.

Social outcomes

Childhood/juvenile absence epilepsy

Social outcome is of concern in typical absence epilepsy, particularly in those without remission of their seizures. In a population-based study comparing long-term psychosocial outcome in young adults who were diagnosed with either CAE/JAE or juvenile rheumatoid arthritis in childhood, Wirrell *et al.* found poorer outcomes in the epilepsy cohort (Wirrell *et al.*, 1997). The mean age at follow-up was 23 years, and significantly more patients with absence epilepsy than juvenile rheumatoid arthritis were in terminal remission (57% *vs.* 28%). Patients with absence epilepsy had greater difficulties in school than those with arthritis. They were more likely to require special educational help ($p < 0.02$), to have below average academic performance ($p < 0.01$) and to repeat a grade ($p < 0.005$). They were also less likely to have graduated from high school ($p < 0.005$) or to have attended college ($p < 0.001$). Regarding behavior, they were more likely to have been labeled as having behavioral problems ($p < 0.001$) and were more likely to report a history of heavy alcohol use ($p < 0.006$). Thirty four percent of women with a history of CAE/JAE had experienced an unplanned pregnancy outside of a stable relationship compared to only 3% of those with arthritis ($p < 0.001$). Difficulties in interpersonal relationships were also more common in absence epilepsy, including poor relationships with siblings ($p < 0.03$) and fewer social outings with friends ($p < 0.04$). Persons with absence epilepsy had lower rates of full time employment ($p < 0.01$), job satisfaction ($p < 0.04$) and were more likely to be working in unskilled labor, as opposed to upper management or professional positions ($p < 0.002$). Most epilepsy-related variables showed no correlation with outcome, however those with cognitive difficulties and those without remission of epilepsy had more concerning psychosocial difficulties.

In a study of 58 young adults with persisting absences, Olsson *et al.*, found greater degrees of social isolation and greater sleep-related problems (Olsson & Campenhausen, 1993). While most subjects were well adjusted regarding family status and employment, they were more likely to be doing manual work and to be overqualified for their jobs.

Juvenile myoclonic epilepsy

While the long-term social outcome of JME has not been well-studied, it has been reported that patients with this disorder are impulsive, irresponsible and immature and, as a result, seizure control may be poor (Janz, 1989). Camfield and Camfield followed a small, population-based cohort of young adults with JME to a mean age of 36 years (Camfield & Camfield, 2009). While educational achievement was favorable, with 87% graduating from high school, and 70% pursuing further education, only 69% were currently employed with enough income to be self-sufficient. One third had previous been suspended from school, and 13% had been previously arrested for a criminal offense, although only 4% were convicted. Eighty percent of pregnancies in the cohort were unplanned and occurred outside of a stable relationship. No significant relationship was found between social outcome and seizure outcome.

■ What are the underlying mechanisms of these comorbidities?

The exact cause(s) of psychosocial and intellectual disability in the idiopathic generalized epilepsies is not clear, however it is likely that several factors play a role including the underlying neurobiologic mechanism leading to the epilepsy, ongoing seizures or frequent epileptiform discharges, antiepileptic medication side effects and stigma of epilepsy.

The idiopathic generalized epilepsies have a predominant genetic etiology with current data suggesting a complex model of inheritance with the interaction of several genes (Berkovic & Scheffer, 2001). The genes identified to date have predominantly affected voltage or ligand-gated ion channels (Helbig et al., 2008). It is possible that ion channelopathies may also predispose to comorbidities.

Studies in rodent models of idiopathic generalized epilepsy suggest that shared neurobiological processes are important, and that effective treatment of seizures or reduction of spike-wave discharges do not necessarily prevent comorbidities. In the WAG/Rij rat absence model, treatment with ethosuximide, levetiracetam and zonisamide reduced spike-wave discharges, but was not linked to a reduced onset of depressive characteristics, as assessed by a forced swimming test (Russo et al., 2011). In another study, Genetic Absence Epilepsy Rats from Strasbourg (GAERS), a model of human absence epilepsy, were compared to non-epileptic control rats. The GAERS strain showed significantly greater levels of both depression and anxiety-like behaviors which both preceded and followed onset of epilepsy (Jones et al., 2008). The fact that these disorders exist before epilepsy onset suggest the comorbidities are related to a common neurobiologic mechanism and are not simply the result of ongoing seizures or medication effects. Similar work in children with new-onset seizures has shown higher rates of behavior problems in the six months preceding the first recognized seizure (Austin et al., 2001).

Neuroimaging studies have documented structural changes in the idiopathic generalized epilepsies that are present early on and which are independent of seizure variables. Caplan et al. (2009) showed significantly smaller gray matter volumes of the left orbitofrontal gyrus and both temporal lobes in children with CAE compared to nonepileptic controls. These regions are important in behavior, cognition and language function. Pulsipher et al. (2011) also showed increased thalamic volume loss and reduced frontal white matter expansion over time in children with new onset idiopathic generalized epilepsy compared to controls. Such alterations in thalamofrontal development may have impact on cognitive function. These same investigators documented that thalamic and frontal abnormalities were related to executive dysfunction in new onset JME (Pulsipher et al., 2009). One study using surface-based morphometry found that children with CAE failed to demonstrate the normal regional age-related decrease in cortical thickness and increase in sulcal depth, suggesting a possible disturbance in pruning (Tosun et al., 2011). These measurements were independent of seizure variables, suggesting they are fixed and unrelated to seizures. Additionally, while children with CAE had both verbal and performance IQs in the normal range, they used different brain regions to perform these cognitive tasks compared to healthy controls. This finding may suggest reorganization of brain development due to neuropathological changes underlying CAE.

In summary, these imaging studies suggest that there are inherent neuropathological changes in the idiopathic generalized epilepsies which are not the result of recurrent seizures. Such abnormalities may result in altered synaptic pruning and brain reorganization, which may impact cognitive, language and behavioral function.

There is also evidence that frequent seizures, and probably very frequent interictal discharges may increase the risk of comorbidity. Distinguishing interictal generalized spike-wave from ictal discharge can be difficult, unless clear behavioral change is documented. However, during exceedingly brief discharge, accurate testing is challenging. Clinicians have suggested that generalized spike-wave discharges lasting longer than two (Sadleir et al., 2009) or three (Holmes et al., 1987) seconds should be considered ictal, rather than interictal, as careful testing suggests alterations in awareness after discharge persists for this duration. However, there is evidence that altered awareness may occur with even briefer discharges, raising the question as to whether these are truly "interictal". In an older study from 1973, the reaction time of patients with absence epilepsy was assessed when stimuli were delivered both at baseline and during generalized discharges (Porter & Penry, 1973). Over half (56%) of reaction times were abnormal when the stimulus was delivered at onset of the generalized paroxysm, and when delivered later in the paroxysm, 81% were abnormal. The term "transitory cognitive impairment" has been defined as "a momentary cognitive deficit during subclinical discharge" (Aarts et al., 1984), and is more common with generalized than focal discharges.

Uncontrolled absence seizures have a negative impact on academic function. Eleven children with newly diagnosed absence epilepsy underwent neuropsychological evaluation during video-EEG monitoring prior to antiepileptic drug treatment (Siren et al., 2007). Both duration of generalized 3 Hz spike-wave discharges and clinical absence seizures correlated significantly with poorer performance on the visual memory task ($p = 0.04$ and $p = 0.02$). Children were then re-evaluated after 10 months of antiepileptic drug therapy, at which point 10/11 were clinically seizure-free and 7/11 had a completely normal video-EEG study. Significant improvements in attention, motor fluency and visual memory were seen, although verbal and performance IQ did not significantly change.

A recent study comparing the cognitive effects of interictal EEG discharges and short nonconvulsive epileptic seizures has shown that frequent interictal discharge (> 1% of the time) has a similar effect to seizures, however it is less pronounced (Nicolai, et al., 2012). Neuropsychological evaluation was performed in 188 children with epilepsy (15% with idiopathic generalized epilepsy) and 41 healthy controls. All children with epilepsy underwent 2 hour EEGs, all of which showed epileptiform discharges +/- subtle seizures. In the epilepsy cohort, the Weschler Intelligence Scale for Children was performed prior to the EEG, but other testing including language and visual-spatial function, attention, speed of central information processing, educational achievement in reading and arithmetic and memory including word and figure recognition were done during EEG monitoring. The epilepsy cohort was divided into those showing subtle seizures on the video-EEG (N = 60) or those with interictal epileptiform discharges alone (N = 128). The group with subtle seizures scored significantly lower on 8/12 tests administered. On block design and reading they scored significantly lower than healthy controls only, but on full scale IQ, auditory reaction time, speed of central information processing, word and figure recognition and block tapping (memory span), they scored significantly lower than both controls and those with interictal discharge alone. Those with only interictal discharge scored significantly lower than controls on 3/12 tests including full scale IQ, figure recognition and reading. To evaluate the impact of interictal discharge frequency, the interictal group was subdivided into two groups, based on whether the interictal epileptiform discharges were present for < 1% or > 1% of the recording. Those with frequent (> 1%) discharges scored significantly lower than the infrequent (< 1%) group on full scale IQ, block design, auditory reaction time, speed of central information processing, block tapping (memory span) and reading. Based on these results, ongoing seizures appear to carry the greatest risk of cognitive concerns, however frequent epileptiform discharges may also have a cost. However, it remains to be proven whether the association between neuropsychological dysfunction and discharges is the result of more severe epilepsy or if the neuropsychological deficits are indeed the result of transitory cognitive impairment due to the epileptiform discharge.

■ Should we treat the patient, the EEG, or both?

The potential negative impact of interictal discharges on cognition raises the question as to whether one should treat these as well as clinical seizures (Binnie, 2003). However, antiepileptic medications may also result in cognitive side effects, with the actual risks dependent on choice of medication and dose. In childhood absence epilepsy, both ethosuximide and valproate have equal efficacy, however the latter is associated with greater attentional dysfunction (Glauser et al., 2010).

Only a small number of studies have evaluated whether treatment of interictal discharges improves neuropsychological functioning. Pressler et al. studied 61 children with mild or well-controlled epilepsy who were randomized to receive either a 13-week trial of lamotrigine followed by a 13-week trial of placebo, or vice versa (Pressler et al., 2005). Interictal epileptiform discharge frequency was assessed by 12-24 hour ambulatory EEG. Behavior was assessed by the parent and teacher Connors Rating scales at baseline, and at the end of each 13-week trial of lamotrigine or placebo. While a significant improvement in behavior was noted in subjects who showed reduction of discharges during the lamotrigine phase, this finding was only seen in the subgroup with focal epilepsy, not generalized epilepsy. Ronen et al. treated 8 children with frequent epileptiform discharge and learning and behavior problems, but without clinical seizures with valproate (Ronen et al., 2000). None of the children showed improvement with valproate therapy, however only half had improvement in their EEG. In a study of 10 patients with frequent interictal discharge (discharges occurring at least every 5 minutes but less than every 10 seconds) treated in a randomized, double-blind, placebo-controlled crossover study with either valproate or clobazam to reduce interictal discharge, Marston et al. found that 80% showed improved global psychosocial function on active drug than placebo, and all responders showed reduction in interictal discharges (Marston et al., 1993). While these results are encouraging, they are confounded by the fact that most patients also had fewer seizures during the active phase. Furthermore, the investigators were unable to document transitory cognitive impairment on a non-verbal memory test in this cohort.

While further research into the impact of brief interictal discharge on cognitive function, particularly in idiopathic generalized epilepsy is needed, the current evidence does not support treating such discharge. Antiepileptic drug treatment of children with idiopathic generalized epilepsy should be aimed at stopping clinical seizures. It is reasonable to repeat the EEG after clinical seizures abate. If generalized spike-wave discharges lasting longer than 2-3 seconds persist or discharges are exceedingly frequent, consideration should be given to adjusting treatment, given that discharges of this duration have been shown to alter response times. Briefer discharges should be treated only if there is evidence during the EEG of impaired cognition during these on careful response testing. If hyperventilation triggers an absence seizure or generalized spike wave discharge longer than 2-3 seconds, medications should also be adjusted (Camfield & Camfield, 2005), although there is little clinical evidence for this practice. Similarly, there is little evidence to guide decisions in a treated patient with JME who shows photosensitive spike-wave discharge on EEG, but is otherwise seizure-free.

EEG is often used to guide decisions regarding weaning of antiepileptic medication, particularly in those patients with self-limited electroclinical syndromes such as CAE, although this practice as not been well studied. It is generally accepted that persisting discharges on EEG reflect a higher risk of recurrent seizures, particularly if antiepileptic drugs are weaned.

■ Concluding remarks

The idiopathic generalized epilepsies comprise a group of well-defined electroclinical syndromes with presumed genetic inheritance. An accurate syndromic diagnosis is essential to define the natural history. Despite frequent pharmacoresponsiveness and achievement of seizure control, intellectual and psychosocial comorbidity is often present and has significant impact on quality of life. Ongoing management of patients with idiopathic generalized epilepsy must address these comorbidities as well as seizure control. The etiology of these comorbidities is not well understood although neuroimaging studies show structural changes in brain regions which may impact on cognitive, language and behavior function, namely frontal, temporal and thalamic regions. However, with the exception of learning disorder and lack of seizure control, epilepsy-related factors are not predictive of these comorbidities. The EEG is often used to guide therapeutic decision-making. While generalized spike-wave bursts lasting longer than 2-3 seconds are correlated with altered awareness, the impact of briefer discharges, particularly if very frequent is less clear and needs further study.

References

- Aarts JH, Binnie CD, Smit AM, Wilkins AJ. Selective cognitive impairment during focal and generalized epileptiform EEG activity. *Brain* 1984; 107 (Pt 1): 293-308.
- Austin JK, Harezlak J, Dunn DW, Huster GA, Rose DF, Ambrosius WT. Behavior problems in children before first recognized seizures. *Pediatrics* 2001; 107: 115-22.
- Bartolomei F, Roger J, Bureau M, Genton P, Dravet C, Viallat D, Gastaut JL. Prognostic factors for childhood and juvenile absence epilepsies. *European Neurology* 1997; 37: 169-75.
- Baykan B, Altindag EA, Bebek N, *et al*. Myoclonic seizures subside in the fourth decade in juvenile myoclonic epilepsy. *Neurology* 2008; 70: 2123-9.
- Berkovic SF, Scheffer IE. Genetics of the epilepsies. *Epilepsia* 2001; 42 (Suppl 5): 16-23.
- Binnie CD. Cognitive impairment during epileptiform discharges: is it ever justifiable to treat the EEG? *Lancet Neurol* 2003; 2: 725-30.

- Bureau M, Tassinari CA. Epilepsy with myoclonic absences. *Brain Dev* 2005; 27: 178-84.
- Callenbach PM, Bouma PA, Geerts AT, et al. Long-term outcome of childhood absence epilepsy: Dutch Study of Epilepsy in Childhood. *Epilepsy Res* 2009; 83: 249-56.
- Camfield C, Camfield P. Management guidelines for children with idiopathic generalized epilepsy. *Epilepsia* 2005; 46 (Suppl 9): 112-6.
- Camfield CS, Camfield PR. Long-term social outcomes for children with epilepsy. *Epilepsia* 2007; 48 (Suppl 9): 3-5.
- Camfield CS, Camfield PR. Juvenile myoclonic epilepsy 25 years after seizure onset: a population-based study. *Neurology* 2009; 73: 1041-5.
- Camfield CS, Camfield PR, Gordon K, Wirrell E, Dooley JM. Incidence of epilepsy in childhood and adolescence: a population-based study in Nova Scotia from 1977 to 1985. *Epilepsia* 1996; 37: 19-23.
- Camfield P, Camfield C. Idiopathic generalized epilepsy with generalized tonic-clonic seizures (IGE-GTC): a population-based cohort with > 20 year follow up fors medical and social outcome. *Epilepsy Behav* 2010; 18: 61-3.
- Caplan R, Siddarth P, Gurbani S, Hanson R, Sankar R, Shields WD. Depression and anxiety disorders in pediatric epilepsy. *Epilepsia* 2005; 46: 720-30.
- Caplan R, Siddarth P, Stahl L, et al. Childhood absence epilepsy: behavioral, cognitive, and linguistic comorbidities. *Epilepsia* 2008; 49: 1838-46.
- Caplan R, Levitt J, Siddarth P, et al. Frontal and temporal volumes in childhood absence epilepsy. *Epilepsia* 2009; 50: 2466-72.
- Chaix Y, Daquin G, Monteiro F, Villeneuve N, Laguitton V, Genton P. Absence epilepsy with onset before age three years: a heterogeneous and often severe condition. *Epilepsia* 2003; 44: 944-9.
- Dravet C, Bureau M, Genton P. Benign myoclonic epilepsy of infancy: electroclinical symptomatology and differential diagnosis from the other types of generalized epilepsy of infancy. *Epilepsy Res* 1992 (Suppl 6): 131-5.
- Geithner J, Schneider F, Wang Z, et al. Predictors for long-term seizure outcome in juvenile myoclonic epilepsy: 25-63 years of follow-up. *Epilepsia* 2012; 53; 1379-86.
- Glauser TA, Cnaan A, Shinnar S, et al.; Childhood Absence Epilepsy Study Group. Ethosuximide, valproic acid and lamotrigine in childhood absence epilepsy. *N Engl J Med* 2010; 362: 790-9.
- Giordano L, Vignoli A, Accorsi P, et al. A clinical and genetic study of 33 new cases with early-onset absence epilepsy. *Epilepsy Res* 2011; 95: 221-6.
- Grosso S, Galimberti D, Vezzosi P, et al. Childhood absence epilepsy: evolution and prognostic factors. *Epilepsia* 2005; 46: 1796-801.
- Helbig I, Scheffer IE, Mulley JC, Berkovic SF. Navigating the channels and beyond: unravelling the genetics of the epilepsies. *Lancet Neurol* 2008; 7: 231-45.
- Holmes GL, McKeever M, Adamson M. Absence seizures in children: clinical and electroencephalographic features. *Ann Neurol* 1987; 21: 268-73.
- Janz D. Juvenile myoclonic epilepsy. Epilepsy with impulsive petit mal. *Cleve Clin J Med* 1989; 56 (Suppl) Pt 1: S23-33; discussion S40-22.
- Jones NC, Salzberg MR, Kumar G, Couper A, Morris MJ, O'Brien TJ. Elevated anxiety and depressive-like behavior in a rat model of genetic generalized epilepsy suggesting common causation. *Experimental Neurology* 2008; 209: 254-60.
- Loiseau P, Duche B, Pedespan JM. Absence epilepsies. *Epilepsia* 1995; 36: 1182-6.
- Marston D, Besag F, Binnie CD, Fowler M. Effects of transitory cognitive impairment on psychosocial functioning of children with epilepsy: a therapeutic trial. *Dev Med Child Neurol* 1993; 35: 574-81.

- Nicolai J, Ebus S, Biemans DP, et al. The cognitive effects of interictal epileptiform EEG discharges and short nonconvulsive epileptic seizures. *Epilepsia* 2012; 53: 1051-9.
- Obeid T. Clinical and genetic aspects of juvenile absence epilepsy. *J Neurol* 1994; 241: 487-91.
- Olsson I, Campenhausen G. Social adjustment in young adults with absence epilepsies. *Epilepsia* 1993; 34: 846-51.
- Panayiotopoulos CP, Koutroumanidis M, Giannakodimos S, Agathonikou A. Idiopathic generalised epilepsy in adults manifested by phantom absences, generalised tonic-clonic seizures, and frequent absence status. *J Neurol Neurosurg Psychiatry* 1997; 63: 622-7.
- Porter RJ, Penry JK. Responsiveness at the onset of spike-wave bursts. *Electroenceph Clin Neurophys* 1973; 34: 239-45.
- Pressler RM, Robinson RO, Wilson GA, Binnie CD. Treatment of interictal epileptiform discharges can improve behavior in children with behavioral problems and epilepsy. *J Pediatr* 2005; 146: 112-7.
- Pulsipher DT, Seidenberg M, Guidotti L, et al. Thalamofrontal circuitry and executive dysfunction in recent onset juvenile myoclonic epilepsy. *Epilepsia* 2009; 50: 1210-9.
- Pulsipher DT, Dabbs K, Tuchscherer V, et al. Thalamofrontal neurodevelopment in new-onset pediatric idiopathic generalized epilepsy. *Neurology* 2011; 76: 28-33.
- Ronen GM, Richards JE, Cunningham C, Secord M, Rosenbloom D. Can sodium valproate improve learning in children with epileptiform bursts but without clinical seizures? *Dev Med Child Neurol* 2000; 42: 751-5.
- Rubboli G, Gardella E, Capovilla G. Idiopathic generalized epilepsy (IGE) syndromes in development: IGE with absences of early childhood, IGE with phantom absences, and perioral myoclonia with absences. *Epilepsia* 2009; 50 (Suppl 5): 24-8.
- Russo E, Citraro R, Scicchitano F, et al. Effects of early long-term treatment with antiepileptic drugs on development of seizures and depressive-like behavior in a rat genetic absence epilepsy model. *Epilepsia* 2011; 52: 1341-50.
- Sadleir LG, Scheffer IE, Smith S, Carstensen B, Farrell K, Connolly MB. EEG features of absence seizures in idiopathic generalized epilepsy: impact of syndrome, age, and state. *Epilepsia* 2009; 50: 1572-8.
- Siren A, Kylliainen A, Tenhunen M, Hirvonen K, Riita T, Koivikko M. Beneficial effects of antiepileptic medication on absence seizures and cognitive functioning in children. *Epilepsy Behav* 2007; 11: 85-91.
- Striano S, Capovilla G, Sofia V, et al. Eyelid myoclonia with absences (Jeavons syndrome): a well-defined idiopathic generalized epilepsy syndrome or a spectrum of photosensitive conditions? *Epilepsia* 2009; 50 (Suppl 5): 15-9.
- Suls A, Mullen SA, Weber YG, et al. Early-onset absence epilepsy caused by mutations in the glucose transporter GLUT1. *Ann Neurol* 2009; 66: 415-9.
- Tosun D, Siddarth P, Toga AW, Hermann B, Caplan R. Effects of childhood absence epilepsy on associations between regional cortical morphometry and aging and cognitive abilities. *Hum Brain Mapp* 2011; 32: 580-91.
- Trinka E, Baumgartner S, Unterberger I, et al. Long-term prognosis for childhood and juvenile absence epilepsy. *J Neurol* 2004; 251: 1235-41.
- Trivisano M, Specchio N, Cappelletti S, et al. Myoclonic astatic epilepsy: an age-dependent epileptic syndrome with favorable seizure outcome but variable cognitive evolution. *Epilepsy Res* 2011; 97: 133-41.
- Vega C, Guo J, Killory B, et al. Symptoms of anxiety and depression in childhood absence epilepsy. *Epilepsia* 2011; 52: e70-4.
- Vega C, Vestal M, DeSalvo M, et al. Differentiation of attention-related problems in childhood absence epilepsy. *Epilepsy Behav* 2010; 19: 82-5.

- Wirrell EC, Camfield CS, Camfield PR, Dooley JM, Gordon KE, Smith B. Long-term psychosocial outcome in typical absence epilepsy. Sometimes a wolf in sheeps' clothing. *Arch Ped Adolesc Med* 1997; 151: 152-8.
- Wirrell EC, Camfield CS, Camfield PR, Gordon KE, Dooley JM. Long-term prognosis of typical childhood absence epilepsy: remission or progression to juvenile myoclonic epilepsy. *Neurology* 1996; 47: 912-8.
- Wirrell EC, Grossardt BR, Wong-Kisiel LC, Nickels KC. Incidence and classification of new-onset epilepsy and epilepsy syndromes in children in Olmsted County, Minnesota from 1980 to 2004: a population-based study. *Epilepsy Res* 2011; 95: 110-8.

Refractory childhood epilepsy: comparing the outcome of medical *versus* surgical treatment

Michael Duchowny

Department of Neurology and Brain Institute, Miami Children's Hospital; Department of Neurology, University of Miami Leonard Miller School of Medicine, Miami, Florida, USA

An impressive array of novel antiepileptic drugs (AEDS) are now used to treat a wide range of epileptic disorders in children including both new-onset and chronic epilepsy. Newer pharmacological agents offer superior efficacy and more beneficial adverse effect profiles but advances in the pediatric surgical therapy for refractory seizures offer the tantalizing possibility of immediate seizure relief. Such an absolute reversal is all the more remarkable as decisive treatment for any chronic and medically intractable neurological symptoms is often elusive.

In recognition of the particular benefits of surgery for children with medically resistant seizures, the ILAE Subcommission for Paediatric Epilepsy Surgery and the Commission of Neurosurgery and Paediatrics issued recommended guidelines for pediatric epilepsy surgery in 2006 (Cross et al., 2006). This consensus summary included a rationale for surgical services, a description of appropriate facilities and a list of childhood-onset disorders amenable to surgical intervention. Outcome assessment included several important postoperative parameters, but the expert panel did not address the need for randomized controlled trials (RCTs) to compare surgical and medical management. Such an omission is understandable as outcomes research, particularly randomized comparative clinical trials comparing surgical and medical treatment, presents many formidable obstacles. The vulnerability of the immature brain to recurrent seizures (Thibeault-Eybalin et al., 2009) and the heterogeneity in clinical presentation of childhood epilepsy are significant obstacles to randomizing subjects or extrapolating the results of outcome analysis for different ages or between disorders. Furthermore, the known poor prognoses of many pediatric epilepsy syndromes argue strongly against undue delay in surgical referral. This latter issue is especially critical in patients with epileptic encephalopathy for whom a delay in definitive treatment is associated with a known potential for permanent brain damage (Shields, 2000).

Despite these challenges, comparisons of medical and surgical treatments for refractory childhood epilepsy have much to offer. Assessing the risks and benefits of each treatment arm can assist clinical decision-making in this difficult patient group and reassure families on an appropriate course of action. RCTs are the gold standard but clinical cohort and cross-sectional cohort studies can provide indirect but important supportive evidence; long-term studies will ultimately be required for a definitive understanding. Given the wealth of evidence that seizure-freedom can be achieved in a significant proportion of selected pediatric epilepsy surgical candidates, Class 1 evidence no longer seems mandatory for continued utilization of surgical intervention.

In this review studies that directly compare or have implications for the medical and surgical management of refractory childhood epilepsy will be presented. Five domains will be examined – seizure control, cognition, quality of life, mortality and economic burden.

■ Seizure control

Evidence supporting the superiority of excisional surgery over medical therapy in chronic epilepsy is largely derived from adult studies. Yet despite numerous studies attesting to the ability of excisional procedures to alleviate or significantly reduce the number of seizures in medically refractory patients, only one RCT has compared the benefits of each treatment arm (Wiebe et al., 2001). This study was made ethically possible by a 1-year waiting list for patients approved for surgical therapy. Of 80 adults with refractory temporal lobe epilepsy selected as surgical candidates, the cumulative percentage of seizure-freedom in the surgical arm at one year was 58% compared to only 8% in the medical arm. Four patients in the surgical group (standard anterior temporal lobectomy) experienced adverse surgical consequences and one patient in the medical group died.

No similar comparison has been undertaken in either adults or children but a recent systematic review and meta-analysis of uncontrolled cohort studies examining the rates of seizure-freedom in medically and surgically treated adult patients yielded confirmatory results (Schmidt & Stavem, 2009). Of 2,734 patients with drug-resistant seizures who underwent predominantly temporal lobe surgery, 719/1,621 (44%) became seizure-free compared to 139/1,113 in the non-operated group. The pooled risk difference of 42% supports the findings of the Wiebe et al. (2001) study and confirms that in appropriately selected patients, surgical treatment is four times more likely to achieve seizure-freedom compared to medical treatment alone. Importantly, the investigators also noted in their outcome analyses that 12% of medical patients who did not undergo surgical intervention also became seizure-free.

The tendency of refractory epilepsy to spontaneously remit or fluctuate has been recognized for many years (Neligan et al., 2011) and suggests that uncontrolled surgical outcome studies may not always provide a true or complete picture. For example, the introduction of a new AED resulted in seizure-freedom for one year or more in 16% of patients with refractory epilepsy and additional worthwhile improvement in 37% (Luciano & Shorvon, 2007). Remarkably, in a small cohort study, 10% of patients who failed to respond to six AEDs became seizure-free with the introduction of a seventh agent (Callaghan et al., 2007). A similar experience was observed in children being evaluated for epilepsy surgery (Gilman et al., 1994). In an uncontrolled observational study, 2 of 21 children referred for surgical therapy became seizure-free or significantly improved after adjusting their medication to achieve maximally tolerated serum levels.

Although the evidence suggests that some patients with refractory epilepsy who are likely to be referred for surgical therapy may become AED treatment-responsive, few studies identify specific patient or treatment-related factors predicting responsivity. Rather, most studies evaluate risk factors that predict initial treatment-resistance and its early identification (Berg et al., 2001; Camfield et al., 1997; Chawla et al., 2002; Kwan & Brodie, 2000; Ohtsuka et al., 2001; Chen et al., 2002). In a recent community-based prospective cohort study of 613 children with non-syndromic epilepsy that began between 1 month and 16 years of age of whom 294 were followed for at least 10 years, Berg et al. (2011) found that 58% achieved complete remission. However, relapses were still possible up to 7.5 years after complete remission.

There is a clear need for additional controlled trials comparing medical and surgical therapy for refractory childhood seizures. A formal prospective RCT such as the Wiebe et al. study (2001) seems unlikely to be performed but more careful attention to pediatric patients deemed surgical candidates but who decline surgery may be more feasible.

■ Cognition

The ability of seizure control to afford significant improvement in cognition may appear axiomatic. However, this issue is complicated by conflicting long-term data and the potential of both medical and surgical therapy to produce undesirable and in some instances unforeseen adverse consequences. For example, medically-induced seizure-freedom based on very high serum AED concentrations could cause serious declines in cognitive function. Alternatively, postoperative seizure freedom could potentially be complicated by anatomic disruption in neural circuits for information processing.

There is a substantial body of evidence showing that uncontrolled adult epilepsy is associated with cognitive decline. In 147 adult patients with newly-diagnosed epilepsy who were compared to healthy volunteers, a decline in intellectual performance was evident one year after diagnosis (Baker et al., 2011). Memory, psychomotor speed and executive function were particularly vulnerable. However studies in children are less clear. The presence of neurobehavioral comorbidities at time of seizure onset is a major predictor of later cognitive impairment (Hermann et al., 2008), and longer-term follow-up of children with newly-diagnosed seizures reveal no change in overall group cognitive or behavioral function but rather instability in individual performance (Oostrom et al., 2005). The investigators in this long-term study concluded that a child's pre-existing cognitive and behavioral profile and parental ability were the main determinants of outcome rather than intrinsic epilepsy-related variables. While the population reported by Oostrom et al. (2005) was MRI-negative (n = 42), their etiologies were either idiopathic (n = 23) or cryptogenic (n = 19). While children in the idiopathic subgroup are unlikely to be surgical candidates, many surgical candidates are cryptogenic and MRI-negative and ultimately found to harbor microscopic dysplastic tissue (Krsek et al., 2008).

In the only comparative cohort analysis of adults with temporal lobe epilepsy followed over 2-10 years, Helmstaedter et al. (2003) found that 50% of medically treated patients and 60% of surgically treated patients evidenced memory decline. The outcome of surgically-treated patients sorted into two sub-populations- memory decline was arrested in surgical patients who obtained seizure control, but unsuccessful surgery, particularly left-sided procedures, appeared to accelerate the memory decline. Thus, rather than being a panacea, temporal lobectomy was a "double-or-nothing" proposition with the potential for harm as well as good.

Despite the inherent complexity of longitudinal studies of cognition in patients with epilepsy, there is mounting evidence that specific subpopulations may be particularly vulnerable to cognitive decline. Chronic temporal lobe epilepsy, especially in surgical candidates constitutes an especially high-risk situation. Longer duration of temporal lobe epilepsy is associated with greater decreases in cognition and is the single most important individual variable predicting decline (Jokeit & Ebner, 2002). Cognitive deficiency, particularly memory and language deficits are established in childhood and subsequently stabilize over the adult lifespan (Baxendale et al., 2010). Prenatal and early acquired dominant temporal lobe lesions demonstrate a particular propensity to disrupt both receptive and expressive language networks compared to similarly-acquired lesions of the dominant frontal lobe (Korman et al., 2010).

Prospective neuroimaging data lend further support to the neuropsychological findings in patients with chronic temporal lobe epilepsy. Hippocampal, amygdala and entorhinal cortex volume loss, cortical thinning and white matter disruptions are associated with a higher seizure frequency and longer duration of epilepsy (Bernasconi et al., 2005; Coan et al., 2009; Kemmotsu et al., 2011), and are more prominent in patients with left-sided seizure onset. In children, chronic temporal lobe epilepsy is associated with reduced brain tissue volume particularly white matter volume-reduction which correlates with reduced cognitive status (Hermann et al., 2002). Reductions in cerebral volumes may also extend to extra-temporal structures.

A comparative cohort study comparing the cognitive outcomes of temporal lobe resection *versus* medical therapy in adults found a more favorable long -term intellectual outcome in surgical patients (Skirrow et al., 2011). However, increases in intelligence were only associated with freedom from seizures and AEDs. Similar findings are described for children with extra-temporal epilepsy (Freitag & Tuxhorn, 2005).

Patients with early seizure onset constitute another vulnerable subpopulation. In a community based cohort study of cognitive outcome in 198 children under age 8 years with new-onset seizures, Berg et al. (2012) found that while as expected, long-term uncontrolled seizures adversely affected cognition, the greatest declines occurred in infancy. Seizure-induced encephalopathy during the formative stages of brain maturation was especially concerning and constituted an important rationale for early surgical intervention with radical procedures if necessary.

In a follow-up cohort study of 58 patients undergoing hemispherectomy for early-onset refractory partial seizures, no child deteriorated and most achieved modest improvement in neurodevelopmental status (Jonas et al., 2004). Improvement correlated with the cessation of seizure activity, shorter preoperative seizure duration and higher preoperative developmental level but not pathological substrate. Stabilization of cognitive decline after hemispherectomy was also observed in a cohort of children operated under age 5 years (Lettori et al., 2008).

In summary, the evidence from limited controlled trials and uncontrolled studies indicates that successful (and only successful) epilepsy surgery has the potential to improve cognitive function or arrest its decline. At the same time, it should be recognized that children with newly diagnosed epilepsy do not always deteriorate and may be influenced by factors unrelated to their intrinsic epilepsy. This group therefore may not require definitive intervention. Furthermore, it is important to bear in mind that unsuccessful surgery is not without risk for further deterioration that might not have otherwise occurred.

■ Quality of life

The high incidence of co-morbid disorders and social stigmatization in patients with chronic epilepsy add a problematic overlay to the fundamental medical problem of epileptic seizures, and the onset of epilepsy in the school-age population is especially likely to negatively impact psychosocial outcome (Shackleton et al., 2003). In a population-based prospective long-term follow-up study of adults with childhood-onset epilepsy, chronic epilepsy rather than AED treatment was shown to be responsible for the increased incidence of concurrent problems including social adjustment and competence issues (Jalava & Sillanpaa, 1996; Jalava et al., 1997). Although diminished quality of life (QOL) is also possible in seizure-free patients on medication, subjects in remission and off medication experience rates of employment and socioeconomic status similar to controls (Sillanpaa et al., 2004).

Cohort studies of adults undergoing epilepsy surgery indicate that successful outcome has a beneficial effect on QOL. In a systematic multi-center review of evidence-based determinants of QOL in adults after epilepsy surgery, Abdel-Hamid et al. (2011) found that 29/32 studies reported a significantly favorable outcome, particularly in the physical, psychological and overall QOL domains. Seizure freedom was highly predictive of positive results but the presence of an aura did not detract from overall gains suggesting that "disabling" seizures were the major determinant. A prospective multi-center study of 396 patients confirmed these findings and further noted that improvement in seizure-free patients was most likely to occur during the first two post-operative years whether or not medication was taken (Spencer et al., 2007).

Similar improvements in QOL are noted for children rendered seizure-free after epilepsy surgery (Sabaz et al., 2006). Gains are reported in overall QOL as well as subscales assessing cognitive, social, emotional, behavioral and physical wellbeing. Children rendered seizure-free also achieve a reduction in the number of postoperative AEDs. A controlled cohort study of QOL in pediatric epilepsy surgery patients compared to matched non-surgical intractable patients and healthy subjects confirmed the superiority of surgical therapy in patients rendered seizure-free (Mikati et al., 2010).

Improvement in QOL is also reported for children undergoing more radical procedures such as hemispherectomy (Griffiths et al., 2007). Children rendered seizure-free after hemispherectomy perceive themselves as more socially competent and having greater self-worth. Remarkably, seizure-free adolescents evidence improved athletic competence and emotional attachment at 2 years postop (van Empelen et al., 2005).

Becoming seizure-free appears pivotal to gains in QOL after surgery. Conversely, postoperative seizure persistence does not confer significant benefit over and above conservative medical management. Seizure persistence in conjunction with postoperative deficits may even worsen quality of life after temporal lobe resection (Langfitt et al., 2007). Diminished QOL has been noted in a sub-group (8%) of patients with persistent seizures and concomitant memory decline. While these individuals represent a small proportion of the overall surgical series, they nevertheless serve as a reminder that improvement or even stability in QOL after epilepsy surgery is not guaranteed.

■ Mortality

Statistical modeling of health-related quality of life data derived from patient data and the medical literature revealed that a prototypical 35 year old medically treated patient with chronic epilepsy has an average life expectancy of 27.3 years compared to an average 44.3 year life expectancy in the general population (Choi et al., 2008). This model also found that anterior temporal resection increased the number of seizure-free years by 15 and reduced the absolute lifetime risk of dying from seizure-related causes by 15%.

An adult cohort study comparing premature mortality in surgical patients and patients assessed for surgery but found to be non-surgical revealed that non-operated patients were 2.4 times more likely to die, and 4.5 times as likely to die a probable epilepsy-related death compared to the surgical cohort (Bell et al., 2010). At one year postop, non-seizure-free patients within the surgical cohort were 4.0 times more likely to die compared to seizure-free patients or patients with simple partial seizures. Mortality rates for postoperative patients rendered seizure-free are indistinguishable from the general population (Sperling et al., 1999). The type of surgical procedure does not influence mortality as long as seizure-freedom is achieved (Sperling et al., 1999). Disturbingly, of the non-seizure-free patients who died, most achieved a substantial reduction in seizure frequency. Mortality during epilepsy surgery is exceedingly rare (Sperling et al., 1999; McClelland et al., 2011).

Similar comparative cohort and modeling data is lacking in childhood epilepsy. However, in a population-based cohort of 245 children with epilepsy followed for 45 years, there were 60 deaths, a rate three times higher than the expected age- and sex-adjusted mortality in the general population (Sillanpaa & Shinnar, 2010). Most of the deaths occurred in adulthood and 48% of patients who died, did not achieve a terminal 5-year remission. Of the 60 deaths, 55% were epilepsy-related including sudden unexplained death in 30%, definite probable seizure in 15% and accidental drowning in 10%.

■ Economic cost

The economics of refractory epilepsy have been assessed in seizure-free and non-seizure-free surgical patients and compared to non-surgical patients. In a multi-center study evaluating the cost of health care two years before and after surgery in adults, total health care expenditures declined 32% at 2 years postop due to decreased AED usage and hospitalization (Langfitt et al., 2007). In comparison, there was no cost savings in patients with seizure persistence whether or not they had undergone surgery.

Two studies examined the cost-effectiveness of pediatric epilepsy surgery. A Canadian study employing a decision analysis model evaluated costs based on literature review and local experience (Keene & Ventureya, 1999). Alternative treatment of chronic childhood epilepsy by AEDs or one-stage surgical resection were calculated based on the aggregate accumulated costs of all services in each cohort, the rates of seizure-freedom after surgery and the projected rates of spontaneous remission in non-surgical patients. The initial costs were found to be initially higher in the surgical population, but equaled the costs of care for medical patients after 14 years and remained lower thereafter.

More recently, Widjaja et al. (2011) used decision analysis to compare the cost-effectiveness of medical *versus* surgical management of children with refractory epilepsy. Surgery had an incremental cost-effectiveness ratio of $36,900 at one year compared to surgically-eligible patients receiving medical therapy, and there was a positive net one-year monetary benefit. Thus, the initial higher costs of surgery were offset by its superior effectiveness at one year. In comparison to the Keene and Ventureya (1999) data, patients undergoing invasive EEG studies were included in the analyses. While these results provide support for the economic benefits of surgical therapy, longer-term data is clearly needed.

Future directions

It is perhaps ironic that one of the least studied aspects of refractory childhood epilepsy is the evidence for deciding on optimal treatment. However, given the collective worldwide experience demonstrating positive benefit from surgically-induced seizure-freedom, class 1 evidence of superiority for surgery over medical therapy may not be necessary. It may be possible to design a clinical trial by comparing patients found to be surgical candidates who then decline operation with matched controls. This group would form a suitable population for a prospective controlled trial. However, due to the heterogeneity of pediatric epilepsy surgical syndromes, subsets of patients would likely be required to compare outcomes more specifically. For some of the less common epileptic disorders associated with refractory seizures, multi-center trials may be the only way to gather sufficient patient numbers.

As the available evidence demonstrates that superiority of surgery over medical therapy occurs only in seizure-free patients, it is not unreasonable to look for ways to both maximize postoperative outcome and compare outcome data at pediatric epilepsy surgical centers worldwide. These issues are politically sensitive and while a full discussion may not be possible, an open dialogue would likely benefit all children with refractory epilepsy.

References

- Abdel-Hamid S, Dhaliwal H, Wiebe S. Determinants of quality of life after epilepsy surgery: systematic review and evidence summary. *Epilepsy Behav* 2011; 21: 441-5.
- Baker GA, Taylor J, Aldenkamp AP. Newly diagnosed epilepsy: cognitive outcome after 12 months. *Epilepsia* 2011; 52: 1084-91.
- Baxendale S, Heaney D, Thompson PJ, Duncan JD. Cognitive consequences of childhood-onset temporal lobe epilepsy across the adult lifespan. *Neurology* 2010; 75: 705-11.
- Bell GS, Sinha S, de Tsi J, *et al*. Premature mortality in refractory partial epilepsy: does surgical treatment make a difference? *J Neurol Neurosurg Psychiatr* 2012; 81: 716-8.
- Berg AT, Shinnar S, Levy SR, Testa FM, Smith-Rapaport S, Beckerman B. Early development of intractable epilepsy in children. A prospective study. *Neurology* 2001; 56: 1445-52.
- Berg AT, Testa FM, Levy SR. Complete remission in non-syndromic childhood-onset epilepsy. *Ann Neurol* 2011; 70: 566-73.
- Berg AT, Zelko FA, Levi SR, Testa FM. Age at onset of epilepsy, pharmacoresistance, and cognitive outcomes. A prospective cohort study. *Neurology* 2012; 79: 1384-91.
- Bernasconi N, Natsume J, Bernasconi A. Progression in temporal lobe epilepsy. Differential atrophy in mesial temporal structures. *Neurology* 2005; 65: 223-8.
- Callaghan B, Anand K, Hauser WA, Hesdorffer D. Likelihood of seizure remission in an adult population with refractory epilepsy. *Ann Neurol* 2007; 62: 382-9.
- Camfield PR, Camfield CS, Gordon K, Dooley JM. If a first antiepileptic drug fails to control a child's epilepsy, what are the chances of success with the next drug? *J Pediatr* 1997; 131: 821-4.

- Chawla S, Aneja S, Kashyap R, Mallika V. Etiology and clinical predictors of intractable epilepsy. *Pediatr Neurol* 2002; 27: 186-91.
- Chen LS, Wang N, Mei-Ing L. Seizure outcome of intractable partial epilepsy in children. *Pediatr Neurol* 2002; 26: 282-7.
- Choi H, Sell RL, Lenert L, Muennig P, Goodman RR, Gilliam FG, Wong JB. Epilepsy surgery for pharmacoresistant temporal lobe epilepsy. A decision analysis. *JAMA* 2008; 300: 2497-505.
- Coan AC, Appenzeller S, Bonilha L, LM, Cendes F. Seizure frequency and lateralization affect progression of atrophy in temporal lobe epilepsy. *Neurology* 2009; 73: 834-42.
- Cross JH, Jayakar P, Nordli D, et al. Proposed criteria for referral and evaluation of children for epilepsy surgery: recommendations of the subcommission for pediatric epilepsy surgery. *Epilepsia* 2006; 47: 952-9.
- Freitag H, Tuxhorn I. Cognitive function in preschool children after epilepsy surgery: Rationale for early intervention. *Epilepsia* 2005; 46: 561-7.
- Gilman J, Duchowny M, Jayakar P, Resnick T. Medical intractability in children evaluated for epilepsy surgery. *Neurology* 1994; 44: 1341-3.
- Griffiths SY, Sherman EM, Slick DJ, Eyri K, Connolly MB, Steinbok P. Postsurgical halth-related quality of life (HRQOL) in children following hemispherectomy for intractable epilepsy. *Epilepsia* 2007; 48:564-70.
- Helmstaedter C, Kurthen M, Lux S, Reuber M, Elger CE. Chronic epilepsy and cognition: a longitudinal study in temporal lobe epilepsy. *Ann Neurol* 2003; 54: 425-32.
- Hermann B, Seidenberg M, Bell B, et al. The neurodevelopmental impact of childhood-onset temporal lobe epilepsy on brain structure and function. *Epilepsia* 2002; 43: 1062-71.
- Hermann BP, Jones JE, Sheth R, et al. Growing up with epilepsy: a two-year investigation of cognitive development in children with new-onset epilepsy. *Epilepsia* 2008; 49: 1847-58.
- Jalava M, Sillanpaa M. Concurrent illnesses in adults with childhood-onset epilepsy: a population-based 35-year follow-up study. *Epilepsia* 1996; 37: 1155-63.
- Jalava M, Silanpaa M, Camfield C, Camfield P. Social adjustment and competence 35 years after onst of childhood epilepsy: a prospective controlled study. *Epilepsia* 1998; 38: 708-15.
- Jokeit H, Ebner A. Effects of chronic epilepsy on intellectual function. *Progress Brain Res* 2002; 135: 455-63.
- Jonas R, Nguyen S, Hu B, et al. Cerebral hemispherectomy: hospital course, seizure, developmental, language and motor outcomes. *Neurology* 2004; 62: 1712-21.
- Keene D, Ventureya ECG. Epilepsy surgery for 5- to 18-year old patients with medical refractory epilepsy- is it cost-efficient? *Child Nerv Syst* 1999; 15: 52-4.
- Kemmotsu N, Girard HM, Bernhardt BC, et al. MRI analysis in temporal lobe epilepsy: cortical thinning and white matter disruptions are related to side of seizure onset. *Epilepsia* 2011; 52: 2257-66.
- Korman B, Bernal B, Duchowny M, et al. Atypical propositional language organization in prenatal and early-acquired lesions. *J Child Neurol* 2010; 25: 985-93.
- Krsek P, Maton B, Jayakar P, et al. Different features of histopathological subtypes of pediatric cortical dysplasia. *Ann Neurol* 2008; 63: 758-69.
- Kwan P, Brodie MJ. Early identification of refractory epilepsy. *NEJM* 2000; 342: 314-9.
- Langfitt JT, Westerveld M, Hamberger MJ, et al. Worsening of quality of life after epilepsy surgery. Effect of seizures and memory decline. *Neurology* 2007; 68: 1988-94.
- Langfitt JT, Holloway RG, McDermott MP, et al. Health care costs decline after successful epilepsy surgery. *Neurology* 2007; 68: 1290-8.
- Lettori D, Battaglia D, Sacco A, et al. Early hemispherectomy in catastrophic epilepsy. A cognitive and epileptic long-term follow-up. *Seizure* 2008; 17: 49-63.

- Luciano AL, Shorvon SD. Results of treatment changes in patients with apparently drug-resistant chronic epilepsy. *Ann Neurol* 2007; 62: 375-81.
- McClelland S, Guo H, Okuyemi KS. Population-based analysis of morbidity and mortality following surgery for intractable temporal lobe epilepsy in the United States. *Arch Neurol* 2011; 68: 725-9.
- Mikati MA, Ataya N, Ferzil J, *et al.* Quality of life after surgery for intractable partial epilepsy in children: a cohort study with controls. *Epilepsy Res* 2010; 90: 207-13.
- Neligan A, Bell GS, Sander JW, Shorvon SD. How refractory is refractory epilepsy? Patterns of relapse and remission in people with refractory epilepsy. *Epilepsy Res* 2011; 96: 225-30.
- Ohtsuka Y, Yoshinaga H, Kobayashi K, *et al.* Predictors and underlying causes of medically intractable localization-related epilepsy in childhood. *Pediatr Neurol* 2001; 24: 209-13.
- Oostrom KJ, van Teeseling A, Smeets-Schouten AC, Peters ACB, Jennekens-Schinkel A. Three to four years after diagnosis: cognition and behavior in children with "epilepsy only". A prospective, controlled study. *Brain* 2005; 128: 1546-55.
- Sabaz M, Lawson JL, Cairns DR, *et al.* The impact of epilepsy surgery on quality of life in children. *Neurology* 2006; 66: 557-61.
- Schmidt D, Stavem K. Long-term seizure outcome of surgery *versus* no surgery for drug-resistant partial epilepsy: A review of controlled studies. *Epilepsia* 2009; 50: 1301-9.
- Shackleton DP, Trenite K-N, de Craen AJM, Vandenbroucke JP, Westendorp RGJ. Living with epilepsy. Long-term prognosis and psychosocial outcomes. *Neurology* 2003; 61: 64-70.
- Shields D. Catastrophic epilepsy in childhood. *Epilepsia* 2000; 41 (Suppl 2): S2-6.
- Sillanpaa M, Haataja L, Shinnar S. Perceived impact of childhood-onset epilepsy on quality of life as an adult. *Epilepsia* 2004; 45: 971-7.
- Sillanpaa M, Shinnar S. Long-term mortality in childhood-onset epilepsy. *NEJM* 363: 2522-9.
- Skirrow C, Cross JH, Cormack F, Harkness W, Vargha-Khadem F, Baldeweg T. Long-term intellectual outcome after temporal lobe surgery in chlildhood. *Neurology* 2011; 76: 1330-7.
- Spencer SS, Berg AT, Vickrey BG, *et al.* Health-related quality of life over time since resective epilepsy surgery. *Ann Neurol* 2007; 62: 327-34.
- Sperling M, Feldman H, Kinman J, Liporace JD, O'Connor J. Seizure control and mortality in epilepsy. *Ann Neurol* 1999; 46: 45-50.
- Thibeault-Eybalin MP, Lortie A, Carmant L. Neonatal seizures: do they damage the brain? *Pediatr Neurol* 2009; 40: 175-80.
- Van Empelen R, Jennekens-Schinkel A, van Rijen PC, Helders PJ, van Nieuwenhuizen O. Health-related quality of life and self-perceived competence of children assessed before and after epilepsy surgery. *Epilepsia* 2005; 46: 258-71.
- Widjaja E, Li B, Schinkel CD, *et al.* Cost-effectivenenss of pediatric epilepsy surgery compared to medical treatment in children with intractable epilepsy. *Epilepsy Res* 2011; 94: 61-8.
- Wiebe S, Blume WT, Girvin JP, Eliasziw M. A randomized controlled trial of surgery for temporal lobe epilepsy. *NEJM* 2001; 345: 311-8.

Adult outcome of childhood-onset, cause unknown (cryptogenic), MRI-negative, focal epilepsy

Carol Camfield, Peter Camfield

Department of Pediatrics, Dalhousie University and the IWK Health Centre, University Ave, Halifax, Nova Scotia, Canada

Many children have focal epilepsy without an identified cause and without an identified lesion on MRI. In the 1989 ILAE classification scheme they would have been identified as "cryptogenic" (ILAE, 1989). "The term cryptogenic refers to a disorder whose cause is hidden or occult. Cryptogenic epilepsies are presumed to be symptomatic, but the etiology is not known. The cryptogenic epilepsies are also age related but often do not have well-defined electro-clinical characteristics." (ILAE, 1989). In 2010, the ILAE commission on Classification and Terminology strongly encouraged the epilepsy community to stop using the term "cryptogenic," because it involved a diagnosis based on a "hunch" rather than a rigorously scientific approach to classification (Berg *et al.*, 2010). The cause is unknown but the clinician thinks that there must be an identifiable lesion but cannot quite identify it. We are sympathetic with the recommendation to change the term to "cause-unknown"; however, we think that there is an important group of children in the old category of cryptogenic who have a good prognosis, those with both normal intelligence and neurological examination. This is the group that forms the basis of this chapter.

Because the term cryptogenic focal epilepsy was so vague and because "cause unknown" does not capture an important concept, we would like to define this group of children as follows. They have: 1) focal seizures; 2) normal intelligence and neurological examinations; 3) no known cause for their epilepsy; 4) normal brain imaging studies; and 5) no well-defined epilepsy syndrome. Well defined epilepsy syndromes include autosomal dominant nocturnal frontal epilepsy (ADNFE), benign rolandic epilepsy (benign focal epilepsy of childhood with centro-temporal spikes) and Panayiotopoulos syndrome (early onset benign occipital epilepsy). The group for consideration has focal epilepsy but we know nothing more!

Obviously, the sophistication of brain imaging studies has improved over time; and, therefore, the group of non-lesional patients has become smaller. When a lesion is found with sophisticated imaging that is congruent with the seizure semiology and EEG findings, then the lesion is presumably the cause of the epilepsy. To say that a patient with focal epilepsy has a negative MRI is to say very little. There is abundant evidence that the technical quality of the MRI, the field strength and the various sequences and modalities used have an important influence on lesion detection. For example, in adults, the addition of diffusion tensor imaging revealed a definite lesion in many who had normal conventional MRI (Rugg-Gunn et al. 2001).

The skill of the neuroradiologist, his interaction with the neurologist and an opportunity to review the MRI together also are important. In our experience, if the initial EEG is normal, the chances of finding a minute lesion on MRI are small. If subsequent EEGs or video-EEG indicate a definite "focus", then MRI review is more likely to reveal a congruent abnormality. Perhaps all focal epilepsy in children will eventually be found to be related to a lesion. Of course, identifying a lesion does not necessarily identify the cause – it may only confirm the anatomical origin of the seizures and histopathology will be needed to establish the cause.

These caveats make outcome studies difficult to interpret and compare. Nonetheless, some important themes have emerged in three large studies (Table I).

Table I. Population-based studies of cryptogenic, cause-unknown, non-lesional epilepsy have similar findings

	Olmstead County N = 359	Connecticut N = 613	Nova Scotia N = 692
% of overall cohort with focal epilepsy	31% Includes 24% with mental or neuro handicap	33% with > 10 yr follow up	19% with > 10 yr follow up
% with cause unknown with terminal remission on or off AEDs	90/111 (81%)	–	110/131 (84%)
% with terminal remission off AEDs	55%	67%	67%
% crypto with cause known and terminal remission	46%	33%	33%
Intractable	7%	Not reported	12%
Benign course	Yes, 32% "smooth sailors"	Yes	Yes, 21% had only 2-5 seizures

■ Olmstead County, Minnesota

All children (n = 359) in Olmstead County who developed epilepsy between 1980 and 2004 were studied (Wirrell et al., 2011). Those with cryptogenic focal epilepsy (N = 111) were compared with those considered symptomatic (N = 95) (identified cause and/or MRI lesion). However, 32% of these 111 children had intellectual disability at diagnosis (9 with moderate to severe disability and 27 with mild mental handicap accompanied by overlapping neurologic abnormalities in 10%). Somewhat surprisingly, these cognitive problems were not strictly statistically associated with poor outcome; however the presence of cognitive problems was "close", $p = 0.06$.

All were followed ≥ 12 months after the diagnosis of epilepsy (median 13 years). At the end of follow up, 82% in the cryptogenic group were seizure-free compared with 50% in the symptomatic group (p < 0.001). Of those who were seizure-free, 67% in the cryptogenic group and 46% of the symptomatic patients had successfully discontinued AED treatment (p = 0.011). Few patients (7%) with cryptogenic cause ended the study with intractable epilepsy compared to 40% in the symptomatic group (p < 0.01). In total, 78 (70%) of the cryptogenic group had an MRI which by definition was normal. Their outcome was very similar to those without an MRI – 77% were seizure-free of whom 60% had discontinued AED treatment and 9% had intractable epilepsy.

Over the clinical course, 32% of the cryptogenic group had "smooth sailing" epilepsy which meant that as soon as AED treatment was started they became seizure-free and were later able to successfully discontinue AEDs (Camfield et al., 1993).

Connecticut

Non-syndromic epilepsy (NSE) was diagnosed prospectively in 347 patients of whom 294 (85%) had a follow up of ≥ 10 years (Berg et al. 2011). Patients (n = 613) were recruited from community-based Pediatric Neurology offices in Connecticut. NSE implied focal onset seizures or convulsions of unclear onset in patients with no identified epilepsy syndrome. Ninety-one children (31%) had an identified brain disorder based on history, examination and/or MRI. An MRI was performed in one setting or another in 89% of the group. For 203 (59%) children with NSE, the cause of the epilepsy was unknown with no clear evidence of an underlying cause for their epilepsy – there was no MRI causative abnormality or intellectual or neurological disability. Of these patients 137 (67%) eventually experienced epilepsy remission (> 5 years seizure-free and no longer taking AEDs). Importantly, only 33 of 91 (36%) with an underlying brain disorder achieved remission. Of the 261 with an MRI, 55 (21%) had an abnormality identified that was thought to be responsible for their epilepsy. Remission occurred in only 33% of those with a causative MRI lesion. In addition, 16 of 43 patients with an abnormal neurologic examination (37%), and 3 out of 11 with intellectual disability (also 37%) achieved remission.

Nova Scotia

This was a population-based study in Nova Scotia for all children with newly diagnosed epilepsy between 1977-1985 and follow up occurring 27.8 ± 5.2 yrs later (Camfield et al., 1993). There were 131 patients with >10 years follow up who fit the criteria for this chapter - focal epilepsy, normal neurological and intellectual function, no identified cause for their epilepsy, and no defined genetic epilepsy syndrome or benign epilepsy syndrome. Brain imaging studies were normal; however, this study was well underway before MRI was invented – imaging was limited to CT scanning in 87% and MRI later in the course of the child's epilepsy in 19%. These patients would be considered to have "cryptogenic epilepsy" by some and "non-syndromic epilepsy" by others. In the cohort there were 55 additional patients who had focal epilepsy, normal intellectual and neurological function, no defined benign or genetic epilepsy syndrome but with a defined cause for their epilepsy (Camfield & Camfield, presented abstract at AES 2012, manuscript in preparation).

In general, patients with unknown cause were more likely to have a favorable epilepsy course and outcome. They were less likely to have partial complex seizures (54% vs. 67%, p = 0.03), less likely to use > 2 AEDs through the clinical course (27% vs. 47%, p = 0.009) and considerably less likely to undergo epilepsy surgery (3% vs. 18%, p = 0.001). They tended to have fewer episodes of status epilepticus (19% vs. 31% p = 0.08) and were somewhat less likely to have > 100 convulsive seizures during the clinical course (14% vs. 25%, p = 0.07). At the end of follow up they were considerably less likely to have either intractable epilepsy or epilepsy surgery (12% vs. 33%, p = 0.001).

On average the longest time seizure-free with or without AED treatment during the entire clinical course was longer in the cause unknown patients (20 ± 9.7 years vs. 14.5 ± 11.4 years, p = 0.001), as was the number of patients with at least 4 years seizure-free (89% vs. 78%, p = 0.001). Cause unknown patients were more likely to attempt to discontinue AED treatment (90% vs. 76%, p = 0.02). Somewhat surprisingly the long-term remission rate was similar when defined as no longer receiving AEDs at the end of follow up (73% vs. 62%, p = ns). However, if remission was defined as seizure-free and off AED treatment, then the cause unknown group had a better chance of remission (67% vs. 53%, p = 0.03).

Over the clinical course, 20% in the cause unknown group had between two to five seizures only. This reflects a very benign disorder, similar to the "smooth sailing" epilepsy of the Omstead County study.

The Nova Scotia study also examined social outcome in the cause unknown and cause known groups. Even though the rate of specific learning disorder, grades repeated and school graduation were essentially the same, people with cause unknown had more favorable social outcomes. As adults they are more likely to be employed (89% vs. 58%, p < 0.00001), married or living common-law (71% vs. 58%, p < 0.0001) and less likely to have incomes in the lowest of three categories (32% vs. 50%, p = 0.05). Those with cause known reported that they were unlikely to have had a romantic relationship for > 3 months (24% vs. 8%, p = 0.002) and more likely to have no close friends (18% vs. 7%, p = 0.01). They were less likely to be involved in a pregnancy (45% vs. 67% p = 0.03). In both groups the proportion of pregnancies outside a stable relationship was the same (48% vs. 32%). Despite all of these findings the two groups had similar rates of visits to a mental health professional (45% vs. 49%) and psychiatric diagnoses other than ADHD (29% vs. 33%).

There were 8 social outcomes that were defined as poor: no high school graduation, a psychiatric diagnosis other than ADHD, at least one visit to a mental health specialist, no close friends, no romantic relationship ever that lasted longer than 3 months, a pregnancy outside a stable relationship (6 months), living alone at the end of follow up and being unemployed. The proportion of patients in each group with at least one unfavorable social outcome was similar (67% vs. 77%) which reflects a high rate of mental health problems in both. The cause known group was nearly twice as likely to have > 1 unfavorable outcome (54% vs. 28%), a finding that was nearly statistically significant (p = 0.06).

When patients with intractable epilepsy were removed from the analysis, remaining patients with cause known continued to have evidence of more severe epilepsy and some of the differences in social outcome persisted. The cause known group was statistically less likely to be married and more likely to be unemployed with lower family income.

Thus, some but not all, of the differences between groups were associated with higher rates of intractable epilepsy in the cause known patients. Psychosocial outcome of childhood-onset epilepsy will be further discussed elsewhere in this book.

■ Other studies

A number of smaller studies have addressed the outcome in "cryptogenic" focal epilepsy. A study from New York ascertained patients from emergency rooms with a first seizure and followed them prospectively (Shinnar et al., 2000). There were 34 patients with cryptogenic partial epilepsy and 82% were in remission after mean follow up of 8.3 years. The very long follow-up study from Turku, Finland identified 32 children with cryptogenic focal epilepsy and after a 25-30 year follow up, 63% were in remission (Sillanpaa et al., 1988).

It is difficult to come to firm conclusions about epilepsy surgery outcomes in children with focal epilepsy with and without a lesion because all publications have been based on small case series (Spooner et al., 2006; Szabó et al., 2001). However, there seems to be a general consensus that the outcome is best with surgery in patients with an MRI lesion, lower in those with no MRI lesion but abnormal histopathology and least favorable when both the MRI and the histopathology are negative. A meta-analysis of adults and children suggested that the chance of successful epilepsy surgery is 2.5 times greater for lesional *vs.* non-lesional cases (Téllez-Zenteno et al., 2010).

■ Concluding remarks

Almost all studies of cryptogenic, cause-unknown, non-lesional epilepsy have similar findings. Therefore, it is safe to conclude that patients with childhood onset epilepsy (excluding benign and other genetic syndromes) with no lesion or no known cause are likely to have relatively mild epilepsy, as compared with similar children with a lesion and/or known cause. The difference in the chance of long term remission is about 65% *vs.* 35% provided that all patients are otherwise intellectually and neurologically normal. Social outcome in this specific group of patients has only been carefully examined in the Nova Scotia study. The findings strongly suggest that patients with unknown cause are more socially successful in adult life with more employment, higher income, more frequent marriage, more children and less social isolation.

References

- Berg AT, Berkovic SF, Brodie MJ, *et al.* Revised terminology and concepts for organization of seizures and epilepsies: report of the ILAE Commission on Classification and Terminology, 2005-2009. *Epilepsia* 2010; 51: 676-85.
- Berg AT, Testa FM, Levy SR. Complete remission in nonsyndromic childhood-onset epilepsy. *Ann Neurol* 2011; 70: 566-73.
- Camfield CS, Camfield PR, Gordon KE, Dooley JM, Smith BS. Predicting the outcome of childhood epilepsy – a population based study yielding a simple scoring system. *J Pediatr* 1993; 122: 861-8.

- Dhamija R, Moseley BD, Cascino GD, Wirrell EC. A population-based study of long-term outcome of epilepsy in childhood with a focal or hemispheric lesion on neuroimaging. *Epilepsia* 2011; 52: 1522-6.
- Geerts A, Arts WF, Stroink H, *et al.* Course and outcome of childhood epilepsy: a 15-year follow-up of the Dutch Study of Epilepsy in Childhood. *Epilepsia* 2010; 51: 1189-97.
- Commission on Classification and Terminology of the International League Against Epilepsy. Proposal for revised classification of epilepsies and epileptic syndromes. *Epilepsia* 1989; 30: 389-99.
- Rantala H, Ingalsuo H. Occurrence and outcome of epilepsy in children younger than 2 years. *J Pediatr* 1999; 135: 761-4.
- Rugg-Gunn FJ, Eriksson SH, Symms MR, Barker GJ, Duncan JS. Diffusion tensor imaging of cryptogenic and acquired partial epilepsies. *Brain* 2001; 124 (Pt 3): 627-36.
- Sillanpää M, Jalava M, Kaleva O, Shinnar S. Long-term prognosis of seizures with onset in childhood. *New Eng J Med* 1998; 338: 1715-22.
- Shinnar S, Berg AT, O'Dell C, *et al.* Predictors of multiple seizures in a cohort of children prospectively followed from the time of their first unprovoked seizure. *Ann Neurol* 2000; 48: 140-7.
- Spooner CG, Berkovic S; Mitchell LA, Wrennall JA, Harvey AS. New-onset temporal lobe epilepsy in children: Lesion on MRI predicts poor seizure outcome. *Neurology* 2006; 67: 2147-53.
- Szabó CA, Rothner AD, Kotagal P, *et al.* Symptomatic or cryptogenic partial epilepsy of childhood onset: fourteen-year follow-up. *Pediatr Neurol* 2001; 24: 264-9.
- Téllez-Zenteno JF, Hernández Ronquillo L, Moien-Afshari F, Wiebe S. Surgical outcomes in lesional and non-lesional epilepsy: a systematic review and meta-analysis. *Epilepsy Res* 2010; 89: 310-8.
- Wirrell EC, Grossardt BR, So EL, Nickels KC. A population-based study of long-term outcomes of cryptogenic focal epilepsy in childhood: cryptogenic epilepsy is probably not symptomatic epilepsy. *Epilepsia* 2011; 52: 738-45.

Focal non-idiopathic epilepsies: does outcome after epilepsy surgery depend on the localization of the epileptogenic zone in frontal and temporal lobe epilepsy?

Ingrid Tuxhorn

Case Western Reserve University, Division Chief Pediatric Epilepsy, Rainbow Babies and Children's University Hospitals, Cleveland, Ohio, USA

In 1955 Wilder Penfield expressed the importance of understanding outcome of surgery to treat epilepsy: "It is not enough to know whether a radical surgical procedure has stopped the attacks or not. We must know its effect upon the patient's behavior, and happiness". And while we have made significant progress in the past 60 years or so there is still much to be learnt especially as it relates to outcome in the pediatric population.

Epilepsy surgery may cure or mitigate seizures in well-selected patients who have a focal area of epileptogenesis that is resectable with minimal or no risk to loss of brain function. It is no longer a treatment of last resort but may be considered "disease modifying" in children who are vulnerable to the progressive effects of active epileptogenesis as their brain is maturing (Aicardi, 1997). Generally presurgical evaluation focuses on defining the epileptogenic zone involving the cortical region that needs to be removed surgically to stop seizures. This chapter will review our current understanding of the variables known to drive favorable as opposed to unfavorable outcome of surgically treated pediatric epilepsy particularly as it relates to localization in the frontal and temporal lobes in the short and long-term. It will focus on a number of recent meta-analyses that have desegregated robust clinical variables predicting outcome. In addition we will discuss insights into the process of epileptogenesis and the dynamic neurobiology of focal epilepsy which may be pertinent to surgical outcome and may need to receive more attention in the clinical management of patients and the outcome literature. Finally we show one illustrative case.

Clinical predictors of post surgical seizure outcome

There is an extensive literature analyzing clinical variables that may predict surgical outcome. The most robust predictor determining good outcome is completeness of resection of the epileptogenic lesion (Paolicchi et al., 2000; Tonini et al., 2004; Sinclair et al., 2003). Completeness of resection has been invariably defined by resection of the MRI visible structural lesion and adjoining area of abnormal interictal and ictal epileptiform activity. Seizure outcome following complete resections has been reported in the 90% range, whereas outcomes following incomplete resections or large multilobar resections only reached the 20-30% seizure free range (Paolocchi et al., 2002).

Positive predictors for a good seizure outcome have included the presence of prior febrile seizures, shorter duration of seizures, abnormal MRI showing a potentially epileptogenic lesion or mesial temporal sclerosis, evidence for EEG and MRI concordance of localization and complete surgical resection of this region (Tonini et al., 2004). The use of intracranial monitoring and electrocorticography has not been predictive for outcome (Gilliam et al., 1997; Tonini et al., 2004; Vachhrajani et al., 2012).

Direct comparisons of various patient series gives limited results due to marked heterogeneity of the patient populations studied. This includes small numbers of patients reported on, the varied underlying conditions causing epilepsy, widely differing surgical approaches and procedures used, biases in patient referrals to the tertiary surgical centers and different methods and tools applied in the presurgical localizing evaluation.

Taking these limitations into consideration, few clinical predictors have been determined. Patient age at surgery and onset is not predictive of seizure outcome after surgery in most series including a recent series of 40 patients with frontal lobe epilepsy from Toronto Children's Hospital (Vachhrajani et al., 2012). Duration of epilepsy, presence of residual spikes on the ECOG, side of resection, lesionectomy versus other types of resections in the frontal lobe, presence of cortical dysplasia over other type of pathologies as well as the volume of tissue resected as judged by a CT or MRI scan all have no clear predictive value for surgical outcome in this recently reported large frontal lobe outcome series (Vachhrajani et al., 2012).

Acute postoperative seizures occurring within the first 24 hours after surgery are seen more frequently after extratemporal resections and are generally a predictor for failed surgery in particular if the semiology is unchanged and patients are less likely to be seizure free after 6-24 months follow-up (Mani et al., 2006). Particularly after hemispherectomy early acute postoperative seizures that have the same semiology as the refractory presurgical seizures are highly likely to predict a failed surgery and an early second surgery should be considered if the reason for failure can be determined and addressed. This may include incomplete resections or disconnections (Mani et al., 2006).

Meta-analyses: temporal lobe epilepsy surgery outcomes are still superior to frontal lobe outcomes in children and adults

The short term efficacy and safety of temporal lobe epilepsy surgery in adults has been verified in a randomized controlled study in addition to a systematic review and meta-analysis of the literature of 32 studies reporting 2,250 patients (Téllez-Zenteno, 2010;

Wiebe et al., 2001; Engel et al., 2003). Overall 65% of patients were seizure free, 21% improved and 14% showed no change. Sub-analysis of smaller datasets show a similar outcome when the follow-up is longer with 63% seizure free in a 2-5-year follow up period.

In a recent 2010 pediatric review the overall seizure control after epilepsy surgery was reported in mixed series of 753 pediatric patients from 1997 to 2008 as Engel I in 67% to 81%, Engel II and III ranging from 5-12% and Engel IV up to 19% (Adhami & Harini, 2010). In this same analysis excellent temporal lobe seizure free outcomes ranged from 72% to 91% at mean durations of follow up over 2 years while extratemporal outcomes consistently ranged lower from 54% to 60% (Gilliam et al., 1997; Cossu et al., 2008; Bourgeois et al., 1999; Benifla et al., 2006; Kan et al., 2008; Kim et al., 2008) (see Table I).

Table I. Summary of selected studies reporting postoperative seizure outcomes (Modified from Adhami and Harini)

Author	Temporal resection		Extratemporal resection	
	n	% seizure free	n	% seizure free
Gilliam (n = 33)	18	72%	15	60%
Massimo (n = 113)	43	91%	70	54%
Kan (n = 58)	33	85%	25	60%
Kim (n = 134)	59	88%	56	55%
Cossu (n = 68)	68	85%		
Liava (n = 53)			53	75%
Benifla (n = 126)			106	72%*

* Benifla: Engel I and II reported together

An extensive meta-analysis of 76 studies reporting on long-term outcome of >5 years published in 2005 by Téllez-Zenteno pooled data on 3895 adult and pediatric temporal lobe patients. Long-term seizure freedom was attained in 66% after temporal lobe surgery (40 studies), 71% in studies using the Engel classification system, 59% in grouped temporal and extratemporal (25 studies of 2334 patients) compared to only 27% seizure free in frontal lobe surgeries (7 studies of 486 patients). While the meta-analysis by Engel in 2003 reported on extratemporal resections in a group, the extratemporal analysis by Téllez-Zenteno et al (2005) looked at outcome per lobar localization. By comparison, hemispherectomy patients (2 studies of 169 patients) had 61% seizure freedom, while parietal and occipital lobe surgeries (82 and 34 patients respectively) each had 46% seizure freedom. The authors highlight that one of the most salient findings of their analysis is that, overall, long-term surgical results were consistently similar to those of short-term studies, including the randomized study by Wiebe. This attests to the sustained benefit of seizure freedom following surgery in general (Téllez-Zenteno et al., 2010). When author defined outcomes were used the seizure free rate was slightly lower in TLE (58% to 66%) than when the Engel I classification was used. Also a narrower range of seizure free rates from 59%-89% was reported compared to extratemporal localizations or resection types.

Studies reporting on frontal lobe resections produced among the worst outcome rates (mean 27%) in the resective surgeries and were also the most heterogeneous in outcomes ranging from 9% to 80%.

The source of heterogeneity was more closely analyzed and in temporal lobe studies included more than 10 years follow up, surgery after 1980, specific etiologies such as tumors and hippocampal sclerosis. In studies of temporal and extratemporal outcomes, potential sources of heterogeneity of outcomes were similar to those in temporal lobe surgery but also included neuronal migration disorders and studied of patients with vascular malformations. Children with vascular malformations had high odds for seizure freedom with follow ups > 10 years and when operated after 1980.

The heterogeneity of seizure free outcome in frontal lobe epilepsy (ranging for 9%-80%) may be related to inability to resect the entire epileptogenic region in proximity to functionally eloquent cortex, an epileptogenic region extending beyond the frontal lobe and rapid extensive seizure spread, differences in outcome assessment, different etiologies (better with tumors), completeness of resection and involvement of the epileptogenic region to adjacent structures beyond the frontal lobe (Englot et al., 2012). There is a suggestion that improvement in patient selection and identification of the seizure focus and surgical techniques have favorably affected outcomes of epilepsy surgery as the two most robust variables predicting good seizure outcome in the large meta-analysis series are if results were published after 1980 and the Engel classification scheme was used (Téllez-Zenteno et al., 2010). The association of more recent surgeries and better outcome may reflect the impact of developments in more precise imaging and seizure mapping techniques. This may play a greater role in frontal lobe epilepsy with more extensive and highly connected areas of epileptogenesis compared to temporal lobe epilepsy where the epileptogenic zone is more confined to the limbic region and adjacent neocortical structure (Vachhrajani et al., 2012).

Overall despite the reported heterogeneity of outcome in various studies which are to a large degree also determined by methodological classifications (outcome assessment is variables, mixed procedures, patient selection bias, different types of presurgical evaluations, no controls, not prospective, consistent patterns of meaningful results are emerging from the numerous types of surgical interventions to treat epilepsy surgically (Téllez-Zenteno et al., 2010) (Tables II and III).

Table II. Factors linked to unfavourable seizure outcomes after temporal lobectomy

Temporal lobe factors linked with unfavourable outcomes
No MRI structural abnormality
Residual tumor or malignant transformation
Emergency temporal lobectomy secondary to complications of invasive presurgical monitoring
Occult or missed dual pathology in same lobe
Bitemporal or extensive unitemporal disease
Missed frontal (basal, mesial, insular) involvement – "temporal plus"

Table III. Factors linked to unfavourable seizure outcomes after extratemporal surgeries

Extratemporal lobe factors linked with unfavourable outcomes
No MRI structural abnormality
More widespread disease than suspected - miss active areas eg dual pathology/multiregional epileptogenesis
Residual tumor and malignant transformation
Multilobar resections
Limited resection in proximity to eloquent cortex
Incomplete lesionectomy
Errors in localization – misinterpretations of data (eg discordant)
Recurring epileptogenesis and propagation
FCD: reorganization due to unique neuronal, receptor properties

■ Patient selection and newer tools – how may they help us to improve surgical outcomes?

Patients with well-delineated focal epilepsy that is refractory to medical and other non-medical therapies are deemed to be the best candidates for epilepsy surgery. Generally a resection or disconnection of the epileptogenic zone sparing eloquent cortex controlling speech, sensory motor, memory or visual functions is performed after the presurgical evaluation has provided this data. The epileptogenic zone has been defined as a hypothetical concept that defines the area of cortex that generates clinical seizures and therefore correlates with the amount of cortical tissue that needs to be resected to make a patient seizure free. A number of EEG biomarkers are used to define the epileptogenic zone including sharp waves and spikes to define the irritative zone and localization of seizure patterns in the surface EEG to define the area of ictal onset. Depth and surface recordings generate more high frequency oscillations in the epileptogenic zone which when resected with areas of spiking appears to improve seizure outcome (Haegelen et al., 2013).

■ Selection of surgical candidates impacts outcome

Referral to an epilepsy centre for pre-surgical evaluation rests with the primary care physician, pediatric neurologist and fortunately to an increasing degree the advocacy initiative taken by parents who will seek a second opinion. A detailed seizure history to assess lateralizing or localizing signs, the burden of epilepsy, treatment gaps, the underlying etiology including febrile seizures, traumatic brain injury (TBI), perinatal and prenatal risk factors, family history to assess genetic dispositions, prior evaluations including EEGs and imaging are some of the useful clinical information that should be gathered. Age of onset and the occurrence of status epilepticus are useful and may point to certain epileptic disorders. Infants and toddlers may have focal and surgically remedial epilepsy even with more generalized appearing seizure semiology and EEG findings. All patients with epileptic encephalopathies associated with structural brain pathology or prominent focal signs (hemiparesis, focal components) should be referred to assess surgical options. Neurologic disorders such as tuberous sclerosis (TSC), Sturge Weber syndrome (SWS), Rasmussen encephalitis, brain malformations, perinatal and postnatal strokes, low grade tumors, vascular anomalies are some of the more common symptomatic etiologies of medically refractory epilepsy and should be referred early in the disease course for a comprehensive epilepsy evaluation by the referring pediatric neurologist. The complexity of cases undergoing evaluation has increased over the years and includes nonlesional, subtle lesional, and multilesional cases as defined by MRI who on further work up may be shown to have a resectable epileptogenic zone and therefore benefit from surgery. The long-term outcome in these patients is as yet unclear and may not fall into a comparably consistent pattern of outcome as example temporal lobe epilepsy.

■ EEG and outcome

Video EEG monitoring with scalp 10-20 and 10-10 electrode placement and additional special electrodes such as sphenoidals in selected cases is performed in most centers to record interictal focal epileptiform abnormalities which define the irritative zone and clinical seizures with the concomitant ictal pattern which defines the ictal onset zone, may be considered the gold standard to lay the framework for the diagnosis of non epileptic *vs.* epileptic paroxysms and generalized *vs.* focal seizures. Seizure semiology with congruent localization of the EEG will allow a first hypothesis to move forward with further steps towards surgical management. Age specific clinical and EEG features may obscure the focal nature of the epilepsy and this will require a high index of suspicion to correctly refer and select these infant and toddlers for surgery. Symptomatic infantile spasms, West syndrome, Lennox Gastaut syndrome (LGS due to cortical dysplasias), early strokes, TSC, etc. may fall into this category.

■ Imaging and outcome

While MRI, PET and SPECT imaging technologies continue to play an important role for defining the epileptic cortical zone as outlined above, advances in structural and functional neuroimaging have led to improved precision in localization of the epileptic focus for surgical planning (Shandal *et al.*, 2012). The identification of a structural abnormality on neuroimaging that may represent the underlying epileptogenic lesion once all the clinical and additional tests have been carefully evaluated for congruence is the single most important factor defining surgical options and outcome prognosis if a complete lesion resection is performed. The typical pathologies that need to be looked for are malformations of cortical development (MCD), low grade tumors, mesial temporal sclerosis, etc. There is sufficient literature pointing to the superior surgical seizure outcome of lesional compared to nonlesional focal epilepsies.

The application of Fluorine-18 deoxyglucose positron emission tomography in the 1980 with symptomatic infantile spasms (IS) due to MCD that was poorly visible on the MRI resolution available at the time demonstrated cortical areas of hypometabolism which had some concordance with focal EEG findings. Surgery was very successful in these cases of catastrophic epilepsy and pathology confirmed cortical dysplasia. Interictal PET continues to be very useful in MRI negative cases suspected of "cryptogenic" focal dysplasias due to subtle lesions.

In addition novel imaging techniques promise to provide a better understanding of the underlying mechanisms and the functional consequences of chronic epilepsy (Luat & Chugani, 2008). PET, fMRI and DTI are being utilized as powerful tools in the in vivo study of epileptic networks. PET scanning using various tracers has identified dysfunctional areas outside the primary epileptic focus which likely reflect remote but interconnected areas (Juhasz, 2012). Similarly primary hypometabolic areas may not be static but undergo dynamic changes depending on stages of chronicity and intractability of seizures. Patients with new onset partial epilepsy will rarely show focal hypometabolic abnormalities on PET and progression of hypometabolism may not be evident for a number of years (Gaillard et al., 2007). Longitudinal changes in the extent of glucose hypometabolism with sequential PET scans in children with partial epilepsy who had normal MRI scans have revealed that the extent of glucose hypometabolism correlated positively with seizure frequency (Benedek et al., 2006). Most patients with persistent or increased seizure frequency showed enlargement of the cortical area of hypometabolism while the extent of glucose hypometabolism remained stable or even decreased when seizures came under control. These findings strongly suggest that persistent seizures and intractable epilepsy may lead to progressively larger areas of neuronal dysfunction on the one hand, while some of the cortical hypometabolism may represent reversible changes in neuronal function as some changes may disappear after seizure control is achieved either medically or surgically. Together these findings suggest that persistent focal seizures in children may progressively recruit larger areas of brain into the seizure network through processes such as secondary epileptogenesis that have been studied in experimental animal models. The development of secondary foci distant from a primary focus associated with a lesion may explain decreased outcome as well as seizure recurrences even after successful resection of the primary focus. This has important implications for the interpretation of the presurgical evaluation, type of surgical treatment and projected prognosis offered to the child and family.

Nonlesional outcomes are clearly less favourable than lesional ones but the reduction of seizures offers an important improvement in seizure control to patients. The reported rates of seizure free outcome range from 37% to 51% and this heterogeneity again most likely reflects non standardized selection criteria and observer biases in each of the studies.

To date the seizure outcome in 360 nonlesional cases have been reported in uncontrolled studies as summarized by Ahdani and Harini in 2010 and the range of seizure freedom is between 25% to 64% seizure freedom while favourable seizure outcome ranged from 58% to 83%. In some of these series subtle pathology was found after resection contributing to better outcome. In summary, the emerging outcome data in nonlesional pediatric cases suggests that a reduction of seizures (Engel II and III) rather than seizure freedom may be an important improvement for high seizure burden patients (palliative).

■ Neurobiology of focal epilepsies – relevance for surgical outcomes?

Epilepsy is a complex group of disorders that follow the perturbation of the normal balance of neuronal excitation and inhibition. The neurobiology of epilepsy may therefore involve diverse mechanisms and the mechanisms underlying epileptogenesis probably are not the same in different types of focal epilepsies which could affect outcome after surgery and require different surgical approaches to achieve a good surgical outcome. A mechanistic approach therefore to a dynamic disease like epilepsy which appears to be caused by multiple mechanisms may severely limit our understanding of all the factors that may impact surgical seizure outcome including genetics, network physiology, etiology and localization.

While seizures and epilepsy have been documented since antiquity, the insight that a seizure is a period of abnormal and synchronous excitation of groups of neurons and subsequent advances in clinical and basic research has opened the door to our understanding the multiple mechanisms underlying clinical seizure and epilepsy manifestations. (Sharfman, 2007) Understanding how seizures are initially produced, what components make up the process of epileptogenesis which refers to the development of the state of the brain underlying epilepsy which again is defined as the state of recurrent, spontaneous seizures offer new avenues for prevention and therapeutic intervention including the surgical treatments. Seizures occur when there is a disruption of the balance between excitation and inhibition of neurons. There are multiple controls at different levels of the nervous system that prevent excessive neuronal firing or enhance neuronal inhibition which will usually prevent seizure activity from occurring. These complex mechanisms may take place at the micro level involving the membrane and ions, cells including circuits and synapses and ultimately at the macro brain level of large scale neuronal networks of the cortex and its connection to subcortical systems (Sharfman, 2007). In the nervous system the ionic milieu and various chemical and electric gradients generate the electrical activity underlying normal brain signaling and function. The normal membrane resting potential of -60 mV is achieved by energy dependent sodium-potassium pumps that maintain a high intracellular potassium concentration and extracellular sodium concentration. Disturbances in these ion concentrations (due to pump immaturity or failure, glial control of ion concentrations) may lead to abnormal depolarization and action potentials and clinical seizures.

These mechanisms also play a role in the pathophysiology of focal epilepsies and conceivably different surgical approaches (*e.g.*, corticectomy, lobectomy, lesionectomy plus, disconnections-hippocampus, fornix, hemispherotomy) may serve to modulate factors that disrupt normal homeostasis with variable outcome.

■ Temporal lobe biology

The mechanism of seizure generation in temporal lobe epilepsy has been quite well elucidated from clinical studies and animal models. In many patients with temporal lobe epilepsy there appears to be an initial insult or injury followed by a lengthy silent period until recurrent seizures begin. Genetic factors may play a role in the susceptibility to the initial insult which then due to various mechanisms may set in motion a process leading to recurrent seizures. The initial injury may take the form of febrile seizures, birth trauma or infections such as meningitis resulting in some form of neuronal injury which appears to be critical to the pathophysiology of temporal lobe epilepsy. A febrile seizure animal model has provided important information about various mechanisms implicated in epileptogenesis after febrile seizures which include the role of proinflammatory cytokines (Scharfman, 2007). Molecular and cellular constituents of neuronal and glial networks are altered setting the stage for subsequent epileptogenesis. Over time the seizure threshold is reduced by increasing hyper-excitability and the risk for seizures increases. These changes may be sufficient to cause epilepsy or seizures or may only be triggered via additional activation by a so-called second hit.

This may come in the form of various environmental factors, emotional stressors, hormones, circadian changes which normally would not trigger seizures but in a brain that has been altered so that there is an underlying state of increased excitability may do so (Scharfman, 2007).

This raises the question of how focal some of these state changes are and whether more widespread changes underlying the mechanisms of epileptogenesis may account for failed surgery in some cases.

Various mechanisms may underlie the seizures of patients with temporal lobe epilepsy including multifocality, *e.g.*, in limbic structures and beyond the temporal boundaries (temporal plus), rather than a single or at least predominant focus. This may explain some of the surgical failures after temporal lobectomy. Further elucidation of these mechanisms may improve the surgical outcome which stays around the 60% to 70% range (except in lesional cases when it may approach the 90% range) despite the use of more refined presurgical diagnostic tests. The biology of frontal lobe epilepsy is much less homogenous and less well understood at this point.

Illustrative case

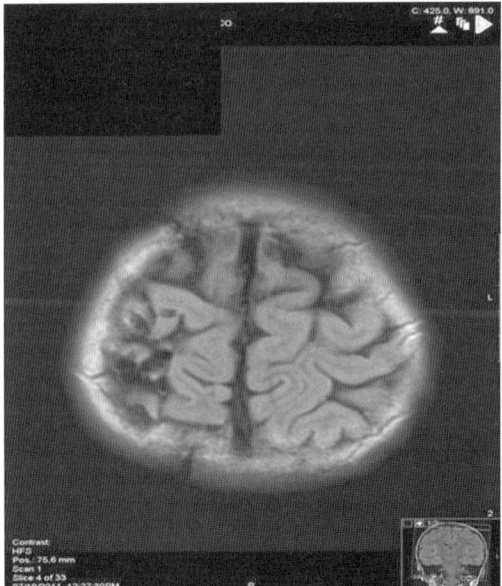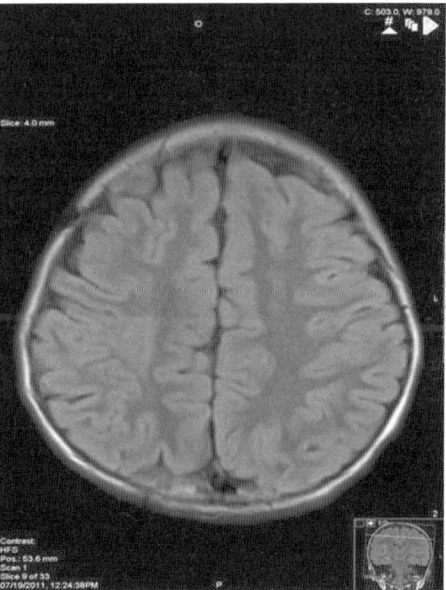

Figure 1. Postoperative MRI shows residual dysplasia located in the right deep central region underlying the resection site.

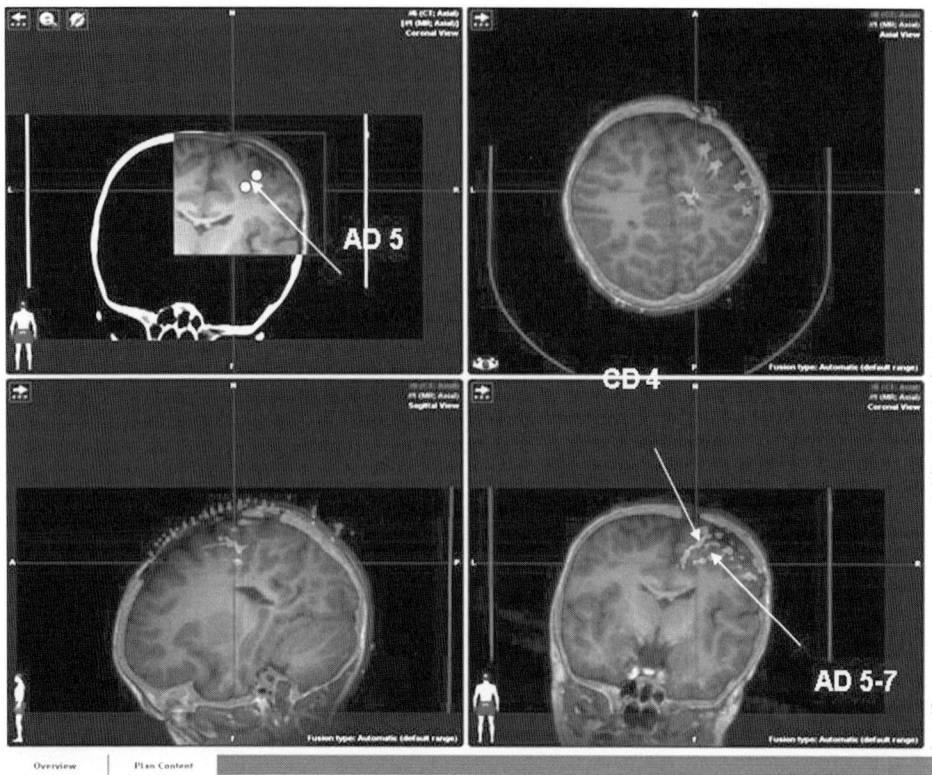

Figure 2. Depth electrodes were placed into the residual lesion to record further EEG to tailor the resection. AD 5 was the active contact.

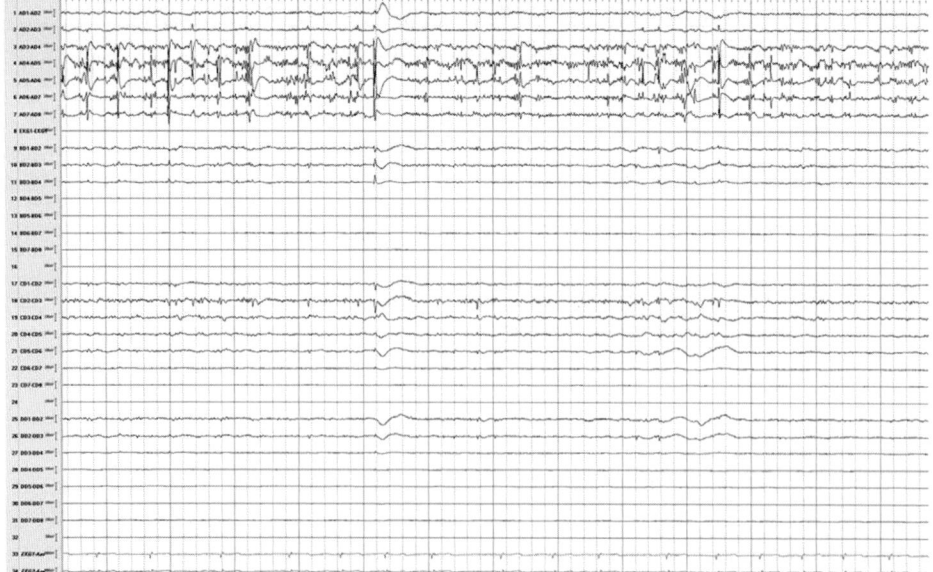

Figure 3. Localized continuous spiking was recorded on EEG from the residual dysplasia. This region was removed in a second surgery and the patient has remained seizure free.

Conclusion

Short and long-term outcome studies support the effectiveness of surgical treatments in refractory childhood epilepsy that is amenable to surgical techniques with an acceptable risk benefit ratio.

However, the results for temporal lobe surgery continue to remain superior to those of frontal lobe epilepsy in adults and children for a number of reasons as outlined above. Temporal lobe surgical seizure remissions are as good in children as in adults and reach the 70-90% range in newer studies with little heterogeneity and a low relapse rate in the long-term. This durable seizure response to surgery supports an aggressive approach to children with suspected temporal lobe epilepsy to offer early seizure remission and minimize secondary deficits in cognitive and psychosocial functions. There is still a clear treatment gap in this group of patients if we consider that temporal lobe epilepsy is a pediatric onset disorder in many adult patients coming for surgical evaluation.

Frontal lobe epilepsy surgical outcomes remain more heterogeneous and have been reported to range from 20-80% averaging a 50% to 60% seizure free outcome range. Variables driving this heterogeneity suggest that there is a trend for improving frontal lobe outcomes in the past few years probably due to more precision in defining the extent of the epileptogenic zone and delineating speech and motor cortex as well as using more tailored surgical approaches. Also the outcome results suggest a sustained and durable long-term outcome in the more recent reported series.

However, if we consider that the seizure free surgical outcome approximates the medical outcome after using two or three antiseizure drugs, a significant number of patients still will not remit with our current therapies. We therefore face continued challenges to find new and innovative therapies in addition to our current modalities that then need to be applied in a multimodal fashion to cure more children with active epilepsy. We are living in exciting times as innovative epilepsy therapies including stem cell therapies are being evaluated in the laboratory and in the near future may translate into better additional therapies for children with epilepsy.

References

- Ahdani S, Harini C. Postoperative seizure control. In: Cataltepe O, Jallo G. *Pediatric Epilepsy Surgery: Preoperative Assessment and Surgical Treatment*. New York-Stuttgart: Thieme Verlag, 2010, pp. 320-31.
- Aicardi J. Pediatric Epilepsy Surgery: how the view has changed. In: Tuxhorn I, Holthausen H, Boenigk H (eds). *Pediatric Epilepsy Syndromes and their Surgical Treatment*. London: John Libbey, 1997.
- Benedek K, Juhász C, Chugani DC, Muzik O, Chugani HT. Longitudinal changes in cortical glucose hypometabolism in children with intractable epilepsy. *J Child Neurol* 2006; 21: 26-31.
- Benifla M, Otsubo H, Ochi A, *et al*. Temporal lobe surgery for intractable epilepsy in children: an analysis of outcomes in 126 children. *Neurosurgery* 2006; 59: 1203-13.
- Bourgeois M Sainte-Rose C, Lellouch-Tuboana A, *et al*. Surgery of epilepsy associated with focal lesions in childhood. *J Neurosurg* 1999; 90: 833-42.
- Cossu M, Lo Russo G, Francione S, *et al*. Epilepsy surgery in children: results and predictors of outcome on seizures. *Epilepsia* 2008; 49: 65-72.

- Engel J Jr, McDermott MP, Wiebe S, et al.; Early Randomized Surgical Epilepsy Trial (ERSET) Study Group. Early surgical therapy for drug-resistant temporal lobe epilepsy: a randomized trial. JAMA 2012; 307: 922-30.
- Englot DJ, Wang DD, Rolston JD, Shih TT, Chang EF. Rates and predictors of long-term seizure freedom after frontal lobe epilepsy surgery: a systematic review and meta-analysis. *J Neurosurg* 2012; 116: 1042-8.
- Gaillard WD, Weinstein S, Conry J, et al. Prognosis of children with partial epilepsy: MRI and serial 18FDG-PET. *Neurology* 2007; 68: 655-9.
- Gilliam F, Wyllie E, Kashden J, et al. Epilepsy surgery outcome: comprehensive assessment in children. *Neurology* 1997; 48: 1368-74.
- Haegelen C, Perucca P, Châtillon CE, et al. High-frequency oscillations, extent of surgical resection, and surgical outcome in drug-resistant focal epilepsy. *Epilepsia* 2013.
- Juhász C. The impact of positron emission tomography imaging on the clinical management of patients with epilepsy. *Expert Rev Neurother* 2012; 12: 719-32.
- Kan P, Van Orman C, Kestle JR. Outcomes after surgery for focal epilepsy in children. *Childs Nerv Syst* 2008; 24: 587-91.
- Kim SK, Wang KC, Hwang YS, et al. Epilepsy surgery in children: outcomes and complications. *J Neurosurg Pediatr* 2008; 1: 277-83.
- Luat AF, Chugani HT. Molecular and diffusion tensor imaging of epileptic networks. *Epilepsia* 2008; 49 (Suppl 3): 15-22.
- Liava A, Francione S, Tassi L, et al. Individually tailored extratemporal epilepsy surgery in children: anatomo-electro-clinical features and outcome predictors in a population of 53 cases. *Epilepsy Behav* 2012; 25 (Suppl 1): 68-80.
- Mani J, Gupta A, Mascha E, et al. Postoperative seizures after extratemporal resections and hemispherectomy in pediatric epilepsy. *Neurology* 2006; 66 (Suppl 7): 1038-43.
- Paolicchi JM, Jayakar P, Dean P, et al. Predictors of outcome in pediatric epilepsy surgery. *Neurology* 2000; 54: 642-7.
- Shandal V, Veenstra AL, Behen M, Sundaram S, Chugani H. Long-term outcome in children with intractable epilepsy showing bilateral diffuse cortical glucose hypometabolism pattern on positron emission tomography. *J Child Neurol* 2012; 27: 39-45.
- Scharfman HE. The neurobiology of epilepsy. *Curr Neurol Neurosci Rep* 2007; 7: 348-54.
- Sinclair DB, Aronyk KE, Snyder TJ, et al. Pediatric epilepsy surgery at the University of Alberta: 1988-2000. *Pediatr Neurol* 2003; 29: 302-11.
- Téllez-Zenteno JF, Hernández Ronquillo L, Moien-Afshari F, Wiebe S. Surgical outcomes in lesional and non-lesional epilepsy: a systematic review and meta-analysis. *Epilepsy Res* 2010; 89: 310-8.
- Tonini C, Beghi E, Berg AT, et al. Predictors of epilepsy surgery outcome: a meta-analysis. *Epilepsy Res* 2004; 62: 75-87.
- Vachhrajani S, de Ribaupierre S, Otsubo H, et al. Neurosurgical management of frontal lobe epilepsy in children. *J Neurosurg Pediatr* 2012; 10: 206-16.
- Wiebe S, Blume WT, Girvin JP, Eliasziw M. Effectiveness and Efficiency of Surgery for Temporal Lobe Epilepsy Study Group. A randomized, controlled trial of surgery for temporal-lobe epilepsy. *N Engl J Med* 2001; 345: 311-8.

Outcome after epilepsy surgery of MRI-negative non-idiopathic focal epilepsies

Thomas Bast

Epilepsy Center Kork, Kehl, Germany

In presurgical epilepsy evaluation, two scenarios represent the most challenging situations regarding the identification of an epileptogenic zone: too many and/or widespread diffuse lesions (*i.e.*, tuberous sclerosis complex, hemispheric or multilobar lesions in patients without neurological impairment) and on the opposite side, no lesion at all or only unspecific changes identified by structural imaging. Without a doubt, MRI is one of the most important diagnostic tools in presurgical evaluation. The proportion of MR-negative (MR-) patients referred for presurgical work-up varies between 16% (Bien *et al.*, 2009) and 32% (Berg *et al.*, 2003). A survey by the ILAE Pediatric Epilepsy Surgery Survey Taskforce revealed that MRI scans were obtained in 99.5% of all operated children (Harvey *et al.*, 2008). MRI was reported to show a definite lesion in 77% of cases and a subtle or suspected lesion in 6%. A total of 17% of children were MR-. The rate of MR- patients within published surgical cohorts varies between 18% and 47% (Berg *et al.*, 2003; Bien *et al.*, 2009; McGonigal *et al.*, 2007; Paolicchi *et al.*, 2000; Scott *et al.*, 1999; Siegel *et al.*, 2001; Tellez-Zenteno *et al.*, 2010). A meta-analysis demonstrated a significantly higher rate of MR- patients in children (31% *vs.* 21% in adults) and in patients with extratemporal lobe epilepsy (ETLE) (Tellez-Zenteno *et al.*, 2010). Thus far, there is no comprehensive and generally accepted concept of how MR- children and adults with pharmacorefractory focal epilepsies should be selected for presurgical evaluation, and which diagnostic tools should be used in identifying candidates for respective modes of epilepsy surgery. Most studies on postsurgical outcome in MR- patients included mainly adults and few data has been reported for exclusively pediatric cohorts (Dorward *et al.*, 2011; Jayakar *et al.*, 2008; Paolicchi *et al.*, 2000; RamachandranNair *et al.*, 2007; Seo *et al.*, 2011). Age-dependent differences are expected since widespread and extratemporal epileptogenesis related to developmentally malformed cortex is more common in children (Jayakar *et al.*, 2008). Differentiation of monofocal and truly multifocal origin of seizures may be complicated in young children. A major reason may be the inconclusive presentation, including an apparently generalized aspect of EEG patterns and seizure semiologies in very young children. Jayakar *et al.*, stated "selection of surgical candidates varies between centers depending on the availability of collective expertise and experience in clinical, neurophysiologic and functional imaging interpretation" (2008).

The rate of operated patients following presurgical evaluation significantly correlates with the presence or absence of a MRI lesion, respectively 81% *vs.* 45% (Berg *et al.*, 2003) and 73% *vs.* 15% (Bien *et al.*, 2009). Decisions for resective surgery following invasive EEG recording (iEEG) have been made more often in MR+ cases, 91% *vs.* 54% in MR- patients (Alarcon *et al.*, 2006).

This report will give an overview on outcomes after epilepsy surgery in MR- patients with a special focus on children. Problems with definitions, the role of established and recently introduced diagnostic tools, and the question of how outcome might be improved in the future will be discussed.

■ Definitions and the role of MRI

The terms "cryptogenic" or "non-lesional" were widely used to characterize patients with epilepsy of unknown cause. However, these terms are imprecise because the methods leading to the categorization remain unclear. "Non-lesional" may be attributed to MR- patients, as well as to those with negative histopathology (Bien *et al.*, 2009; Tellez-Zenteno *et al.*, 2010). A negative MRI does not automatically mean that the etiology will remain unclear after resection. About one third to two thirds of all resective specimens of MR- patients show specific pathological lesions that are commonly related to epileptogenicity (Alarcon *et al.*, 2006; Bell *et al.*, 2009; Bien *et al.*, 2009; Chapman *et al.*, 2005; Cukiert *et al.*, 2001; Hong *et al.*, 2002; Lee *et al.*, 2005; McGonigal *et al.*, 2007; Siegel *et al.*, 2001; Sylaja *et al.*, 2004). Methods of imaging have failed to detect the underlying structural cause of epilepsy in these cases. Most studies found focal cortical dysplasia (FCD) to be the most frequent identifiable etiology in MR- ETLE (Bien *et al.*, 2009; Brodbeck *et al.*, 2010; Chapman *et al.*, 2005; Cukiert *et al.*, 2001; Lee *et al.*, 2005; RamachandranNair *et al.*, 2007; Seo *et al.*, 2011; Wu *et al.*, 2012). Because pathology is available only after resection, the term "non-lesional" is not practical for the decision to operate. During evaluation, structural MRI is the gold standard in identifying clear candidates for epilepsy surgery. Complicated cases requiring extensive and multimodal work-up are exempt from this group. It is proposed here to use the term "MRI negative" to characterize this challenging subgroup of focal epilepsies.

However, the definition of "MR-" is controversial. The rate of positive findings depends on the techniques used. These should be established, reported and eventually compared. In addition, the experience of the reviewer plays a vital role which cannot easily be controlled or compared. This especially applies to studies on new diagnostic methods. Compared to the 1990s, the MRI technique is currently under rapid development with the introduction of high-field 3T MRI in clinical routine and the application of new methods (diffusion tensor imaging (DTI), voxel based post-processing, etc.). Presumably, patients with a previous MR- classification may actually be MR+. Therefore, a comparison between previous and current MR- patients may be inaccurate or even impossible.

The problem of MRI negativity was highlighted by a study from Bonn (von Oertzen *et al.*, 2002). Non-experts found lesions in routine MRI in only 39% of patients with a histopathological substrate. The rate of MR+ increased to 50% when the same routine MRIs were reviewed by experts. Epilepsy dedicated high-resolution MRI had a sensitivity of 91%. A MRI lesion was detected in 85% of standard MR- patients. The number of MR+ patients increases in post-hoc analysis compared to presurgical evaluation if the reviewer knows about the underlying pathological substrate. With the knowledge of the pathological substrate, Bien et al. carefully re-analyzed MRI after surgery and detected the underlying lesion in eight out of nine previously MR- patients (2009).

Although 3T MRI has become the standard in presurgical epilepsy evaluation, few data exist on its potential superiority over 1.5T in identifying candidates. Most important would be an improvement in the surgical outcome but this has yet to be demonstrated. Knake et al. applied 3T phase array MRI in 23 patients with previously negative 1.5T MRI and found lesions in 15 (65%) (Knake et al., 2005). One significant shortcoming was that 1.5T MRIs were analyzed only by the radiologists of the referring centers and not by a central, blinded reviewer. In addition, effects from phase array and 3T field techniques could not be differentiated. Other studies reported lower rates (5.6% to 20%) of newly detected lesions in 3T MRI (Nguyen et al., 2010; Strandberg et al., 2008). Interestingly, 3T is not necessarily the superior MRI (Zijlmans et al., 2009). Two experienced blinded neuroradiologists reevaluated 1.5T and 3T MRI with phased-array coils of 37 patients considered ineligible for surgery. One found 22 lesions in both 1.5T and 3T, and surprisingly the other detected more lesions in 1.5T (28 *vs.* 20 in 3T).

Methods of postprocessing may increase the rate of MR+ patients in presurgical evaluation. Voxel-based morphometric postprocessing of 3D-T1 data may detect lesions independently from the experience of the reviewer (Huppertz et al., 2005). The method was compared to visual evaluation in 91 patients with defined FCD type 2 (FCD2a 17, FCD2b 74) (Wagner et al., 2011). Whereas both approaches detected FCD2b in the same high proportion (92% *vs.* 91%), morphometric analysis was superior in detecting FCD2a (82% *vs.* 65%). Most importantly, the combination of morphometry with visual inspection was significantly more sensitive as compared to visual evaluation alone (98% *vs.* 86%). Voxel-based analysis based on 3T FLAIR may lead to even higher rates of FCD detection (Riney et al., 2012). FLAIR morphometry was correct in 7/8 cases compared to 3/8 for T1. DTI has been shown to provide additional information in patients with MR- ETLE in a multimodal diagnostic setting (Thivard et al., 2011). It is difficult to detect discrete malformations in infants under the age of two because of their immature myelination. Before 6 months of age, MRI may detect FCD with a typically low T2 signal. Thereafter, lesions may become less apparent or even disappear during maturation before myelination is complete (Duprez et al., 1998, Eltze et al., 2005). MRI negativity under two years of age requires repetition in later life.

Advanced techniques may detect abnormalities in about 50% of patients with a previously negative MRI (Koepp and Woermann 2005). However, these abnormalities do not necessarily correlate with the epileptogenic zone as revealed by functional methods. Increasing sensitivity of imaging methods may unintentionally increase the number of innocuous lesions. At best, these lesions confuse the neurologist. At worst, the placement of invasive electrodes or even resections may be incorrect.

Thus, interpretation of structural imaging requires a context of clinical findings and information from functional studies.

■ Seizure outcome after surgery of MRI-negative focal epilepsy

Many studies reported on the postoperative outcome in MR- cohorts of adults and some children (Table I). Some studies were intended to demonstrate the clinical value of new diagnostic methods. Only few studies exclusively focused on children and adolescents.

The largest group of 102 operated MR- children and adolescents (age 0.5 to 21 years, mean 10.7 years; 93 patients < 18 years) was reported by the Miami group (Jayakar et al., 2008). Eighty out of 102 underwent extra-operative long-term invasive EEG recording (iEEG). Seizure freedom rates after 2, 5 and 10 years were 44%, 44% and 38%, respectively. A seizure reduction of at least 90% was achieved in 58%, 59% and 68%. Dorward et al. investigated 33 children that underwent surgery for MR- ETLE (2011). Procedures included resections and multiple subpial transections (MST). Engel 1 outcome was achieved in 42.4%. Seven of 14 MR- children who underwent multimodal functional imaging and resections between 2006 and 2009 became seizure-free (Seo et al., 2011). During this period a total of 25 MR- children were operated at this center with 12 (48%) rendered seizure-free. RamachandranNair et al. investigated the impact of magnetoencephalography (MEG) and invasive EEG (iEEG) on operations in 22 MR- children (2007). Eight (36%) became seizure-free and 17 (77%) had at least an Engel 3a outcome.

A recent review and meta-analysis compared surgical outcome for lesional and non-lesional epilepsy (Tellez-Zenteno et al., 2010). Ninety-two articles published from 1995 to 2007 were summarized and 40 entered the meta-analysis. The analysis compared results from 697 patients with non-lesional epilepsy to 2,860 patients with lesional epilepsy. Absence of a lesion was a clear negative predictor regarding a seizure-free outcome. There were no significant differences between children and adults. It made no difference whether a non-lesional status was based on MRI or histopathology.

The rate of seizure-free MR- patients was 46% (95% CI 39-46) compared to 70% (95% CI 68-73) of MR+ patients. The odds ratio for seizure-free outcome in MR+ patients was 2.4 (95% CI 1.8-3.2). In ETLE, a seizure-free outcome was achieved in 60% (54-66) of MR+ patients compared to 35% (27-42) of MR- patients. The results of children were not significantly different. In children, only results for non-lesional cases with a classification based on either MRI or histopathology were reported. The seizure freedom rate was 45% (35-55) in 93 children without a lesion compared to 74% (69-79) in 317 lesional cases.

A methodological shortcoming of this meta-analysis is the inability to separate contributive factors like type of MRI, results of invasive recordings and functional imaging, type of surgery and many others. Only one study included in the review exclusively reported on children (Paolicchi et al., 2000). The study included 75 out of 83 operated children under the age of 12. All 35 MR- and 20 out of 40 MR+ cases underwent iEEG with subdural electrodes. The high rate of MR- patients may be attributed to the local characteristics of the center in Miami with corresponding referrals. A high rate of children was investigated with only 0.5 T MRI. A total of 59% became seizure-free after surgery without a significant difference between 35 MR- and 40 MR+ cases (56% vs. 70%). A seizure reduction of > 90% was observed in 80% in MR+ and 67% in MR- children.

The lack of a MRI lesion led to a significantly lower seizure freedom rate (38% vs. 66% in MR+) in 29 MR- and 736 MR+ patients operated upon at the Epilepsy Center in Bonn (Bien et al., 2009). While 7/9 MR- patients with definite histopathological lesions became seizure free, the rate was only 4/20 in patients with normal or unspecific pathology. McGonigal et al. (2007) reported on the outcome in 60 patients operated after evaluation by

Table I. Seizure outcomes in MR patients

First author	Year of publication	Cohort	Aim of study	N	Period of recruitment	Follow-up (y)	Seizure free outcome (%)	Outcome Engel 1 (%)	Outcome other (%)
Tellez-Zenteno	2010	C+A	Meta-analysis for comparing MR+ anc MR-	398	1995-2007	≥ 1	43		
Bell	2009	C		93			45		
Bien	2009	C+A	Outcome MR- TLE	40	1997-2005	≥ 1	60		
Chapman	2005	C+A	Outcome MR+ and MR-	29	2000-2006	≥ 0.5	38	45	
Cukiert	2001	C+A	Outcome MR-	24	1994-2001	≥ 1	37	45	
Dorward	2011	C+A	Outcome and iEEG n MR-/diffuse MRI	10	1997-2000	≥ 1	90		
Jayakar	2008	C	Outcome in MR- ET_E	22	1994-2007	≥ 2		36	
Krsek	2009	C(+A)	Outcome MR-	102	?	≥ 2	44		
Lee	2005	C (+A)	FCD study	26	1986-2006	≥ 2		54	
McGonigal	2007	C+A	Outcome MR-	89	1995-2002	≥ 2	47		
Park	2002	C+A	iEEG	20	2000-2006	1	55		
Ramachandran Nair	2007	C+A	iEEG	18	1995-2000	≥ 1			> 90% seizure reduction: 44
Schneider	2012	C	Functional imaging	22	1998-2005	≥ 0.75	36		< Engel 3a:77
Seo	2011	C+A	Functional imaging	18	2008-2010	≥ 2	56		
Siegel	2001	C	Functional imaging	25	2006-2009	≥ 1	48		
Thivard	2011	A	MR- outcome	24	1992-1999	≥ 2		83	
Wetjen	2009	A	(Functional) imaging	12	2003-2006	N.R.		67	
Wu	2012	C+A	iEEG and MR- outcome	28	1992-2002	> 1	36	50	
Zhang	2012	A	Functional imaging	18	1990-2009	≥ 1	22		Engel 1+2: 55
	2011	C+A	Functional imaging	20	2006-2009	≥ 1	35		

N: number of patients; C: children; A: adults; (A): young adults; iEEG: invasive long-term EEG recording; Number: number of operated MR cases; N.R.: not reported stereo-EEG. Seizure freedom rates did not differ between the MR- and MR+ group (MR-11/20 = 55%, MR+ 21/40 = 53%). In the context of a MEG study, Zhang et al. reported 20 MR- and 23 MR+ operated patients (Zhang et al., 2011). The seizure freedom rate was significantly lower in MR- patients (35%) compared to MR+ cases (65.2%).

The outcome after surgery for MR- frontal lobe epilepsy is inconclusive. While some studies reported a poorer outcome compared to MR+ cases (Jeha et al., 2007; Elsharkawy et al., 2008), a recent study found no differences in seizure control between MR- (15/26 = 58% seizure-free) and MR+ (17/32 = 53%) cases (Lazow et al., 2012).

■ Subgroup of focal cortical dysplasia

FCD is the most common histopathological finding in children surgically treated for epilepsy (Harvey et al., 2008). Up to 25% of pathologically confirmed FCD in adults remains MR- (Widdes-Walsh et al., 2006). Data from studies comparing postoperative outcomes in MR+ and MR- FCD are inconclusive. Some studies found a significantly poorer outcome in MR- cases (Cossu et al., 2008; Siegel et al., 2001; Phi et al., 2010), while others did not find any differences (Hader et al., 2004; Krsek et al., 2009; Park et al., 2006; Siegel et al., 2006; Widdes-Walsh et al., 2007).

Park et al. studied 30 children, ages 1.5 to 18.3 years, with FCD (2006). Six patients had dual pathology with a tumor and FCD. Engel outcome 1 was achieved in 67% of children. Six out of 8 MR-patients had a favorable outcome (Engel 1 and 2), not differing from MR+ patients. Krsek et al. investigated 144 children and adolescents (< 20 years) and 5 young adults (20-25 years) who were operated at Miami Children's Hospital (2009). Presurgical MRIs (108 1.5 T, 41 0.5 T) were re-evaluated. The MRI was negative in 26 patients. One hundred patients including all MR- children underwent iEEG. Seizure outcome did not differ between patients that were MR- (Engel 1 in 54%) and MR+ (55%). In contrast to these studies, Phi et al. from Seoul found a significant difference in univariate analysis regarding seizure outcome between MR- and MR+ histopathologically proven FCD (2010). Out of 41 children with FCD, 49% became seizure-free one year after surgery and 33% remained seizure free after 5 years. The exact rate of seizure-free outcome in 19 MR- children was not specified in the text.

■ How can outcome be predicted and potentially improved?

In the subgroup of MR- patients with a histopathological substrate, advances in structural MRI are crucial for improving their outcome. Cases with negative pathology represent a different entity of epilepsies and an improvement of only structural imaging will most likely not influence their outcome (Bien et al., 2009). The underlying pathophysiological mechanisms may be related to disturbed network connections and functions acting on a submicroscopic level. There is hope that multimodal functional imaging may improve selection of patients and postsurgical outcome in both MR- patients with and without a lesion in histopathology. Different methods have been studied. Most studies were observational and monocentric leading to a bias in recruitment of patients. The outcome of surgery may be better when only patients with positive results of a specific diagnostic method are included.

Higher rates of seizure-free outcome have been demonstrated in patients with unifocal clusters of interictal MEG-dipoles and complete resection of the identified zone compared to multifocal or widespread activity and/or incomplete resection (RamachandranNair, 2007; Schneider et al., 2012; Wu et al., 2012; Zhang et al., 2011). Electrical source imaging (ESI) in EEG from dense array surface electrodes was applied in 10 MR- patients (Brodbeck et al., 2010). Resection covered the interictal spike zone identified by ESI in 8 patients and the outcome was favorable in all of them. The other two patients had outcome Engel 1 and Engel 4.

Fluoro-2-desoxy-D-glucose positron emission tomography (FDG-PET) may contribute crucial information in young children with severe epileptic encephalopathies (Chugani et al., 1990). Resection of hypometabolic areas revealed by FDG-PET may (Lee et al., 2005) or may not (Dorward et al., 2011) correlate with a better outcome in MR- cases.

Ictal single-photon emission computed tomography (SPECT) and especially subtracted ictal–interictal SPECT (SISCOM) (coregistered with MRI) may add substantial information in MR- cases. High concordance of areas with ictal hyperperfusion and the epileptogenic zone, as defined by iEEG has been demonstrated (Seo et al., 2011). A higher rate of seizure-free outcome in cases with complete resection of the areas of hyperperfusion has been described (Bell et al., 2009). Discordance of SISCOM results was related to poor outcomes in MR- patients (Bien et al., 2009). However, some studies did not find any correlation between SPECT results and the outcome (Chapman et al., 2005, Jayakar et al., 2008, Lee et al., 2005).

The vast majority of the patients with MR- epilepsy have to be investigated by invasive recordings before a final decision for and a tailoring of resection is possible. Complete resection of the seizure-onset zone as defined by invasive recordings leads to higher seizure freedom rates (Blume et al., 2004, RamachandranNair et al., 2007, Schneider et al., 2012, Wetjen et al., 2009). There is some evidence that resection of seizure zones presenting with high-frequent oscillations as onset activity may be associated with better outcome compared to other types of ictal activity (Park et al., 2002, Wetjen et al., 2009). In patients with frontal lobe epilepsies, success rates in localizing seizure onset by stereo-EEG were identical in MR- and MR+ cases (McGonigal et al., 2007).

Convergent results of several non-invasive functional studies in a multimodal approach may avoid the necessity of iEEG in some patients (Jayakar et al., 2008). In this study, 20/102 children underwent resective surgery for MR- epilepsy without invasive recordings. The outcome also correlated with the presence of focal interictal spike discharges on the scalp EEG convergent with the resected area. Whereas SPECT was not correlated with the outcome, a favorable outcome was more frequent in cases with a complete resection of the epileptogenic zone as defined by the combination of SPECT and focal interictal spikes. Bien et al., analyzed the value of semiology, interictal and ictal surface EEG, PET, SPECT, SISCOM and MRI postprocessing in MR- patients (Bien et al., 2009). Postprocessing and semiology rarely provided localization information, but when they did, positive and negative predictive values were high. Concordant information from semiology, interictal surface EEG and MRI postprocessing were predictive for a good outcome whereas discordance from semiology, interictal surface EEG, MRI postprocessing and SISCOM predicted poor seizure outcome. Seo et al., scored concordance of MEG, PET and SISCOM with iEEG in MR- children and found a tendency towards better outcomes in patients with higher cumulative scores (Seo et al., 2011). A combination of lack of contralateral interictal spikes with complete resection of the

SISCOM-identified zone of hyperperfusion and unspecific MRI findings correlated with a high rate of seizure-free patients with MR- temporal lobe epilepsies (Bell et al., 2009). Thivard et al., compared sensitivity and specificity of PET (visual and statistical analysis), DTI and voxel-based morphometry in 20 MR- patients (Thivard et al., 2011). Unblinded visually analyzed PET had the highest sensitivity. However, DTI was superior in ETLE and had the overall highest specificity. A combination of PET with DTI resulted in an increase of sensitivity in mesial temporal lobe epilepsy and frontal lobe epilepsy, but not in lateral temporal lobe epilepsy.

The diagnostic value of each non-invasive method and the optimal combination in multimodal work-up remain unclear. It should be noted that concordant results of two or more repeated presurgical evaluations may be a useful approach to selecting appropriate candidates for surgery and may help to avoid invasive procedures in unpromising cases (Lee et al., 2005; Jayakar 2008).

■ Risks of surgery in cases with normal pathology?

Resection of a pathologically proven lesion should not be related to a higher risk of neurocognitive impairment following surgery when comparing MR- and MR+ focal epilepsies. However, normal histopathology can be found in one third to two thirds of the specimens. Helmstaedter et al. hypothesized that temporal lobe resections in MR- adults with normal histopathology may result in a more severe loss of memory function compared to lesional cases (Helmstaedter et al., 2011). They compared 15 MR- patients with normal pathology to 15 matched controls (MR+, positive histopathology). While preoperative memory functions were significantly better in patients with normal histopathology, these patients experienced a marked decrease in function after resection. Postoperative performance was comparably low in both groups. The authors conclude that surgery should be considered with caution in temporal lobe epilepsy patients with normal MRI and normal memory function.

There is no comparable study in children. Dorward et al. analyzed seizure and neurocognitive outcome in 33 patients after surgery for MR- ETLE (Dorward et al., 2011). Pre- and postoperative neuropsychological assessments were conducted in 23 children. Intellectual functioning measured by full-scale IQ was stable. Children with left-sided resection demonstrated significant improvements in performance IQ and performance on a measure of nonverbal reasoning. Other tested domains remained unchanged. A shortcoming is the inclusion of patients with different kinds of surgical procedures among which a considerable number of multiple subpial transections (MST) with or without resection. Potential differences between 14 children with normal pathology and 18 with a histopathological substrate were not tested.

■ Conservative treatment of MR- focal epilepsy

Wirrell et al. reported the long-term outcome of childhood onset focal epilepsies (2011) and noticed a seizure free period of at least 12 months before the end of the follow-up was in 81% out of 215 patients with non-idiopathic focal epilepsies. 77% MR- patients became seizure free. This is in concordance with other reports on the outcome in non-idiopathic focal that are summarized in chapter "Outcome after non-surgical treatment of MRI-negative non-idiopathic focal epilepsies" by C. Camfield.

It has been shown in adults that etiology of focal epilepsies is a major prognostic factor (Semah et al., 1999). In this hospital based study from Paris, a total of 2,200 adult outpatients were included in an observational survey. Partial epilepsies were diagnosed in 62%. Seizure control (> 1 year) was achieved in 45% of 408 patients with cryptogenic focal epilepsies compared to 35% of 535 with symptomatic etiology. However, seizure control required polytherapy in the majority of patients.

These rates of seizure control in cryptogenic focal epilepsies markedly differ from reported outcomes following epilepsy surgery in MR- patients. However, the cohorts are all but comparable with respect to the quality of applied imaging. It is of importance that only patients with drug resistance enter presurgical programs and thus represent a complicated subset of patients with cryptogenic epilepsies. There is only one study comparing seizure outcome between operated and conservatively treated MR- patients who all underwent presurgical work-up (Bien et al., 2009). In the years 2000-2006 a total number of 1,192 patients (children > 0.5 years and adults) underwent presurgical evaluation at the Epilepsy Center in Bonn. A clear MRI lesion was found in 1,002 patients. Surgery was performed on 736 of them. From the MR- group, 29 out of 190 patients underwent surgery. Conservative treatment led to a significantly lower rate of seizure freedom in MR- cases (19/120 with documented follow-up, 16%) compared to surgically treated MR- patients (38%). The response to antiepileptic drugs was comparable to conservatively treated MR+ patients (22/142 with documented follow-up, 15%).

Despite the difficulties in diagnostic work-up and the higher rate of evaluations not resulting in surgery, these results clearly demonstrate the value of epilepsy surgery in this challenging population.

Concluding remarks

Epilepsy surgery should be considered in children with pharmacorefractory non-idiopathic focal epilepsies even in the absence of a potentially epileptogenic lesion in structural MRI. It seems that epilepsy surgery is superior to further antiepileptic treatment in this challenging group of patients with pharmacoresistant epilepsy.

References

- Alarcón G, Valentín A, Watt C, et al. Is it worth pursuing surgery for epilepsy in patients with normal neuroimaging? *J Neurol Neurosurg Psychiatr* 2006; 77: 474-80.
- Bell ML, Rao S, So EL, et al. Epilepsy surgery outcomes in temporal lobe epilepsy with a normal MRI. *Epilepsia* 2009; 50: 2053-60.
- Berg AT, Vickrey BG, Langfitt JT, et al. The multicenter study of epilepsy surgery: recruitment and selection for surgery. *Epilepsia* 2003; 44: 1425-33.
- Bien CG, Szinay M, Wagner J, Clusmann H, Becker AJ, Urbach H. Characteristics and surgical outcomes of patients with refractory magnetic resonance imaging-negative epilepsies. *Arch Neurol* 2009; 66: 1491-9.
- Brodbeck V, Spinelli L, Lascano AM, et al. Electrical source imaging for presurgical focus localization in epilepsy patients with normal MRI. *Epilepsia* 2010; 51: 583-91.
- Camfield P, Camfield C. Epileptic syndromes in childhood: clinical features, outcomes, and treatment. *Epilepsia* 2002; 43 (Suppl 3): 27-32.

- Chapman K, Wyllie E, Najm I, et al. Seizure outcome after epilepsy surgery in patients with normal preoperative MRI. *J Neurol Neurosurg Psychiatr* 2005; 76: 710-3.
- Chugani HT, Shewmon DA, Shields WD, et al. Surgery for intractable infantile spasms: Neuroimaging perspectives. *Epilepsia* 1993; 34: 764-71.
- Cukiert A, Buratini JA, Machado E, et al. Results of surgery in patients with refractory extratemporal epilepsy with normal or nonlocalizing magnetic resonance findings investigated with subdural grids. *Epilepsia* 2001; 42: 889-94.
- Dorward IG, Titus JB, Limbrick DD, Johnston JM, Bertrand ME, Smyth MD. Extratemporal, nonlesional epilepsy in children: postsurgical clinical and neurocognitive outcomes. *J Neurosurg Pediatr* 2011; 7: 179-88.
- Elsharkawy AE, Alabbasi AH, Pannek H, et al. Outcome of frontal lobe epilepsy surgery in adults. *Epilepsy Res* 2008; 8: 97-106.
- Focke NK, Symms MR, Burdett JL, Duncan JS. Voxel-based analysis of whole brain FLAIR at 3T detects focal cortical dysplasia. *Epilepsia* 2008; 49: 786-93.
- Hader WJ, Mackay M, Otsubo H, et al. Cortical dysplastic lesions in children with intractable epilepsy: role of complete resection. *J Neurosurg* 2004; 100 (2 Suppl Pediatrics): 110-17.
- Harvey AS, Cross JH, Shinnar S, Mathern BW; ILAE Pediatric Epilepsy Surgery Survey Taskforce. Defining the spectrum of international practice in pediatric epilepsy surgery patients. *Epilepsia* 2008; 49: 146-55.
- Helmstaedter C, Petzold I, Bien CG. The cognitive consequence of resecting nonlesional tissues in epilepsy surgery-results from MRI- and histopathology-negative patients with temporal lobe epilepsy. *Epilepsia* 2011; 52: 1402-8.
- Hong KS, Lee SK, Kim JY Lee DS, Chung CK. Pre-surgical evaluation and surgical outcome of 41 patients with non-lesional neocortical epilepsy. *Seizure* 2002; 11: 184-92.
- Huppertz HJ, Grimm C, Fauser S, et al. Enhanced visualization of blurred graywhite matter junctions in focal cortical dysplasia by voxel-based 3D MRI analysis. *Epilepsy Res* 2005; 67 (1-2): 35-50.
- Jayakar P, Dunoyer C, Dean P, et al. Epilepsy surgery in patients with normal or nonfocal MRI scans: integrative strategies offer long-term seizure relief. *Epilepsia* 2008; 49: 758-64.
- Jeha LE, Najm I, Bingaman W, Dinner D, Widdess-Walsh P, Lüders H. Surgical outcome and prognostic factors of frontal lobe epilepsy surgery. *Brain* 2007; 130: 574-84.
- Knake S, Triantafyllou C, Wald LL, et al. 3T phased array MRI improves the presurgical evaluation in focal epilepsies: a prospective study. *Neurology* 2005; 65: 1026-31.
- Koepp MJ, Woermann FG. Imaging structure and function in refractory partial epilepsy. *Lancet Neurol* 2005; 4: 42-53.
- Krsek P, Maton B, Jayakar P, et al. Incomplete resection of focal cortical dysplasia is the main predictor of poor postsurgical outcome. *Neurology* 2009; 72: 217-23.
- Kuba R, Tyrlíková I, Chrastina J, et al. "MRI-negative PET-positive" temporal lobe epilepsy: invasive EEG findings, histopathology, and postoperative outcomes. *Epilepsy Behav* 2011; 22: 537-41.
- Lazow SP, Thadani VM, Gilbert KL, et al. Outcome of frontal lobe epilepsy surgery. *Epilepsia* 2012; 53: 1746-55.
- Lee SK, Lee SY, Kim KK, Hong KS, Lee DS, Chung CK. Surgical outcome and prognostic factors of cryptogenic neocortical epilepsy. *Ann Neurol* 2005; 58: 525-32.
- McGonigal A, Bartolomei F, Regis J, et al. Stereoelectroencephalography in presurgical assessment of MRI-negative epilepsy. *Brain* 2007; 130: 3169-83.
- Nguyen DK, Rochette E, Leroux JM, et al. Value of 3.0 T MR imaging in refractory partial epilepsy and negative 1.5 T MRI. *Seizure* 2010; 19: 475-8.

- Paolicchi JM, Jayakar P, Dean P, et al. Predictors of outcome in pediatric epilepsy surgery. *Neurology* 2000; 54, 642-7.
- Park SA, Lim SR, Kim GS, et al. Ictal electrocorticographic findings related with surgical outcomes in nonlesional neocortical epilepsy. *Epilepsy Res* 2002; 48: 199-206.
- Park CK, Kim SK, Wang KC, et al. Surgical outcome and prognostic factors of pediatric epilepsy caused by cortical dysplasia. *Childs Nerv Syst* 2006; 22: 586-92.
- Phi JH, Cho BK, Wang KC, et al. Longitudinal analyses of the surgical outcomes of pediatric epilepsy patients with focal cortical dysplasia. *J Neurosurg Pediatr* 2010; 6: 49-56.
- RamachandranNair R, Otsubo H, Shroff MM, et al. MEG predicts outcome following surgery for intractable epilepsy in children with normal or nonfocal MRI findings. *Epilepsia* 2007; 48: 149-57.
- Riney CJ, Chong WK, Clark CA, Cross JH. Voxel based morphometry of FLAIR MRI in children with intractable focal epilepsy: implications for surgical intervention. *Eur J Radiol* 2012; 81: 1299-305.
- Schneider F, Alexopoulos AV, Wang Z, et al. Magnetic source imaging in non-lesional neocortical epilepsy: additional value and comparison with ICEEG. *Epilepsy Behav* 2012; 24: 234-40.
- Scott CA, Fish DR, Smith SJ, et al. Presurgical evaluation of patients with epilepsy and normal MRI: role of scalp video-EEG telemetry. *J Neurol Neurosurg Psychiatr* 1999; 66: 69-71.
- Semah F, Picot MC, Adam C, et al. Is the underlying cause of epilepsy a major prognostic factor for recurrence? *Neurology* 1998; 51: 1256-62.
- Seo JH, Holland K, Rose D, et al. Multimodality imaging in the surgical treatment of children with nonlesional epilepsy. *Neurology* 2011; 76: 41-8.
- Shinnar S, O'Dell C, Berg AT. Distribution of epilepsy syndromes in a cohort of children prospectively monitored from the time of their first unprovoked seizure. *Epilepsia* 1999; 40: 1378-83.
- Siegel AM, Jobst BC, Thadani VM, et al. Medically intractable, localization-related epilepsy with normal MRI: presurgical evaluation and surgical outcome in 43 patients. *Epilepsia* 2001; 42: 883-8.
- Siegel AM, Cascino GD, Meyer FB, Marsh WR, Scheithauer BW, Sharbrough FW. Surgical outcome and predictive factors in adult patients with intractable epilepsy and focal cortical dysplasia. *Acta Neurol Scand* 2006; 113: 65-71.
- Sillanpaa M, Jalava M, Kaleva O, Shinnar S. Long-term prognosis of seizures with onset in childhood. *N Engl J Med* 1998; 338: 1715-22.
- Strandberg M, Larsson EM, Backman S, Källén K. Pre-surgical epilepsy evaluation using 3T MRI. Do surface coils provide additional information? *Epileptic Disord* 2008; 10: 83-92.
- Sylaja PN, Radhakrishnan K, Kesavadas C, Sarma PS. Seizure outcome after anterior temporal lobectomy and its predictors in patients with apparent temporal lobe epilepsy and normal MRI. *Epilepsia* 2004; 45: 803-8.
- Téllez-Zenteno JF, Hernández Ronquillo L, Moien-Afshari F, Wiebe S. Surgical outcomes in lesional and non-lesional epilepsy: a systematic review and meta-analysis. *Epilepsy Res* 2010; 89: 310-8.
- Thivard L, Bouilleret V, Chassoux F, Adam C, Dormont D, Baulac M, et al. Diffusion tensor imaging can localize the epileptogenic zone in nonlesional extra-temporal refractory epilepsies when [(18)F]FDG-PET is not contributive. *Epilepsy Res* 2011; 97: 170-82.
- Von Oertzen J, Urbach H, Jungbluth S, Kurthen M, Reuber M, Fernández G, et al. Standard magnetic resonance imaging is inadequate for patients with refractory focal epilepsy. *J Neurol Neurosurg Psychiatr* 2002; 73: 643-7.
- Wagner J, Weber B, Urbach H, Elger CE, Huppertz HJ. Morphometric MRI analysis improves detection of focal cortical dysplasia type II. *Brain* 2011; 134: 2844-54.
- Wang ZI, Jones SE, Ristic AJ, et al. Voxel-based morphometric MRI post-processing in MRI-negative focal cortical dysplasia followed by simultaneously recorded MEG and stereo-EEG. *Epilepsy Res* 2012; 100: 188-93.

- Wetjen NM, Marsh WR, Meyer FB, et al. Intracranial electroencephalography seizure onset patterns and surgical outcomes in nonlesional extratemporal epilepsy. Clinical article. *J Neurosurg* 2009; 110: 1147-52.
- Widdess-Walsh P, Diehl B, Najm I. Neuroimaging of focal cortical dysplasia. *J Neuroimaging* 2006; 16: 185-96.
- Widdess-Walsh P, Jeha L, Nair D, Kotagal P, Bingaman W, Najm I. Subdural electrode analysis in focal cortical dysplasia: predictors of surgical outcome. *Neurology* 2007; 69: 660-7.
- Wirrell EC, Grossardt BR, So EL, Nickels KC. A population-based study of long-term outcomes of cryptogenic focal epilepsy in childhood: cryptogenic epilepsy is probably not symptomatic epilepsy. *Epilepsia* 2011; 52: 738-45.
- Wu XT, Rampp S, Buchfelder M, et al. Interictal magnetoencephalography used in magnetic resonance imaging-negative patients with epilepsy. *Acta Neurol Scand* 2012 [Epub ahead of print].
- Zhang R, Wu T, Wang Y, et al. Interictal magnetoencephalographic findings related with surgical outcomes in lesional and nonlesional neocortical epilepsy. *Seizure* 2011; 20: 692-700.
- Zijlmans M, de Kort GAP, Witkamp TD, et al. 3 T versus 1.5 T phased-array MRI in the presurgical work-up of patients with partial epilepsy of uncertain focus. *J Magn Reson Imaging* 2009; 30: 256-62.

Outcome when malformations of cortical development (MCD) are the cause

Hans Holthausen[1], Tom Pieper[1], Manfred Kudernatsch[2], Ingmar Blümcke[3]

[1] *Neuropediatric Clinic and Clinic for Neurorehabilitation, Epilepsy Center for Children and Adolescents, Schön-Klinik Vogtareuth, Germany*
[2] *Neurosurgery Clinic and Clinic for Epilepsy Surgery, Schön-Klinik Vogtareuth, Germany*
[3] *Neuropathological Institut, University Tübingen, Germany*

Focal cortical dysplasias (FCD) are subtypes of malformations of cortical development (MCD). In the Barkovich-classification of the MCDs, FCD type II (FCD II) are listed in the "full classification scheme" in the category "cortical dysgenesis with abnormal cell proliferation but without neoplasia" and FCD type I (FCD I) in the category" focal cortical dysplasias (without dysmorphic neurons) due to late developmental disturbances" (Barkovich *et al.*, 2012). This classification system, which is regularly updated, tries to incorporate genetic, imaging and neuropathological aspects – as well as hypothetical considerations in order to create the best possible classification of all kinds of MCDs. Classification systems exclusively for FCD and dealing more directly with epilepsy surgery issues have been in use for many years (Tassi *et al.*, 2002; Palmini *et al.*, 2004), and have recently been revised by an "*ad-hoc* Task Force of the ILAE Diagnostic Methods Commission" (Blümcke *et al.*, 2011). This revised classification has rapidly become widely accepted (*Table I*).

The prevalence of FCD in the pediatric population with focal epilepsy is not exactly known because earlier publications, in which were listed the underlying etiologies of medically treated cohorts, did not report FCD separately from other types of MCD. The percentage of children with "disorders of cortical development" in a large population-based study of children with epilepsy from Italy was 14,7% (Alexandre Jr. *et al.*, 2012). Considering that FCD are certainly heavily represented in this etiology group, the estimation by Bast *et al.* (2006) of a prevalence of 5%-10%, based on their review of the literature, is certainly not too high. Seizures caused by FCD are more difficult to control by medication than is the case in most other etiologies of focal epilepsies; a lower response rate is seen only in mesial temporal lobe epilepsy (Stephen *et al.*, 2001). FCD are the cause in about 50% of children operated on because of drug-resistant seizures (Harvey et al., 2008; Lerner et al., 2009; Hemb et al., 2011; Kessler-Uberti et al., 2011; D'Argenzio et al., 2012) – in contrast to epilepsy surgery for adults where FCD come on third place, after mesio-temporal sclerosis (MTS) and benign tumors (Lerner et al., 2009; Blümcke et al., 2009; Blümcke & Spreafico, 2012). Seventy five percent of MCD in pediatric surgical series are FCD (Blümcke et al., 2009).

Table I. The new ILAE-classification of FCDs (with permission from Blumcke et al., Epilepsia, 2011)

FCD type I (isolated)	Focal cortical dysplasia with abnormal radial cortical lamination (FCD type Ia)	Focal cortical dysplasia with abnormal tangential cortical lamination (FCD type Ib)	Focal cortical dysplasia with abnormal radial and tangential cortical lamination (FCD type Ic)	
FCD type II (isolated)	Focal cortical dysplasia with dysmorphic neurons (FCD type IIa)		Focal cortical dysplasia with dysmorphic neurons and balloon cells (FCD type IIb)	
FCD type III (associated with principal lesion)	Cortical lamination abnormalities in the temporal lobe associated with hippocampal sclerosis (FCD type IIIa)	Cortical lamination abnormalities adjacent to a glial or glioneuronal tumor (FCD type IIIb)	Cortical lamination abnormalities adjacent to vascular malformation (FCD type IIIc)	Cortical lamination abnormalities adjacent to any other lesion acquired during early life, e.g., trauma, ischemic injury, encephalitis (FCD type IIIc)

FCD type III (not otherwise specified, NOS): if clinically/radiologically suspected principal lesion is not available for microscopic inspection.
Please note that the rare association between FCD type IIa and IIb with hippocampal sclerosis, tumors, or vascular malformations should not be classified as FCD type III variant.

Average age at onset of epilepsy in pediatric FCD surgical series is usually before school age, many times in the first year of life (Kloss et al., 2002; Lerner et al., 2009; Krsek et al., 2009a, b). In our experience, children with FCD I are on average somewhat younger than those with FCD II (Krsek et al., 2009b; Blümcke et al., 2010), but this was not true for children with FCD I from UCLA and from the Miami Children's Hospital (Krsek et al., 2009a; Lerner et al., 2009). The average age at onset of epilepsy is somewhat older, usually at school age, in adult FCD surgical series (Hong et al., 2000; Urbach et al., 2002; Cohen-Gadol et al., 2004; Siegel et al., 2005; Tassi et al., 2010; Bien et al., 2012). Because of this, it would not be a rational approach for an analysis of factors influencing surgical outcome in children with FCD to take only the data from pediatric series and leaving out data form adult series. Therefore, data from pediatric and adult series are considered together in the following paragraphs; to discuss mental and developmental outcome only data dealing with children are reviewed.

Surgical outcome with respect to seizures: children do not differ from adults

Overall around 50-60% of patients with FCD become seizure-free after surgery and outcome figures in children are as good as in adults. This has been shown in publications from single centers where operations in both children and adults are performed (Alexandre Jr. et al., 2006), and in two meta-analyses of predictors of seizure outcome after epilepsy surgery for patients with drug-resistant seizures caused by FCD (Chern et al., 2010; Rowland et al., 2012).

Postoperative outcome and reliability of outcome data in FCD type II vs. FCD type I

The pathological changes in FCD IIa and FCD IIb (for the distinction, see *Table I*) have been well known to neuropathologists for a long time and there is a great inter-observer consensus with respect to the classification of these changes, when investigators are blinded for all other data of the patients (Chamberlain et al., 2009). The confidence in the classification of these changes as FCD II is reflected by the fact that the criteria for the diagnosis of FCD II were not changed in the recently revised ILAE classification (Blümcke et al., 2011).

In contrast, the correct classification of cortical changes like cortical dyslamination, the presence or absence of giant neurons, etc, has always been less certain. Most confusion has been created by different labeling of changes that are frequently seen in the temporal pole of patients with amygdalohippocampal sclerosis (AHS). A center judging most of these changes as FCD I will, not surprisingly because of the generally good outcome of patients with AHS, report a better outcome after surgery in patients with FCD I (Fauser et al., 2004) whereas most other centers report better outcomes in patients with FCD II (meta-analysis by Rowland et al., 2012).

The creation of a group *type III FCD* within the revised ILAE classification, for FCD found in association with primary lesions, is a major step forward for a better transparency in the comparison of outcome figures of the various studies. Recent publications, using the revised classification, show that the outcome for patients with isolated FCD I is worse in comparison to FCD II – in adults and in children (Krsek et al., 2009a, b; Tassi et al., 2010). However, there is one study in which outcome of patients with "mild FCD" (FCD I) was better than of those with "severe FCD" (FCD II; Lerner et al., 2009).

The new ILAE classification is at first glance very suggestive of having solved the uncertainties with respect to a proper judgment and classification of "mild" changes, which might be labeled as FCD Ia, Ib or Ic. But in fact inter-observer agreement was only moderate for FCD Ib and poor for FCD Ic (Coras et al., 2012). Changes labeled as FCD Ib in patients with AHS might really be acquired lesions of sclerotic rather than of dysplastic nature (Thom et al., 2009). It has also been suggested that, in contrast to epilepsies caused by FCD II, describing epilepsies as caused by FCD I without presenting additional clinical and electrophysiological information, may not be sufficient for rational group comparisons, in particular with respect to postoperative seizure outcome (Blümcke et al., 2010). Epilepsies caused by FCD I are indeed more variable than epilepsies caused by FCD II (Krsek et al., 2009a, b). No center has reported figures about the exact anatomical distribution of the different subclasses of isolated FCD I so far. Not surprisingly, postoperative seizure outcome is worst in children with large multilobar or hemispheric isolated FCD I, when hemispherectomy is not performed, *e.g.*, because patients do not have a pre-existing hemiparesis (Krsek *et al.*, 2009b), and better in (older) children and adults with more circumscribed lesions, *e.g.*, within the frontal lobe or with fronto-temporal location (Krsek *et al.*, 2009a; Tassi *et al.*, 2010). But even in these series less than 50% of the patients with FCD I became seizure-free.

In contrast, patients with FCD II outside eloquent cortical areas have a 70-90% chance of becoming seizure-free after surgery (Kloss *et al.*, 2002; Hader *et al.*, 2004; Chern *et al.*, 2010; Lerner *et al.*, 2009; Rowland *et al.*, 2012). When outcome is reported separately for FCD IIa and FCD IIb, results are better for patients with FCD IIb (Urbach *et al.*, 2002, Colombo *et al.*, 2003; Hader *et al.*, 2004; Kim *et al.*, 2009; Krsek *et al.*, 2009a,b; Colombo *et al.*, 2012). Less favorable results in FCD IIa may be explained by the fact that this type is less clearly visible on MRI than FCD IIb, and often cannot be exactly delineated. The lesion may even be completely invisible on MRI and be diagnosed only pathologically (Colombo *et al.*, 2012).

Factors associated with postoperative seizure outcome other than subtypes of FCD

Complete resection of the lesion as it is seen on MRI is the most important factor to render patients seizure-free. Further variables associated with a more favorable seizure outcome are a positive MRI, focal seizures (*vs.* generalized seizures) and a temporal location (Rowland *et al.*, 2012). The main reason for incomplete resection is overlap with or close vicinity to eloquent cortical areas. More than 70% of children with frontal and temporal FCD became seizure-free in the series reported by Kloss *et al.*, (2002) but less than 40% with lesions within the central and parieto-occipital areas. In most studies results are better in more circumscribed lesions and in lobar resections in comparison to multilobar resections. Surprisingly, the meta-analysis by Rowland *et al.* (2012) found that "identification of an ictal-onset zone did not appear to make any difference with respect to seizure outcome at last follow up". However, the authors did not evaluate the predictive value of complete vs. incomplete resection of cortical areas generating the specific EEG pattern called variously ictal-like pattern (Palmini *et al.*, 1994), continuous epileptiform discharges (Gambardella *et al.*, 1996), FEDOIS (frequent epileptiform discharges on irregular slow activity – Holthausen *et al.*, 1997) or polyspike brushes (Tassi *et al.*, 2012). There is no doubt that a complete resection of the cortical area generating this peculiar pathological pattern is a prerequisite for a good seizure outcome.

Long-term outcome of FCD patients who are seizure-free after surgery

An increasing number of publications is dealing with long-term postoperative seizure outcome in patients with FCD – and most reports show relatively stable percentages over a longer period of time (Kloss *et al.*, 2002; Cohen-Gadol *et al.*, 2004; Krsek *et al.*, 2010). This is very gratifying because this is not seen in all pathologies. In the recent report from the Epilepsy Center Bonn (dealing with 1,721 children and adults), with an average follow-up of five years, only patients with benign tumors (61% seizure-free) had a better long-term seizure outcome than patients with FCD (57.6% seizure free); the rate for patients with AHS was down to 49.4% (Bien *et al.*, 2012). Jehi *et al.* (2009) from the

Cleveland Clinic have also shown in their longitudinal study of "posterior cortex epilepsy surgery" that patients with tumors or FCD had a better chance to remain seizure-free than patients with other etiologies. According to Krsek *et al.* (2009a), seizure outcome in children with FCD remains stable after the second postoperative year in around 75%. Jehi *et al.* (2010) analyzed data from 276 patients (out of 915 patients with all kinds of etiology, operated on between 1990 and 2007) who had one or more seizures beyond the immediate postoperative period, and found that 2 unprovoked seizures within 6 months after surgery and ipsilateral spikes on an EEG at six months after surgery are very strong predictors of epilepsy recurrence.

Stable percentages, however, do not imply that all patients remain in the same outcome class for ever: changes are occurring in both directions, although in a minority of patients only. Most interesting is the observation by Krsek *et al.* (2008), that almost all FCD II patients who changed outcome after the second year either recurred or worsened, and that on the other hand a significant proportion of MCD and FCD I patients, if there was a change, improved. This implied that outcome differences seen at two years follow-up (favoring FCD II) disappeared at five and ten years follow-up. This finding is of interest with respect to the question whether different types of FCD have different mechanisms of epileptogenicity and / or different degrees of epileptogenicity, or if various pathological changes could, after a cascade of abnormal electrophysiological or neurochemical events, at the end create one common and decisive electrophysiological condition, from which seizures would set off (see next paragraph).

Completeness of resection of the lesion as visible on MRI is the most important variable also for long-term seizure freedom. But FCD I lesions are often not seen on MRI and when they are, it may be impossible to identify clear margins. And in children with early-onset severe epilepsies caused by extended multilobar, sub-hemispheric or hemispheric FCD, a reliable determination of the epileptogenic zone is often not possible. The EEG is often misleading, e.g., because of circumscribed ictal-onset zones over much bigger dysplastic areas (not visible on MRI), or is not helpful because it shows a generalized seizure pattern. The UCLA group doubts whether children with onset of severe epilepsy within the first year of life caused by extended FCD have a fair chance of long-term seizure freedom by surgical procedures other than hemispherectomy or hemispherotomy. They do not perform temporo-parieto-occipital resections anymore, whether children have a pre-existing hemiparesis or not. With this change of their approach, 70% were seizure-free at six months follow-up and 60% remained in remission after five years. In their previous series, which contained a larger number of tailored resections, the rate of seizure recurrence was much higher (Hemb *et al.*, 2010). In a consecutive series of 24 patients with extended FCD I from our center, none of them having a hemiparesis, a hemispherotomy was performed only once and only 21% became seizure-free, whereas 22% were in Engel's Class II (Krsek *et al.*, 2009b). Since then we have not given up to perform multilobar or sub-hemispheric resections in these challenging patients (and results are getting better; Pascher *et al.*, 2011) but we have also learned under which circumstances proposals other than a hemispherectomy or hemispherotomy are just wishful thinking.

■ A considerable number of patients become seizure-free despite incomplete resection

Incomplete resections are done on purpose in patients in whom the lesion is overlapping with or adjacent to eloquent cortical areas in order to prevent neurological damage but can also occur unintentionally. From the numerous publications dealing with seizure outcome in patients with FCD one can estimate that on average 20% become seizure-free despite incomplete resection. A better understanding of the reasons why a minority of patients becomes seizure-free despite incomplete resection is very urgent because this would be of great help in the planning of operations in which a complete resection would definitely lead to severe permanent neurological deficit and help in the counseling of patients or parents. A step forward in this direction may come from recent findings that areas containing balloon cells are less, and areas containing more dysmature interneurons ("cytomegalic neurons having features similar to immature neurons") more epileptogenic (Boonyapisit et al., 2003; Cepeda et al., 2005, 2006; André et al., 2010). A varying distribution of pathological cell types of different epileptogenicity could also explain the puzzling observation that in tuberous sclerosis complex (TSC) only a minority of tubers showing the typical signal changes and the characteristic transmantle sign of FCD IIb are epileptogenic. Indeed, Cepeda et al. (2010) found that in TSC, balloon cells outnumbered (abnormal) cytomegalic pyramidal neurons in some tubers, while in in FCD II the reverse was found. These (and other) cell types are, therefore, not homogeneously distributed across these tubers, but probably also not within FCD IIb lesions. This could explain why complete resection of FCD IIb is desirable but not always an absolute must for a seizure-free outcome. It may be expected that in the future, with "fine-tuning" of invasive recording, more sophisticated fiber tracking, very precise neuro-navigation and the application of tools like MEG and source imaging, more patients with FCD IIb that overlap with or are very adjacent to eloquent cortical areas, will benefit from epilepsy surgery. Extremely helpful for the planning of operations that carry a higher risk of neurological complications, is the result of the study published by Wagner et al. (2011) that the "tail" – this is the transmantle sign in FCD IIb – does not need to be resected to achieve seizure freedom.

Whether areas containing FCD I are resected completely or not is difficult to judge or can very often not be decided at all, because pre-operative MRI in many of these cases is interpreted as normal. The two hallmarks in the neuroradiological diagnosis of this type of lesion, regional reduction of the volume of the white matter and slightly increased white-matter signals on T2-weighted images and FLAIR (Colomobo et al., 2003, 2009; Krsek et al., 2009a, b; Tassi et al., 2010) are not suitable for giving an answer to this question. Although it remains unknown which epileptogenic mechanisms generate seizures in patients with FCD I, we have learned from patients who underwent re-operations, that the pathological micro-columnar architecture as seen in FCD Ia cannot be the cause of the epilepsy (own unpublished data). To summarize, there is no data that allow a rational discussion regarding the chances for seizure-free outcome with limited resections in cases with FCD I. However, there is the experience of the Miami Children's hospital group that some patients with FCD I, who continued to have seizures after surgery, remitted after two or more years after surgery (Krsek et al., 2008). More observations of this kind are needed before one can draw conclusions under which conditions patients with FCD I may have a chance to become seizure-free on long-term follow up despite resections that are intentionally limited in order to prevent neurological deficits.

Early surgery might not be early enough for the prevention of permanent mental retardation

So far, we have dealt with the results of surgery for the occurrence of seizures at short- and long-term follow-up. But, especially in young children, the delay of mental development occurring during the course of the epilepsy is a very important outcome parameter, too. There is no reason why children with FCD II should have better or worse mental outcome than children with other pathologies undergoing epilepsy surgery because of drug-resistant seizures. There are no remote other factors that could influence mental outcome: the ipsilateral brain regions outside the areas containing FCD II and the contralateral hemisphere are usually normal. Like for all patients, the main risk factors for mental retardation are onset of epilepsy below the age of 2 years and duration of epilepsy (Freitag & Tuxhorn, 2005). Onset within the first year of life is an even greater risk than onset within the second year of life (Cormack et al., 2007). Not rarely, children with FCD may present with the alarming sign of infantile spasms. Early cessation of spasms and hypsarrhythmia are a prerequisite for a more or less normal psychomotor development, in TSC (Muzykewicz et al., 2009; Jozwiak et al., 2011) and other affections causing West syndrome. The deleterious effect of a long delay of treatment in children with West syndrome has been underpinned recently by the results of the KISS-study (O'Callaghan et al., 2011).

One cannot exclude that a subgroup of children with FCD I has a poor prognosis regarding mental outcome because of the nature of the disease, although this is far from clear. Krsek et al. (2009b, 2010) found an overrepresentation of pre- and perinatal adverse events in children with FCD I (not in FCD II). It is hypothesized that the neuropathological changes as seen in children with early-onset severe epilepsy caused by FCD I may be the result of a compromised brain development during pregnancy, delivery or early postnatal development (Blümcke et al., 2010). A logical question is whether children with FCD I and a history of a perinatal adverse advent can have such compromised brain development restricted to one region or one hemisphere, or if one has to assume more generalized subtle damage, with one side more affected than the other. But in our series, children with a history of such events were only a small minority among the unfortunately large group with severe mental retardation at the time of surgery. None of 27 consecutive children with FCD I operated on at the Epilepsy Center Vogtareuth had a normal IQ; 55% had an IQ less than 35. Location of the FCD type I was in the posterior or posterior plus anterior regions; at least two lobes were always affected (Krsek et al., 2009b). We have not yet analyzed in detail the results of the postoperative neuropsychological tests but our impression is that the majority of children with FCD I, who presented with a severe mental retardation prior to surgery (and many of them with features of autistic disorder), remain severely mentally retarded and autistic. As already mentioned in the paragraph on long-term follow-up, at UCLA, the special group of children with extensive FCD I is now operated upon at younger and younger age in order to prevent lasting severe mental retardation. Moreover, they do not perform large multilobar posterior resections any more but hemispherectomies instead (Hemb et al., 2010). Follow-up investigations showed that 55% of their patients with hemi-cortical dysplasia = large FCD I and II, who had undergone a hemispherectomy or hemispherotomy, had IQs of 50 and higher (Jonas et al., 2005). The reported negative correlation between duration of epilepsy and immediate postoperative IQ at one hand, as well as the postoperative gains in terms of mental performance with shorter durations of epilepsy are impressive.

With all the experience from recent years that onset of epilepsy within the first year of life is such a dramatic risk factor for a lasting severe mental retardation and that duration of epilepsy is another one, it would be highly consistent to keep the duration of epilepsy with onset in the first year of life as short as possible. This is indeed done at some centers now, with promising results *(Table II)*.

Table II. Cognitive changes after surgery in relation to age at surgery and duration of epilepsy

No changes	Positive changes	Remarks
Devlin et al., 2001 (London) (hem)		Relativity old at operation and long duration
Pulsifer et al., 2004 (Baltimore) (hem)		Relativity old at operation and long duration
Dunkley et al., 2010 (London) (infants)		Young at operation and short duration
	Jonas et al., 2004, 2005 (UCLA) (hemispherectomy)	Young at operation and short duration
	Loddenkemper et al., 2007 (Cleveland Clinic Foundation)	Young at operation and short duration
	Honda et al., 2012 (Tokyo) (hemimegalencephaly)	Young at operation and short duration

Young: within the first year of life; patients had predominantly dysplasias

■ (Re-)organization of sensorimotor functions is virtually never seen in patients with circumscribed central FCD II nor in children with extended FCD I

Ipsilateral (re-)organization of sensorimotor functions is a well-known phenomenon to occur under a variety of circumstances: porencephalic cysts, Sturge-Weber syndrome, hemispheric polymicrogyria, HME and others, but apparently not in circumscribed central FCD II. We are not aware of any study investigating this more systematically. Paresis in patients with central FCD II should be taken as a sign of dysfunction (with an anatomical substrate or functionally in the sense of a Todd's paralysis) and one should not have too much hope that sensorimotor functions of the affected limbs are located in the ipsilateral rolandic area and that motor functions will be unchanged after an extended resection in the central area. FCD II lesions seem to cause a displacement of functions (Barba et al., 2012) rather than to exert pressure on the brain to preserve uncrossed corticospinal tracts during development *(Figure 1)*. What can be said, however, is that in FCD IIb the areas with the brightest signal changes most likely do not contain functions (Marusic et al., 2002; Janzky et al., 2003).

We perform fMRI and fiber-tracking (DTI) each time when a FCD II is located within or very close to the central area but we have never seen (re-)organization of sensorimotor functions within the opposite hemisphere.

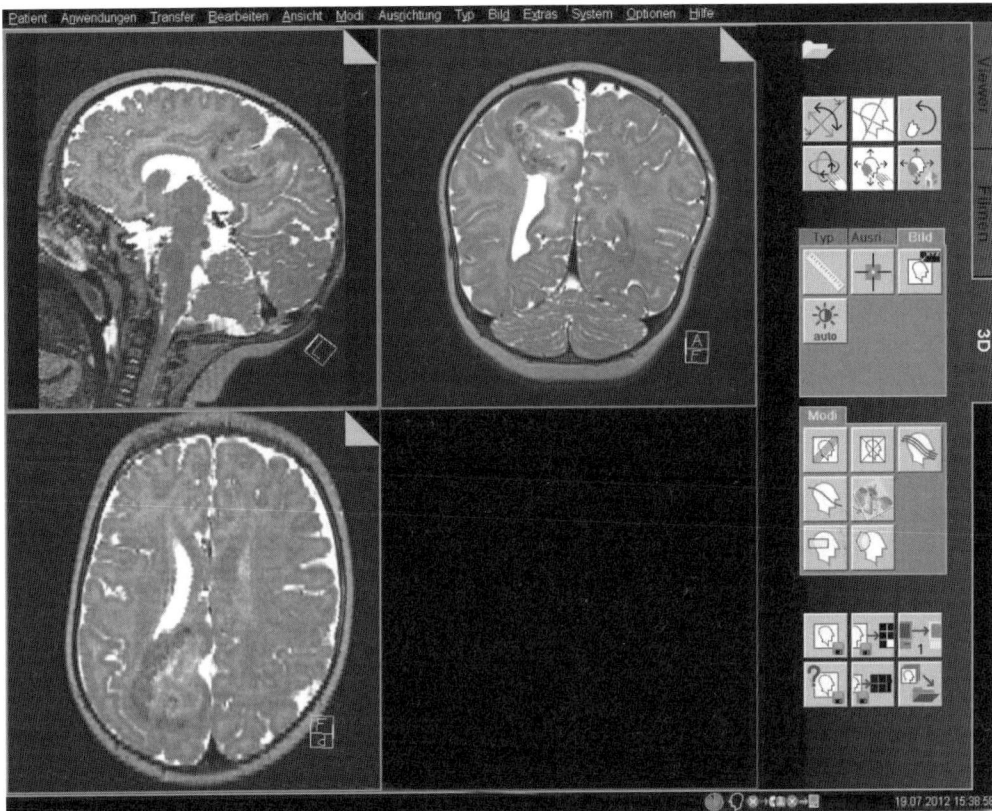

Figure 1. Large FCD IIb with calcifications within the central area; displacement of sensory-motor functions was detected and no (re-)organization of sensory-motor functions within the contra-lateral hemisphere.

Gross architecture is normal in FCD I. This fact might already be sufficient to explain why it is unrealistic to expect that a (re-)organization of motor functions takes place within the contralateral hemisphere in children with FCD type I – and because of this there is also no reason to assume that motor functions could be displaced (Janzky et al., 2003). Mono- or hemiparetic signs in infants and children with FCD type I, in whom imaging and electrophysiology are pointing to the posterior quadrant, may be taken as a hint that the lesion is more extended and that the child might not become seizure-free by a tailored resection, but might need a hemispherectomy/ hemispherotomy. However, these neurological signs, which are subtle most of the time, can also be the result of frequent seizure spread to the central area. When hemispherectomies/ hemispherotomies are performed under these circumstances, a worsening of function is almost regularly seen after surgery. Nevertheless, it makes a huge difference whether such a new deficit, as a price a child has to pay for a better perspective with respect to mental outcome, is created in an infant who is not yet able to walk (or may even not be able to sit without support), or in a young child already enjoying walking around and running.

■ There is no reorganization of visual functions after resection of visual cortex and/or dissection of the visual tract but many children compensate almost perfectly

A hemifield-cut as a complication of the operation in patients who have a normal intelligence has dramatic consequences because in most countries patients will not get a driver's license afterwards. One can almost be sure that hemifield cuts as a result of unintentional resections of the Meyer's loop have decreased since the advent of fiber-tracking and neuronavigation (Diehl et al., 2010). Kuzniecky et al. (1997) were surprised to find a low frequency of pre- and postoperative deficits in patients with "occipital lobe developmental malformations" and speculated "that some degree of cortical visual reorganization may occur in patients with occipital lobe malformations". But there is no such re-organization for visual functions with early lesions as it is the case for sensory-motor functions. Instead, children with early epileptogenic occipital lesions who have visual field cuts but appear unaffected in daily life compensate by a much faster "scanning" of the entire visual field with their eyes than this is the case in persons without a hemifield cut. We investigated the relevance of hemifield cuts (preexisting or as result from surgery) in activities of daily life in 47 children and found a tendency for pathological EEG-changes as being more predictive for the presence of such a (wishful) compensatory mechanism than the presence of clear-cut lesions within the posterior areas (Eitel et al., 2005).

■ Language functions before and after surgery in children with focal cortical dysplasia – when plasticity really matters

There is no data comparing language functions before or after epilepsy surgery in a larger number of children with FCD. "Developmental lesions" do not displace language cortex to the same extent as is seen e.g. in children with acquired pre-, peri-, or early postnatal lesions (Duchowny et al., 1996; Gaillard et al., 2007), but nevertheless unusual language representations are found far more often than in controls (Wilke et al., 2011). Early onset of epilepsy is another predictor for a higher rate of atypical language functions (Gaillard et al., 2007) – and an important one because the great majority of children with severe epilepsies caused by FCD have seizure onset in the first two years of life.

There are no reports about children with FCD who have become aphasic after surgery. This is astonishing considering how difficult it often is in children to localize and lateralize language functions (a discussion on the diagnostic yield of the different methods for the determination of localizing and lateralizing language functions is beyond the scope of this chapter). There are also no data on how often surgery has been postponed because of uncertainties in terms of the localization or even lateralization of language areas. Whenever surgery should be postponed in a young child with FCD for one or another reason, one has to bear in mind that one is giving up the advantage of the enormous plasticity for language representations in young children. To make a decision later on when language representations are still not clear and cannot be established by tests because of a child's mental or behavioral status, is far more stressful in particular when the child has meanwhile acquired at least language functions. These aspects are, however, not different from considerations in children with difficult to treat epilepsies caused by other etiologies than FCD.

References

- Alexandre V Jr, Walz R, Bianchin MM, et al. Seizure outcome after surgery for epilepsy due to focal cortical dysplastic lesions. Seizure 2006; 15: 420-7.
- Alexandre Jr V, Capovilla G, Fattore C, et al. Characteristics of a large population of patients with refractory epilepsy attending tertiary referral centers in Italy. Epilepsia 2010; 51: 921-5.
- Andre VM, Cepeda C, Vinters HV, Huynh M, Mathern GW, Levine MS. Interneurons, GABA currents, and subunit composition of the GABAA receptor in type I and type II cortical dysplasia. Epilepsia 2010; 51 (Suppl 3): 166-70.
- Barba C, Montanaro D, Frijia F, et al. Focal cortical dysplasia type IIb in the rolandic cortex: functional reorganization after early surgery documented by passive task functional MRI. Epilepsia 2012; 53: 141-5.
- Barkovich AJ, Guerrini R, Kuzniecky RI, Jackson GD, Dobyns WB. A developmental and genetic classification for malformations of cortical development: update 2012. Brain 2012: 1-22.
- Bast T, Ramantani G, Seitz A, Rating D. Focal cortical dysplasia: prevalence, clinical presentation and epilepsy in children and adults. Acta Neurol Scand 2006; 113: 72-81.
- Bien CG, Raabe AL, Schramm J, Becker A, Urbach H, Elger CE. Trends in presurgical evaluation and surgical treatment of epilepsy at one centre from 1988-2009. J Neurol Neurosurg Psychiatry 2013; 84: 54-61.
- Blümcke I. Neuropathology of focal epilepsies: a critical review. Epilepsy Behav 2009; 15: 34-9.
- Blümcke I, Pieper T, Pauli E, et al. A distinct variant of focal corticaldysplasia type I characterised by magnetic resonance imaging and neuropathological examination in children with severe epilepsies. Epileptic Disord 2010; 12: 172-80.
- Blümcke I, Thom M, Aronica E, et al. The clinicopathologic spectrum of focal cortical dysplasias: a consensus classification proposed by an ad hoc Task Force of the ILAE Diagnostic Methods Commission. Epilepsia 2011; 52: 158-74.
- Boonyapisit K, Najm I, Klem G, et al. Epileptogenicity of focal malformations due to abnormal cortical development: Direct electrocorticographic-histopathologic correlations. Epilepsia 2003; 44: 69-76.
- Cepeda C, Andre VM, Flores-Hernandez J, et al. Pediatric cortical dysplasia: correlations between neuroimaging, electrophysiology and location of cytomegalic neurons and balloon cells and glutamate/GABA synaptic circuits. Dev Neurosci 2005; 27: 59-76.
- Cepeda C, Andre VM, Levine MS, et al. Epileptogenesis in pediatric cortical dysplasia: The dysmature cerebral development hypothesis. Epilepsy Behav 2006; 9: 219-35.
- Chamberlain WA, Cohen ML, Gyure KA, et al. Interobserver and intraobserver reproducibility in focal cortical dysplasia (malformations of cortical development). Epilepsia 2009; 50: 2593-8.
- Chern JJ, Patel AJ, Jea A, Curry DJ, Comair YG. Surgical outcome for focal cortical dysplasia: an analysis of recent surgical series. A review. J Neurosurg Pediatrics 2010; 6: 452-8.
- Cohen-Gadol AA, Ozduman K, Bronen RA, Kim JH, Spencer DD. Long-term outcome after epilepsy surgery for focal cortical dysplasia. J Neurosurg 2004; 101: 55-65.
- Colombo N, Tassi L, Galli C, et al. Focal cortical dysplasias: MR imaging, histopathological, and clinical correlations in surgically treated patients with epilepsy. Am J Neuroradiol 2003; 24: 724-33.
- Colombo N, Salamon N, Raybaud C, Ozkara C, Barkovich AJ. Imaging of malformations of cortical development. Epileptic Disorders 2009; 11: 194-205.
- Colombo N, Tassi L, Deleo F, et al. Focal cortical dysplasia type IIa and IIb: MRI aspects in 118 cases proven by histopathology. Neuroradiology 2012; 54: 1065-77.
- Cormack F, Cross JH, Isaacs E, et al. The development of intellectual abilities in pediatric temporal lobe epilepsy. Epilepsia 2007; 48: 201-4.

- D'Argenzio L, Colonnelli MC, Harrison S, *et al.* Seizure outcome after extratemporal epilepsy surgery in childhood. *Dev Med Child Neurol* 2012; 5: 995-10.
- Devlin AM, Cross JH, Harkness W, *et al.* Clinical outcomes of hemispherectomy for epilepsy in childhood and adolescence. *Brain* 2003; 126: 556-66.
- Diehl B, Tkach J, Piao Z, *et al.* Diffusion tensor imaging in patients with focal epilepsy due to cortical dysplasia in the temporo-occipital region: electro-clinico-pathological correlations. *Epilepsia* 2010; 90: 178-87.
- Duchowny MS, Jayakar P, Harvey AS, *et al.* Language cortex respresentation: effects of developmental *versus* acquired pathology. *Ann Neurol* 1996; 40: 31-8.
- Dunkley C, Kung J, Scott RC, *et al.* Epilepsy surgery in children under 3 years. *Epilepsy Res* 2003; 93: 96-106.
- Freitag H, Tuxhorn I. Cognitive function in preschool children after epilepsy surgery: rationale for early intervention. *Epilepsia* 2005; 46: 561-7.
- Gaillard WD, Berl MM, Moore EN, *et al.* Atypical language in lesional and nonlesional complex partial epilepsy. *Neurology* 2007; 30: 1761-71.
- Gambardella A, Palmini A, Andermann F, *et al.* Usefulness of focal rhythmic discharges on scalp EEG of patients with focal cortical dysplasia and intractable epilepsy. *Electroencephalogr Clin Neurophysiol* 1996; 98: 243-9.
- Hader WJ, Mackay M, Otsubo H, *et al.* Cortical dysplastic lesions in children with intractable epilepsy: role of complete resection. *J Neurosurg (Pediatrics 2)* 2004; 100: 110-7.
- Harvey AS, Cross JH, Shinnar S, Mathern BW, ILAE Pediatric Epilepsy Surgery Survey Taskforce. Defining the spectrum of international practice in pediatric epilepsy surgery patients. *Epilepsia* 2008; 49: 146-55.
- Hemb M, Velasco TR, Parnes MS, *et al.* Improved outcomes in epilepsy surgery: The UCLA experience, 1986-2008. *Neurology* 2010; 74: 1768-75.
- Holthausen H, Teixeira VA, Tuxhorn I, *et al.* Epilepsy surgery in children and adolescents with focal cortical dysplasia. In: Tuxhorn I, Holthausen H, Boenigk H (eds). *Paediatric Epilepsy Syndromes and their Surgical Treatment*. London: John Libbey &Company Ltd, 1997a, pp. 199-215.
- Honda R, Kaido T, Takahashi A, *et al.* Long-term outcome of hemimegalencephaly after hemispherectomy in infancy. Platform presentation during the 5th International Epilepsy Colloquium, Pediatric Epilepsy Surgery, Lyon; May 20-23, 2012.
- Jehi L, Sarkis R, Bingaman W, Kotagal P, Najm I. When is a postoperative seizure equivalent to "epilepsy recurrence" after epilepsy surgery? *Epilepsia* 2010; 51: 994-1003.
- Jehi LE, Silveira DC, Bingaman W, Najm I. Temporal lobe epilepsy surgery failures: predictors of seizure recurrence, yield of reevaluation, and outcome following reoperation. *J Neurosurg* 2010; 113: 1186-94.
- Jonas R, Nguyen S, Hu B, *et al.* Cerebral hemispherectomy: hospital course, seizure, developmental, language, and motor outcomes. *Neurology* 2004; 62: 1712-21.
- Jonas R, Asarnow RF, LoPresti C, *et al.* Surgery for symptomatic infant-onset epileptic encephalopathy with and without infantile spasms. *Neurology* 2005; 64: 746-50.
- Jozwiak S, Kotulska K, Doman'ska-Pakieła D, *et al.* Antiepileptic treatment before the onset of seizures reduces epilepsy severity and risk of mental retardation in infants with tuberous sclerosis complex. *Eur J Paediatr Neurol* 2011; 15: 424-31.
- Kesler-Uberti S, Pieper T, Eitel H, *et al.* 12 years of pediatric epilepsy surgery – The Vogtareuth experience. *Neuropediatrics* 2011; 42 *(abstract)*: S32-S33.
- Kim DW, Lee SK, Chu K, *et al.* Predictors of surgical outcome and pathologic considerations in focal cortical dysplasia. *Neurology* 2009; 72: 211-6.
- Kloss S, Pieper T, Pannek H, Holthausen H, Tuxhorn I. Epilepsy surgery in children with focal cortical dysplasia (FCD): Results of longterm seizure outcome. *Neuropediatrics* 2002; 33: 21-6.

- Krsek P, Maton B, Korman B, et al. Different features of histopathological subtypes of pediatric focal cortical dysplasia. *Ann Neurol* 2008; 63: 758-69.
- Krsek P, Pieper T, Karlmeier A, et al. Different presurgical characteristics and seizure outcomes in children with focal cortical dysplasia type I or II. *Epilepsia* 2009a; 50: 125-37.
- Krsek P, Maton B, Jayakar P, et al. Incomplete resection of focal cortical dysplasia is the main predictor of poor postsurgical outcome. *Neurology* 2009b; 72: 217-23.
- Krsek P, Jahodova A, Maton B, et al. Low-grade focal cortical dysplasia is associated with prenatal and perinatal brain injury. *Epilepsia* 2010; 51: 2440-8.
- Loddenkemper T, Holland KD, Stanford LD, Kotagal P, Bingaman W, Wyllie E. Developmental outcome after epilepsy surgery in infancy. *Pediatrics* 2007; 119: 930-5.
- Kuzniecky R, Murro A, King D, et al. Magnetic resonance imaging in childhood intractable partial epilepsies: pathologic correlations. *Neurology* 1993: 681-7.
- Lerner JT, Salamon N, Hauptman JS, et al. Assessment and surgical outcomes for mild type I and severe type II cortical dysplasia: A critical review and the UCLA experience. *Epilepsia* 2009; 50: 1310-35.
- Marusic P, Najm IM, Ying Z, et al. Focal cortical dysplasias in eloquent cortex: functional characteristics and correlation with MRI and histopathologic changes. *Epilepsia* 2002; 43: 27-32.
- Muzykewicz DA, Costello DJ, Halpern EF, Thiele EA. Infantile spasms in tuberous sclerosis complex: Prognostic utility of EEG. *Epilepsia* 2009; 50: 290-6.
- O'Callaghan FJ, Lux AL, Darke K, et al. The effect of lead time to treatment and of age of onset on developmental outcome at 4 years in infantile spasms: evidence from the United Kingdom Infantile Spasms Study. *Epilepsia* 2011; 52: 1359-64.
- Palmini A, Gambardella A, Andermann F, et al. Operative strategies for patients with cortical dysplastic lesions and intractable epilepsy. *Epilepsia* 1994; 35 (Suppl 6): S57-S71.
- Palmini A, Najm I, Avanzini G, Babb T, et al. Terminology and classification of the cortical dysplasias. *Neurology* 2004; 62: S2-S8.
- Pascher B, Pieper T, Kessler-Uberti S, et al. "Everything but motor (EBM)" – subtotal hemispherectomy sparing the primary sensori-motor region in children with hemispheric epilepsies but without hemiparesis (abstract). *Neuropediatrics* 2011; 42: S32.
- Pulsifer MB, Brandt J, Salorio CF, Vining EP, Carson BS, Freeman JM. The cognitive outcome of hemispherectomy in 71 children. *Epilepsia* 2004; 45: 243-54.
- Rowland NC, Englott DJ, Cage TA, Sughrue ME, Barbaro NM, Chang EF. A meta-analysis of predictors of seizure freedom in the surgical management of focal cortical dysplasia. *J Neurosurg* 2012; 116: 1035-41.
- Stephen LJ, Kwan P, Brodie MJ. Does the cause of localization related epilepsy influence the response to antiepileptic drug treatment? *Epilepsia* 2001; 42: 357-62.
- Tassi L, Colombo N, Garbelli R, et al. Focal cortical dysplasia: neuropathological subtypes, EEG, neuroimaging and surgical outcome. *Brain* 2002; 125: 1719-32.
- Tassi L, Garbelli R, Colombo N, et al. Type I focal cortical dysplasia: surgical outcome is related to histopathology. *Epileptic Disorders* 2010; 12: 181-91.
- Tassi L, Garbelli R, Colombo N, et al. Electroclinical, MRI and surgical outcomes in 100 epileptic patients with type II FCD. *Epileptic Disord* 2012; 14: 257-66.
- Urbach H, Scheffler B, Heinrichsmeier T, et al. Focal cortical dysplasia of Taylor's balloon cell type: a clinicopathological entity with characteristic neuroimaging and histopathological features, and favorable postsurgical outcome. *Epilepsia* 2002; 43: 33-40.
- Wagner J, Weber B, Urbach H, Elger CE, Huppertz HJ. Morphometric MRI analysis improves detection of focal cortical dysplasia type II. *Brain* 2011; 134: 2844-54.
- Wilke M, Pieper T, Lindner K, et al. Clinical functional MRI of the language domain in children with epilepsy. *Hum Brain Mapp* 2011; 32: 1882-93.

Timing of antiepileptic drug withdrawal after pediatric epilepsy surgery

Kees P.J. Braun, Kim Boshuisen

Rudolf Magnus Institute of Neuroscience, University Medical Center Utrecht, The Netherlands

---

In 2008, a pivotal debate article listed the arguments in favor of, and against postoperative drug discontinuation (Cole & Wiebe, 2008). Its title – "Should antiepileptic drugs be stopped after successful epilepsy surgery?" – harbored an intrinsic paradox: whether or not epilepsy surgery has been truly successful can only be judged after antiepileptic drugs (AEDs) are stopped and seizure freedom persists. As summarized in their debate, withdrawing AEDs would prevent ongoing adverse events, cognitive side effects, costs, and affirmation of the sick role. Proof of the protective effect of continuing AEDs was lacking, and no studies had unequivocally shown that the declining rate of seizure freedom with increasing postoperative follow-up duration was negatively influenced by drug withdrawal, or that post-withdrawal recurrences predisposed to the recurrence of intractable epilepsy (Cole & Wiebe, 2008). Nevertheless, recurrent seizures after postoperative drug withdrawal may have important clinical, social or psychological consequences and not all patients regain seizure control after restarting AEDs. In the era of evidence-based medicine, it was argued that clinical practice recommendations could not be supported with the methodologically weak class IV studies on the topic that were available at that time (Cole & Wiebe, 2008).

Not unexpectedly, many of us still recommend to continue AEDs for at least one to two years after having reached postoperative seizure freedom, based on the experience in non-surgical cohorts. In a survey among US. adult epileptologists, 71% said they would stop medication only after two or more years of seizure-freedom, or even never (Berg *et al.*, 2007). More recently, Canadian epileptologists expressed a more aggressive AED withdrawal approach. Only 3% of them would require more than two years of postoperative seizure-freedom before start of AED reduction in patients that use two or more drugs. In patients treated with only one AED and in whom the intent is to withdraw all medication, 24% of epileptologists would wait with AED reduction for more than two years (Tellez-Zenteno *et al.*, 2012). Interestingly, drug withdrawal policies were more conservative in children who were operated upon in UCLA after 1997, compared to those who underwent surgery before 1997 (Hemb *et al.*, 2010). Is prolonged continuation of AEDs justified in children, who may be more vulnerable to cognitive side effects of medication, and in whom the psychosocial consequences of recurrence may be less pronounced compared to adults? Recent studies have provided new insights in the benefits, safety, and timing of postoperative AED withdrawal in children.

■ Cognitive benefits of AED withdrawal

Antiepileptic medication, generally suppressing neuronal excitability or enhancing inhibitory neurotransmission, often affects cognitive functions, among which vigilance, attention, psychomotor speed, memory and learning (Mula & Trible, 2009). Children, more than adults, probably are at risk of permanent cognitive impairment after long-term AED use. First, because the cumulative consequences of even small cognitive adverse effects during this critical period of life can affect educational progress and thereby eventual academic achievements (Mula & Trible, 2009). Second, AEDs can interfere with normal brain development during the first few years of life, not only prenatally (Ikonomidou & Turski, 2010), and their influence on e.g., cell proliferation, apoptosis, and synaptogenesis may permanently affect the child's cognitive potential.

In our experience, most parents report improved alertness, attention or behavior of their child after postoperative discontinuation of AEDs. Surprisingly few studies have looked at the improvement of cognitive functions after drug discontinuation. In a non-surgical cohort of seizure-free adults on monotherapy who were randomized to withdraw or continue their medication, discontinuation led to a significant improvement of cognitive processing under time pressure (Hessen et al., 2006). Although IQ scores did not significantly improve after cessation of AEDs in seizure-free medically treated children (Chen et al., 2001), psychomotor speed increased, and parents reported improved alertness and activation (Aldenkamp et al., 1993, 1998). In children who underwent temporal lobe surgery, cessation of AEDs was the strongest predictor of long-term postoperative IQ increase (Skirrow et al., 2011). We recently found that seizure free children who discontinued at least one AED after surgery improved significantly more on cognitive tests for reaction time and fine motor speed than those who stayed on AEDs (unpublished data). In conclusion, it is reasonable to assume that, particularly in young children who underwent anticipated curative epilepsy surgery, postoperative withdrawal of AEDs improves at least some of their cognitive functions and reduces the long-term and cumulative risks of cognitive impairments.

■ Safety of AED withdrawal

Seizure recurrences after discontinuation of AEDs in patients who initially were seizure free after surgery are not necessarily caused by withdrawal itself. We know that, independent of medication policy, postoperative seizure-freedom rates decline with increasing follow-up duration (Schmidt et al., 2004; Cole & Wiebe, 2008; Hemb et al., 2010). In many retrospective adult cohort studies, patients who became seizure-free after surgery almost always at some point started AED reduction, whereas the majority of patients who did not reach seizure-control never withdrew (e.g., Park et al., 2010). Thus, the safety of withdrawal itself can never be properly assessed. The few studies performed so far (listed below), dealt largely or exclusively with adults. They compared – often retrospectively – recurrence rates between seizure-free patients in whom it was decided to discontinue AEDs, and those who reached seizure-control but stayed on medication. In one retrospective series, 19% of the 180 patients who reduced or discontinued AEDs after epilepsy surgery had seizure recurrences within the first five years, as opposed to 7% of 30 seizure-free patients who did not alter AED treatment (Schiller et al., 2000). In their analysis of 301 patients who achieved 1-year postoperative seizure remission, Berg et al. (2006) found that relapse rates were higher in the group of patients who continued medication (45%), compared to those who reduced AEDs (32%). In a prospective controlled study, adults who were seizure-free one year after surgery were proposed to withdraw AEDs (Kerling et al., 2009). Of those who decided to maintain medication unchanged (n = 26), 62% remained seizure-free five years after surgery, compared to 76% in the withdrawal group (n = 34). A retrospective analysis of patients who underwent anterior temporal lobectomy revealed that complete discontinuation of AEDs after two years of postoperative seizure freedom did not increase recurrence risk (McIntosh et al., 2004).

These results all suggest that AED withdrawal, at least in adults, does not significantly increase the risk of seizure recurrence, although there are severe methodological limitations; the experimental set-up will inevitably cause a selection bias that influences differences in seizure outcome. When withdrawal is considered, surgical success is more often anticipated than in patients who stay on AEDs, implying that there are inherent differences between the groups that are equally or even more likely to affect outcome – such as completeness of resection, pathology, and surgical procedure – than withdrawal alone. To reliably appreciate whether or not drug discontinuation itself increases the risk of seizure recurrence, randomized controlled studies are needed, assuring patient groups that only differ in terms of medication policy. These, however, are lacking.

Patients and doctors may fear that discontinuing AEDs in patients who initially were seizure-free after surgery can lead to permanent loss of seizure-control. In a pooled analysis, 64% of adults who had a recurrence after AED reduction, regained seizure-control following restart of medication (Schiller et al., 2000; Schmidt et al., 2004; Berg et al., 2006; Kerling et al., 2009, Park et al., 2010; Rathore et al., 2011; Menon et al., 2012). Importantly, in the other 36% loss of seizure freedom is not necessarily attributed to AED withdrawal. As Berg et al. (2006) illustrated, the number of patients who regained seizure-freedom after restart of medication in the postoperative AED withdrawal group (63%) was even somewhat higher than in patients who had recurrences while maintaining all drugs, of whom only 51% experienced a subsequent remission. These and similar findings from the prospective study of Kerling et al. (2009), suggest that seizure recurrence during or after medication withdrawal might be regarded as relatively benign, and that it is not withdrawal itself that causes permanent loss of seizure-freedom.

What is known about safety of AED withdrawal in children? Until recently, drug policies after paediatric epilepsy surgery had been specifically addressed in four retrospective studies (Hoppe et al., 2006; Sinclair et al., 2007; Lachhwani et al., 2008; Boshuisen et al., 2009). Study populations are difficult to compare, some studies describing seizure outcome only in children who withdrew medication, others including all patients who underwent surgery. When pooling the results from these cohorts, 62% of all children who were operated upon, discontinued medication (Hoppe et al., 2006; Boshuisen et al., 2009), 18% of all children who withdrew AEDs had seizure recurrences, and of these patients 80% regained seizure freedom after restart of medication (Hoppe et al., 2006; Sinclair et al., 2007; Lachhwani et al., 2008; Boshuisen et al., 2009). Of the documented group of children who stayed on drugs after surgery, 53% had ongoing or recurring seizures (Hoppe et al., 2006; Boshuisen et al., 2009).

Although, again, safety of AED withdrawal cannot be proven from these studies, results suggest that seizure outcomes are good in children who discontinue medication, and that recurring seizures are sensitive to restart of medication. Cognitive side effects may be more pronounced in children, and the psychosocial consequences of seizure recurrence probably are less dramatic than in adults, who can fear loss of driving or occupational abilities. Therefore, especially in children, the ultimate goal of surgery should be to "cure" the epilepsy, defined as reaching freedom from both seizures and medication. It is not surprising that a systematic review of the literature revealed that "cure" was reached more often in children (27%) than in adults (19%, Tellez-Zenteno et al., 2007). The question remains at which point in time after surgery start of AED withdrawal and complete discontinuation of medication can be safely considered.

■ Timing of AED withdrawal

In patients, mainly adults, who underwent surgery for mesial temporal lobe epilepsy (TLE) (Lee et al. 2008), or neocortical epilepsy (Park et al., 2010), early AED reduction, before 10 or 9 months respectively, increased the risk of seizure recurrence after withdrawal. Others, however, have shown that the interval to complete discontinuation of medication was identical in patients with mesial TLE who did, and those who did not, relapse after attempted drug withdrawal (Rathore et al., 2011). Results of these studies should be interpreted with caution, because early withdrawal was not compared with late reduction in a controlled and randomized fashion, and other differences between groups could explain the differences in relapse rate. Available data cannot support the idea that early withdrawal itself is the cause of seizure recurrence. Most importantly, patients who start to reduce AEDs later have had a longer time to prove surgical success than those who withdraw early. Since AED withdrawal is generally not considered in patients who have ongoing or recurring seizures after surgery, and many postoperative recurrences occur early, the cohort of patients who start to reduce soon, inherently will reveal more surgical failures than those in whom a longer period of seizure-freedom preceded the attempt to reduce medication.

Timing of withdrawal in children had, until recently, been addressed in only three studies (Lachhwani et al., 2008; Boshuisen et al., 2009; Hemb et al., 2010). Although we showed in a small series that children who withdrew very early had good seizure outcomes (Boshuisen et al., 2009), Lachwani et al. (2008) suggested that discontinuing AEDs earlier than 6 months following surgery was associated with a higher risk of breakthrough seizures, compared to children who continued drugs for more than 6 months. If a cutoff point of 12 or 24 months was used, analyses did not reveal differences between withdrawal and continuation groups. The UCLA team compared children who were operated upon before 1997 with those who underwent surgery between 1998 and 2008 (Hemb et al., 2010). The seizure-freedom rate was significantly higher in the more recently operated cohort, as was the number of seizure-free children still on AEDs two years after surgery. Cure rates were therefore lower in the post-1997 cohort at two years postoperatively, but were equal between cohorts at five years after surgery. A multivariate logistic regression analysis revealed that drug use at two years was associated with a higher chance of seizure freedom. These two studies may suggest that later withdrawal improves seizure outcome in children. However, continuing AEDs will hide incomplete surgical success, implying that the earlier drugs are withdrawn, the sooner it becomes evident that the epilepsy is not cured. That does not mean that the chance of eventual seizure freedom is affected by early withdrawal, neither does it prove that recurrences after early withdrawal have less chance of responding to restart of medication than relapses that occur after late withdrawal. Further studies were warranted to really establish how timing of withdrawal affects not only the risk of seizure recurrences, but also – and even more importantly – the chance of eventual seizure freedom and cure in children after epilepsy surgery.

We therefore conducted a retrospective multicenter European cohort study within the frame of the European Taskforce for Epilepsy Surgery in Children ("U-task"), the "TimeToStop Study" (Boshuisen et al., 2012). Fifteen centers participated, allowing the inclusion of 766 children, operated between 2000 and 2008, in whom AED reduction was started after having reached postoperative seizure-freedom. The interval between surgery and start of AED withdrawal (time to reduction, TTR) was highly variable, with a median duration of 12.5 months. The median time to complete discontinuation (TTD), which could be achieved in a subgroup of 444 patients, was 28.8 months. As expected, several of the known predictors of postoperative seizure outcome were found to determine the timing of AED withdrawal. Being potential confounders of the relation between timing and outcome, we corrected statistical analyses for these independent predictors of timing, such as aetiology, type of surgery, multifocal MRI lesions, completeness of resection, and the number of drugs used at time of surgery. The main findings of the study are listed in Table I. In short, timing of start (TTR) and completion (TTD) of AED withdrawal

Table I. Main results from the TimeToStop study (adapted from Boshuisen et al., 2012)

Outcome measures	Seizure recurrence (during or after withdrawal)	Seizure freedom at end of study (Engel 1 > 1yr)	"Cure" at end of study (Engel 1+AED-free > 1yr)
Determinants	HR (95% CI), p-value	HR (95% CI), p-value	HR (95% CI), p-value
Timing variables			
TTR (per 3 months)	0.94 (0.89-1.00), 0.05	*0.97 (0.90-1.07), 0.55 NS*	*0.97 (0.97-1.03), 0.84 NS*
TTD (per 3 months)	0.90 (0.83-0.98), 0.02	*1.03 (0.93-1.14), 0.55 NS*	*0.98 (0.94-1.02), 0.31 NS*
Independent significant predictors			
Total withdrawal group (n = 766)*			
Multifocal MRI lesions	2.27 (1.23-4.20), 0.01	NS	NS
Nr of AEDs at surgery	NS	0.63 (0.41-0.97), 0.04	0.81 (0.70-0.94), 0.01
Hemispherectomy	2.28 (1.03-5.04), 0.04	NS	1.70 (1.01-2.85), 0.04
Previous surgery	2.28 (1.02-5.10), 0.04	NS	0.60 (0.36-1.00), 0.05
Epileptic EEG abnrl.	1.84 (1.15-2.96), 0.01	NS	NS
Incomplete resection[&]	2.61 (1.58-4.33), < 0.0001	0.40 (0.17-0.93), 0.03	0.64 (0.47-0.88), 0.01
Complete discontinuation group (n = 444)[#]			
Rasmussen's encephalitis	NS	NS 0.18 (0.05-0.73), 0.02	0.09 (0.03-0.33), < 0.0001
Incomplete resection[&]	4.9 (2.08-11.52), < 0.0001		0.37 (0.20-0.71), < 0.0001

The relation between time to start of AED reduction (TTR), time to complete discontinuation of AEDs (TTD) and the three seizure outcome measures was analyzed with Cox proportional hazard regression models, adjusted for potential confounders (variables that determined timing of withdrawal). Other variables that were shown to be related to outcome are listed. * Multivariable Cox regression analysis with TTR in the entire cohort, and [#]> with TTD in the subgroup that completely discontinued AEDs. HR: hazard ratio; *NS*: not significantly related. [&] Proven incomplete resection of the anatomical lesion.

significantly related to seizure recurrence; shorter intervals increased the risk of relapse with 2-3% per month. However, and more importantly, timing intervals did not relate to the chance of regaining seizure-freedom after restart of medication following a recurrence. Therefore, the eventual seizure outcome measures, *i.e.*, seizure freedom and "cure" for at least 1 year at latest follow-up, were not affected by timing of start or completion of AED withdrawal *(Table I, Figure 1)*. Factors that negatively influenced eventual seizure outcomes were previous surgery, the number of drugs used, and incomplete resection of the anatomical lesion *(Table I,* Boshuisen *et al.*, 2012).

Figure 1. Cumulative survival curve for eventual seizure freedom at latest follow up (Engel I/ILAE I for at least 1 year and followed for > 1 year since start of AED withdrawal). For the purpose of this graph, time to start of AED reduction (TTR) was categorized as < 6, 6-12, 12-24, and > 24 months after surgery. TTR was not related to seizure freedom. Results were similar for time to complete discontinuation (TTD), and for "cure" as primary outcome measure (not shown).

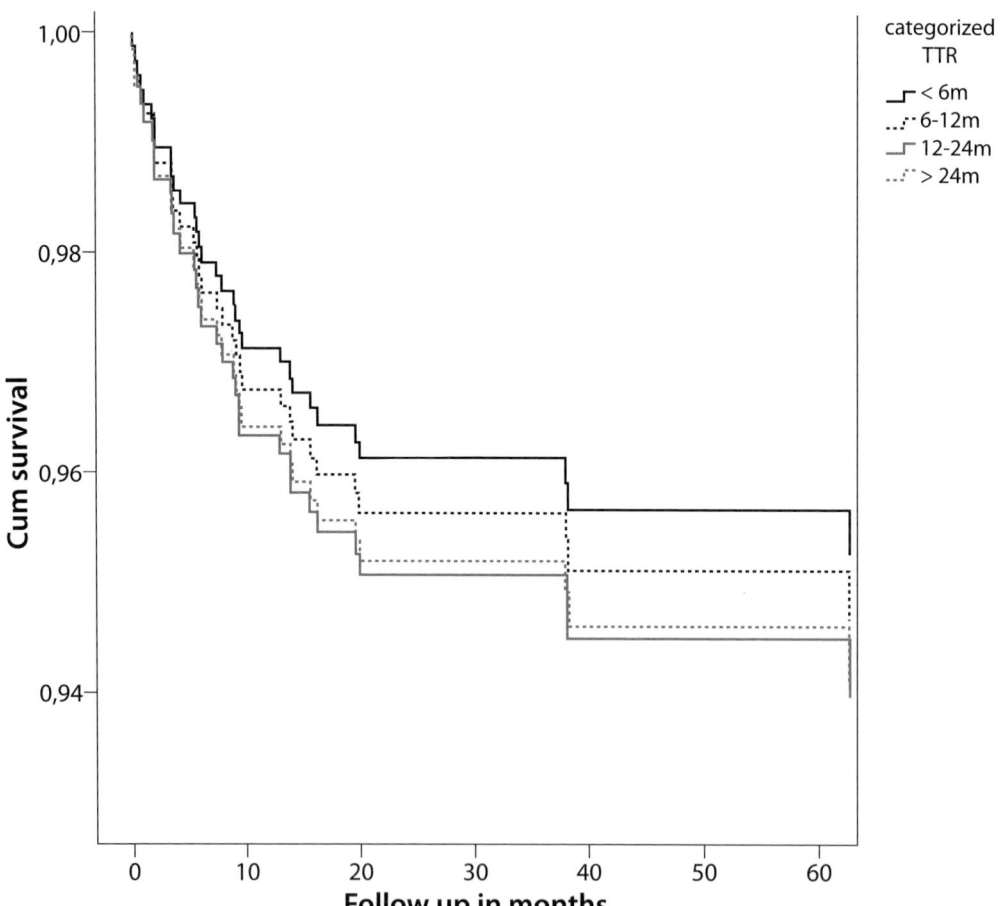

Concluding remarks

In children, antiepileptic drugs have cognitive side effects that may be cumulative, affecting learning and eventual academic achievements. Withdrawal of medication often improves at least some aspects of cognitive functioning. Although in few patients surgical treatment is offered from a palliative perspective, most children undergo epilepsy surgery with the intention to reach "cure", *i.e.*, being both seizure- and medication-free. Safety of postoperative drug discontinuation, in terms of seizure recurrence and eventual seizure status, has never been proven by randomized controlled studies in seizure-free cohorts of patients. Nevertheless, retrospective series in adults and children suggest that AED withdrawal itself does not cause an unfavorable long-term outcome. Seizure recurrences in children probably have less psychosocial consequences than in adults, and the vast majority of children who relapse after drug withdrawal regain seizure control after restart of medication. Therefore, AED reduction and discontinuation is reasonable in children who reach postoperative seizure freedom, provided that strong predictors of unfavorable seizure outcome are absent. Early start and completion of withdrawal does not affect the chance of reaching eventual seizure-freedom and cure, nor does it influence the probability of regaining seizure-freedom after restart of AEDs following a relapse. The small increase in seizure recurrence risk after earlier withdrawal is inherent to the fact that there is shorter proof of surgical success. Early withdrawal merely unmasks continuing drug-dependency sooner in children whose surgery was not completely successful, preventing unnecessary long-term continuation of medication in many others. The cognitive benefits of early withdrawal will be assessed in a future randomized controlled study.

Acknowledgements

We gratefully appreciate the help and support of the TimeToStop study group members. Both authors were financially supported by the Dutch National Epilepsy Fund (NEF 08-10).

References

- Aldenkamp AP, Alpherts WC, Blennow G, *et al.* Withdrawal of antiepileptic medication in children – effects on cognition: the multicenter Holmfrid study. *Neurology* 1993; 43: 41-50.
- Aldenkamp AP, Alpherts WC, Sandstedt P, *et al.* Antiepileptic drug-related cognitive complaints in seizure-free children with epilepsy before and after drug discontinuation. *Epilepsia* 1998; 39: 1070-4.
- Berg AT, Langfitt JT, Spencer SS, Vickrey BG. Stopping antiepileptic drugs after epilepsy surgery: a survey of U.S. epilepsy center neurologists. *Epilepsy Behav* 2007; 10: 219-22.
- Boshuisen K, Braams O, Jennekens-Schinkel A, Braun KP, Jansen FE, van Rijen PC, van Nieuwenhuizen O. Medication policy after epilepsy surgery. *Pediatr Neurol* 2009; 41: 332-8.
- Boshuisen K, Arzimanoglou A, Cross JH, *et al.*, for the TimeToStop study group. Timing of antiepileptic drug withdrawal and long-term seizure outcome after paediatric epilepsy surgery (TimeToStop): a retrospective observational study. *Lancet Neurol* 2012; 11: 784-91.
- Chen Y, Chow JC, Lee I. Comparison of the cognitive effect of antiepileptic drugs in seizure-free children with epilepsy before and after drug withdrawal. *Epilepsy Res* 2001; 44: 65-70.
- Cole AJ, Wiebe S. Debate: Should antiepileptic drugs be stopped after successful epilepsy surgery? *Epilepsia* 2008; 49 (Suppl. 9): 29-34.

- Hemb M, Velasco TR, Parnes MS, et al. Improved outcomes in pediatric epilepsy surgery: the UCLA experience, 1986-2008. Neurology 2010; 74: 1768-75.
- Hessen E, Lossius MI, Reinvang I, Gjerstad L. Influence of major antiepileptic drugs on attention, reaction time, and speed of information processing: results from a randomized, double-blind, placebo-controlled withdrawal study of seizure-free epilepsy patients receiving monotherapy. Epilepsia 2006; 47: 2038-45.
- Hoppe C, Poepel A, Sassen R, Elger CE. Discontinuation of anticonvulsant medication after epilepsy surgery in children. Epilepsia 2006; 47: 580-3.
- Ikonomidou C, Turski L. Antiepileptic drugs and brain development. Epilepsy Res 2010; 88: 11-22.
- Kerling F, Pauli E, Lorber B, Blumcke I, Buchfelder M, Stefan H. Drug withdrawal after successful epilepsy surgery: how safe is it? Epilepsy Behav 2009; 15: 476-80.
- Lachhwani DK, Loddenkemper T, Holland KD, et al. Discontinuation of medications after successful epilepsy surgery in children. Pediatr Neurol 2008; 38: 340-4.
- McIntosh AM, Kalnins RM, Mitchell A, Fabinyi GC, Briellmann RS, Berkovic SF. Temporal lobectomy: long-term seizure outcome, late recurrence and risks for seizure recurrence. Brain 2004; 127: 2018-30.
- Mula M, Trible MR. Antiepileptic drug-induced cognitive adverse effects. Potential mechanisms and contributing factors. CNS Drugs 2009; 33: 121-37.
- Lee S, Lee J, Kim DW, Lee S, Chun CK. Factors related to successful antiepileptic drug withdrawal after anterior temporal lobectomy for medial temporal lobe epilepsy. Seizure 2008; 17: 11-8.
- Park K, Lee SK, Chu K, et al. Withdrawal of antiepileptic drugs after neocortical epilepsy surgery. Ann Neurol 2010; 67: 230-8.
- Rathore C, Panda S, Sarma SP, Radhakrishnan K. How safe is it to withdraw antiepileptic drugs following successful surgery for mesial temporal lobe epilepsy? Epilepsia 2011; 52: 627-35.
- Schiller Y, Cascino GD, So EL, Marsh WR. Discontinuation of antiepileptic drugs after successful epilepsy surgery. Neurology 2000; 54: 346-9.
- Schmidt D, Baumgartner G, Loscher W. Seizure recurrence after planned discontinuation of antiepileptic drugs in seizure-free patients after epilepsy surgery: a review of current clinical experience. Epilepsia 2004; 45: 179-86.
- Sinclair DB, Jurasek L, Wheatley M, et al. Discontinuation of antiepileptic drugs after pediatric epilepsy surgery. Pediatr Neurol 2007; 37: 200-2.
- Skirrow C, Cross JH, Cormack F, Harkness W, Vargha-Khadem F, Baldeweg T. Long-term intellectual outcome after temporal lobe surgery in childhood. Neurology 2011; 76: 1330-7.
- Tellez-Zenteno JF, Dhar R, Hernandez-Ronquillo L, Wiebe S. Long-term outcomes in epilepsy surgery: antiepileptic drugs, mortality, cognitive and psychosocial aspects. Brain 2007; 130: 334-45.
- Tellez-Zenteno JF, Ronquillo LH, Jette N, Burneo JG, et al. Discontinuation of antiepileptic drugs after successful epilepsy surgery. A Canadian survey. Epilepsy Res 2012; May 15 [Epub ahead of print].

Anxiety and depression in children with epilepsy

Julianne Giust, David W. Dunn

Departments of Psychiatry and Neurology, Indiana University School of Medicine, Indianapolis, USA

In this chapter, we will focus on two major behavioral problems, depression and anxiety. The successful outcome of childhood epilepsy includes not only control of seizures but prevention of serious cognitive and behavioral co-morbidities. There are several reasons for emphasizing depression and anxiety. First, an elevated prevalence of depression and anxiety in children with epilepsy (CWE) has been repeatedly found in both epidemiological and clinical surveys. Second, depression and anxiety may increase the risk of subsequent epilepsy. Third, depression and anxiety have also been associated with compromise of quality of life in children with epilepsy and are often overlooked and undertreated in pediatric epilepsy clinics. In addition, there are modifications of treatment for depression and anxiety that should be made in children with epilepsy.

Do depression and anxiety differ in children with epilepsy compared to children in the general population? We will review the evidence for distinct features of depression and anxiety in CWE. If depression and anxiety in the CWE is a sequel or dependent on epilepsy, there should be distinctive clinical phenomenology, demographic characteristics, and risk factors for the occurrence of depression and anxiety associated with childhood epilepsy. There may be distinctive genetic factors, family environment, and psychosocial variables associated with these behavioral problems in the child with epilepsy. Finally, there may be an expectation that depression and anxiety might have unique response to treatment, specific clinical course, and outcome when compared to children without epilepsy.

■ Prevalence of anxiety and depression in children with epilepsy

A first major difference between depression and anxiety in CWE compared to those in the general population is the prevalence of the symptoms. Children with epilepsy are at increased risk for behavioral and cognitive disorders. Using data from the National Survey and Children's Health (NSHC, 2007), a cross-sectional analysis of 91,605 children demonstrated a lifetime prevalence of epilepsy/seizure disorder was about 1%. The survey also examined socio-demographics, patterns of co-morbidity, and functioning of CWE. In comparison to children without a seizure disorder, significantly more children with a seizure disorder had reported mental health and developmental concerns, including depression (8% vs. 2%), anxiety (17% vs. 3%), attention deficit/hyperactivity (ADHD) (23% vs. 6%), conduct difficulties (16% vs. 3%), developmental delay (51% vs. 3%), and autism spectrum disorders (16% vs. 1%). Children with a former seizure disorder also more frequently reported to experience depression (7% vs. 2%), anxiety (9% vs. 3%), ADHD (16% vs.%6), conduct disorder (8% vs. 3%), developmental delay (17% vs. 3%), and autistic spectrum disorder (7% vs. 1%) highlighting the importance of screening and treatment of psychiatric co-morbidities in both children with current and former seizure disorders (Russ et al., 2012). In addition, the cross- sectional analysis showed children with current seizures experience an impact on functioning with increased risk of grade failure, social competency issues, parent aggravation, and limitations in activities. Importantly, these children were also at higher risk of having unmet mental health needs suggesting a need to reexamine the current system of care (Russ et al., 2012).

Other epidemiological studies have found an increased risk of anxiety and depression in CWE. Davies et al. (2003) reported emotional problems in 16-17% of CWE compared to 6.4% in children with diabetes mellitus, and 4.2% of healthy controls. Another community-based survey from the United Kingdom noted emotional problems in 34% by parent report and in 13% using self-report from adolescents > 11 years of age and depression in 40% by parent report and 23% by self-report (Turky et al., 2008). Alfstad et al. (2001) found emotional problems in 31.5% of CWE compared to 19.4% of controls. Berg et al. (2007) reported clinically significant scores for affective disorders in 20% and anxiety disorders in 24% of CWE. At a 9-year follow up, they found that 13% of the CWE had depression and 5% anxiety (Berg et al., 2011). In comparison, in the general population, the prevalence of Major Depressive Disorder in childhood is 2% in children and 4-8% in adolescents. By 16 years of age, approximately 10% of children and adolescents will have experienced an anxiety disorder (Costello et al., 2003).

Cross sectional studies of clinic samples have found a range of prevalence figures (see Hermann & Jones, 2013; Dunn et al., 2009; Roeder et al., 20009). Eight studies reported depression in 9.6-36.5% of CWE with 5 of the studies finding a prevalence of 20-29%. The prevalence figures for anxiety range from 16-48% with 4 of 7 studies reporting a prevalence of 27-36%. Most studies have reported prevalence figures for anxiety without separation into subtypes. In a sample of CWE of at least 6 months duration, Dunn et al. (2009) found separation anxiety in 6%, generalized anxiety 2%, specific phobia in 35%, social phobia in 2%, obsessions in 35%, and compulsions in 9%. Symptoms of panic attacks and post-traumatic stress disorder were reported in 36% and 34% respectively, but the diagnoses could not be confirmed on follow up structures interviews.

Demographic variables differ somewhat in CWE compared to controls. In the general population, depression is more common in adolescents than in younger children. The specific type of anxiety disorder varies by age. Gender differences are not present in younger children but by adolescence, more girls than boys experience internalizing disorders. In CWE, the prevalence of depression may increase with age but very few studies have found gender differences in either anxiety or depression.

Depression and anxiety may be major contributors to the increased risk of suicidal ideation in children with epilepsy. In a group of 171 CWE with a mean age of 10.3, 20% of the children experienced suicidal ideation in comparison to a multi-variant analysis of the general population showing 8% of 12 to 15 year old youths experienced suicidal ideation (Caplan et al., 2005; Caplan et al., 2010; Peter et al., 2008).

■ Symptoms of anxiety and depression in youth

As in adults, the diagnosis of depression and anxiety in youth is made through the DSM-IV-TR criteria or the ICD-10. While the symptoms are overall similar, there are some differences in how a youth may present with depression, reflecting developmental processes. Children may present with more irritability, poor frustration tolerance, behavioral outburst, social withdrawal, and somatic complaints; whereas, adolescents may have more suicidality and melancholic features. These differences in presentation may complicate early diagnosis and treatment diagnosis, especially in preadolescent children (Birmaher & Brent, 2010; Lewinsohn et al., 2003; Luby et al., 2004).

Anxiety also varies by age. Fears and worry are developmentally normal. Normal children may report one or two fears that are not functionally interfering; whereas, children with anxiety disorders have more symptoms and more functional impairment. Children are more likely to develop separation anxiety disorder or specific phobia. Panic disorder and social phobia are more likely to begin in adolescence. Some children with anxiety disorders may recover but others may have either depression or anxiety disorders as adults.

Children frequently have difficulty understanding their emotional world and verbalizing their symptoms. Often they will present with externalizing behaviors, such as tantrums, aggression, and oppositionality (Birmaher & Brent, 2010; Luby et al., 2004). These symptoms may lead the parents, teachers, and physicians to believe that the child has a behavioral disorder, when, in fact, they may be experiencing a depressive episode causing the problems. In this situation, it is helpful to educate the child, family, and school that these behaviors are due to an underlying depression and the child is not labeled as a "bad" child. Also, as mentioned above, some children will present with somatic complaints, such as stomach upset or headaches. After confirming that there is not an underlying illness, the parent and child should be reassured that this is part of his/her depression in order to prevent further limitation of his/her functioning.

Data from the Centers for Disease Control and Prevention 2007 showed that suicide was the third leading cause of death in youth in 2005 in the United States. As mentioned above, CWE have an increased rate of suicidal ideation. Multiple risk factors should be assessed in patients with suicidal ideation, including the quality of suicidal ideation, previous suicidality, availability of lethal means, psychological factors (such as hopelessness, impulsive aggression, neuroticism), psychiatric disorders, parent/family mental health, and medical disorders (Goldstein & Brent, 2010). In addition to assessing for suicidal ideation, children with mood disorders should be examined for homicidal ideation. Homicidal ideation can be present with suicidal ideation. In one study, a third of adolescent suicide victims experienced homicidal ideation in the week before suicide (Goldstein & Brent, 2010; Brent et al., 1993).

There does not seem to be any data to suggest that the phenomenology of depression in CWE is different from that seen in the general pediatric population (Plioplys, 2003). Vega et al. (2011) compared children with absence seizures to healthy controls for reported items on anxiety and depression subscales. On item analysis, they found that children with absence seizures had more symptoms of worrying, rumination, sadness, and easy upset than healthy controls. There was no comparison group with anxiety or depression but the symptoms seem to be that found in general population children with depression or anxiety. The one area of difference in phenomenology may be in worries associated with having epilepsy. Approximately one-third of children with new onset seizure report fears of having another seizure and worries about telling others about their epilepsy (McNelis et al., 1998).

■ Considerations in evaluation of CWE: seizure specific risk factors for depression and anxiety

During the evaluation for anxiety and depression in a CWE, many factors have to be sorted through to identify potential causes. Seizure-related factors that have been examined for possible association with internalizing problems include age at onset, seizure type and syndrome, seizure severity, and additional cognitive problems. The role of antiepileptic drugs (AEDs) and seizure effects on mood needs to be considered in the differential. Additionally, as with children without epilepsy, a timeline for symptoms of depression and the role of psychosocial stressors, such as family stress, school issues, and peer issues, should be identified. Such stressors may point to a diagnosis of adjustment disorder instead of depression and can be important areas to be addressed in treatment.

Recent reviews found limited evidence for the association of epilepsy-related variables with depression or anxiety (Ekinci et al., 2009; Reilly et al., 2011). An early age of onset has been associated with cognitive problems but rarely with behavioral problems. Though a few studies found focal seizures associated with depression, most found no association. Rates of psychopathology appear to be higher in children with persistent seizures than in those whose seizures resolve (Berg et al., 2007; Austin et al., 2011; Russ et al., 2012). Poor control of seizures was a risk factor in only a couple of studies (Oğuz et al., 2002; Adewuya & Ola, 2005). There is limited information on the association of cognitive function and internalizing problems. Buelow et al. (2003) found more symptoms of depression in children with lower IQ scores and Caplan et al. (2005) found that lower verbal IQ scores were associated with internalizing disorders. Austin et al. (2011) showed that a progressive decrease in processing speed was associated with increasing symptoms of depression 3 years after the onset of seizures.

When a CWE appears to have depression, it is important to examine the current medication regimen, in particular the antiepileptic drugs (AEDs). Symptoms of depression or emotional dysregulation have been associated with several AEDs. Mood changes at the time of AED initiation or dosage changes may be alleviated by a change in AED; therefore, it is imperative that the potential for depression on these AEDs be discussed with the parent and CWE for early intervention. AEDs associated with depression include: phenobarbital, tiagabine, vigabatrin, and to a lesser extent, zonisamide, topiramate, and levetiracetam (Kanner et al., 2012; Kanner & Dunn, 2004). In comparison to depression, anxiety has less often been reported as a side effect of medication. There are reports of felbamate, levetiracetam, and zonisamide triggering anxiety or nervousness, and Weintraub et al. (2007) reported a nonsignificant increase in anxiety in adults receiving tiagabine. In contrast, other studies have found an anxiolytic effect from tiagabine, gabapentin, and pregabalin (Mula & Sander, 2007).

Additionally, when a CWE presents with mood changes, the physician should review with the parent and patient the patient's seizure control. Children and adolescents do not seem to have episodes of ictal or postictal depression but may experience prodromal anxiety or fear during the aura or beginning of a seizure originating from the temporal lobe. Since reducing the rate of seizures may improve depression and reduce anxiety in a CWE, it is helpful to assess the effectiveness of the AED and patient compliance to the AED and seizure hygiene (Kanner et al., 2012; Barry et al., 2008).

As in others with anxiety or depression, a CWE and an internalizing disorder should have a full investigation of his/her psychosocial stressors, including the impact of having epilepsy on the patient and the family. In a meta-analysis, Rodenburg et al. (2005a) found similar rates or internalizing problems in children with epilepsy compared to children with other chronic illnesses. Several studies found a significant association between family variables, including lack of confidence in managing epilepsy, limited support, and poor communication, and internalizing problems in children with epilepsy (Dunn et al., 1999; Austin et al., 2004; Rodenburg et al., 2006; Austin et al., 2010).

It is possible that both seizures and psychiatric problems may be due to a common underlying disorder. Studies have shown that depression and anxiety are risk factors for the subsequent development of seizures (Hesdorffer et al., 2006; Adelów et al., 2012). Hesdorrfer et al. (2012) have found a familial clustering of uncomplicated epilepsy and behavioral disorders. Austin et al. (2001) noted an increase in symptoms of depression and anxiety in children with new-onset seizures compared to siblings.

■ Treatment of anxiety and depression in youth examining the general population and CWE

Treatment of anxiety and depression in CWE can involve therapy, an antidepressant (AD), or a combination of the two. There is very limited data on treatment of anxiety and depression in CWE and the provider will need to use approaches developed for children without seizures. Initial therapies for the treatment of mild to moderate anxiety and depression may include psychoeducation, supportive therapy, family involvement, and school interventions. With more moderate to severe anxiety or depression, the above therapies may not be adequate. In these cases, an AD and specific types of therapy, such as cognitive-behavioral therapy (CBT) or interpersonal therapy (IPT), may be selected for a more robust treatment (AACAP practice parameter).

Psychoeducation about depression educates the patient and family about mood symptoms, causes, course, treatment, and risk. Psychoeducation appears to improve compliance to treatment and reduce the symptoms of depression (AACAP practice parameter 2007; Brent et al., 1993; Renaud et al., 1998). In addition to education about depression, the parents of CWE will benefit from an increase in knowledge about seizure disorders, the associated stigma, learning problems, and AEDs (Barry et al., 2008). One study of 220 CWE suggested that patients with less knowledge of epilepsy were more likely to have a worse self-concept and to be depressed (Hirfanoglu et al., 2009). Another intervention in the treatment of depression is supportive therapy. Supportive therapy includes listening and reflecting, development of problem solving and coping skills, and encouraging continued participation in treatment (AACAP practice parameter, 2007).

In addition to psycho-education and supportive therapy, a family approach is essential in managing depression. The family plays a significant role in identification of symptoms, motivation or barrier to treatment, and monitoring progress and safety (AACAP practice parameter). Also, parent-child conflict is associated with prolongation, relapse, and recurrence of depressive episodes in children (AACAP practice parameter, 2007; Birmaher et al., 2000).

As in most childhood illness, family adjustment and parent's mental health are important to developing or preventing psychopathology in CWE. For example, when seizure-related factors and family/child characteristics are controlled for in CWE, parenting style and the parent-child relationship are demonstrated to be significant components to the child developing problems (Austin et al., 2004; Rodenburg et al., 2005b). In a study of 340 parents of CWE, the prevalence and determinants of parental anxiety and its effect on the child's quality of life (QOL) were examined. The study found that 56% of the parents reported significant anxiety on the questionnaire Hospital Anxiety and Depression (HAD) with predominant contributing factors which included seizure frequency, finances, and parent's knowledge of epilepsy. Also, the children's QOL examined through the use of the questionnaires for Quality of Life in Childhood Epilepsy (QOLCE) showed a significant correlation to the parental anxiety (Li et al., 2008).

Depression is common in mothers of children with new onset seizure disorders. It is associated with a decrease in quality of life in CWE, and negatively affects the child's health related quality of life (HRLQ) (Adewuya 2006; Wood et al., 2008; Yong et al., 2006). Another study demonstrated maternal depression to affect the HRQOL significantly during the first 24 months after new-onset of epilepsy in a negative way (Ferro et al., 2011). Also, maternal depressive symptoms are positively correlated with behavior problems in CWE (Ferro et al., 2011; Rodenberg et al., 2006; Yong et al., 2006). Similarly, maternal anxiety has been found to be related to impaired adaptive function and lower quality of life in CWE (Chapieski et al., 2005; Ferro et al., 2011). It has also been shown that a reduction in maternal symptoms of depression significantly reduced child symptoms of depression (Kanner et al., 2012; Pilowsky et al., 2008). These studies suggest the possibility of intervention at the family level for promotion of improved outcomes.

An additional way to intervene is through the child's school environment. The school may accommodate CWE and depression by monitoring symptoms and providing support through the counselor. As mentioned earlier, CWE also have increased learning problems. Also seizures have a negative impact on school attendance, which may increase academic problems (Aguiar et al., 2007). These are issues that can be addressed by the school. In addition, one study of 220 CWE showed that poorer self-concept and increased symptoms of depression were associated with a perceived lack of social support and peer stigmatization (Hirfanoglu et al., 2009). School may be able to impact feelings of stigmatization by increasing peer and teacher knowledge and positive attitudes toward epilepsy through epilepsy education programs (Bozkaya et al., 2010).

In children with more than a single episode of mild depression, CBT or IPT and/or pharmacological intervention may be recommended. CBT works on the thoughts and behaviors leading to feelings of depression; whereas, IPT works on depression through discussion of relationships, role transitions and loss (AACAP practice parameter, 2007). There is limited data specific to the effectiveness of these treatments in CWE. In one RCT examining adolescents with epilepsy, CBT was found to be beneficial in preventing depression (Kanner et al., 2012; Martinovic et al., 2006). More severe depression will generally require treatment with antidepressants (AACAP practice parameter, 2007). The Treatment for Adolescents with Depression Study (TADS) showed that combined CBT and medication is more optimal treatment than CBT or medication alone in children and adolescents with more severe depression (March et al., 2004).

The first-line antidepressant for youth population is generally a selective serotonin reuptake inhibitor (SSRI). The typical SSRIs used to treat youth depression include fluoxetine, citalopram, escitalopram, and sertraline. Fluoxetine is the only medication for treatment of adolescent and child depression that is approved by the US Food and Drug Administration (FDA). In randomized controlled trials (RCTs) with venlafaxine or mirtazapine, no effect difference was seen against placebo in treatment of youth. Secondary analysis demonstrated that there may be an age effect with venlafaxine, showing it effective in depressed adolescents (AACAP practice parameter, 2007; Bridge et al., 2007; Cheung et al., 2005; Emslie et al., 2007; Wagner, 2005). Another treatment of depression in adults is tricyclic antidepressants (TCAs) and buproprion. For these two psychotropics, clinical efficacy compared to placebo has not been established in children (Barry et al., 2008; Hazell et al., 2002). In addition, treatment of depression with TCAs or buproprion is not recommended in CWE due to the risk of lowering the seizure threshold.

Barriers to treatment

A major concern is the limited number of CWE and internalizing problems that receive mental health treatment. Between 20 and 33% of CWE and depression or anxiety receive therapy (Caplan et al., 2005, Hanssen-Bauer et al., 2007; Caplan et al., 2008). This could be either a failure of diagnosis or inability or unwillingness to seek care. Ettinger et al., (1999) noted that none of the CWE and symptoms of depression or anxiety had received a prior diagnosis. Roeder et al., (2009) informed families of CWE that their child had evidence of an internalizing problem, but only 36% subsequently were enrolled in mental health clinics.

There are many barriers to diagnosis of depression in CWE. As mentioned above the presentation of depression is affected by the developmental age of a patient and can appear quite different than in an adult. Because of this some physicians may feel uncomfortable in making the diagnosis early diagnosis of depression. Unfortunately, many patients may not report symptoms of depression without prompting from medical staff. In a cross-sectional study of 579 adult patients on AEDs, 0% spontaneously reported feeling depressed. With questioning, 24% of patients on monotherapy and 39% on polytherapy endorsed symptoms of depression when given a checklist (Kanner et al., 2012, Carreno et al., 2008), reaffirming the importance of screening. In addition to difficulties with the screening for depression in patients, providers may also worry about the potential problems with prescribing an antidepressant, including risk and necessary follow up time required (Kanner et al., 2012; Cotterman-Hart, 2010).

Concluding remarks

Anxiety and depression are common co-morbidities in children and adolescents with epilepsy. The prevalence of both disorders is higher than seen in the general population. Symptoms are similar to that seen in the general population but age and gender differences are less pronounced. There are no risk factors that reliably predict anxiety or depression in CWE, although cognitive impairment, seizure severity, and family disruption may be important. Genetic factors may be of significance, as studies have demonstrated an increased risk of seizures in individuals that have anxiety or depression and family studies have shown a clustering of seizures and behavioral problems. Certain antiepileptic drugs may precipitate symptoms in individual patients. There is limited data on the long-term natural history of these co-morbidities but persistence of seizures seems to be associated with more mental health symptoms. The standard treatments of anxiety and depression require minimal modification for CWE. The main current barrier to successful treatments is lack to recognize symptoms and reluctance or inability to find adequate mental health services.

References

- Adelów C, Andersson T, Ahlbom A, Tomson T. Hospitalization for psychiatric disorders before and after onset of unprovoked seizures/epilepsy. *Neurology* 2012; 78: 396-401.
- Adewuya AO. Parental psychopathology and self-rated quality of life in adolescents with epilepsy in Nigeria. *Dev Med Child Neurol* 2006; 48:600-3.
- Adewuya AO, Ola BA. Prevalence of and risk factors for anxiety and depressive disorders in Nigerian adolescents with epilepsy. *Epilepsy Behav* 2005; 6: 342-7.
- Aguiar BV, Guerreiro MM, McBrian D, Montenegro M. Seizure impact on the school attendance in children with epilepsy. *Seizure* 2007; 16: 698-702.
- Alfstad KÅ, Clench-Aas J, Roy BV, Mowinckel P, Gjerstad L, Lossius MI. Psychiatric symptoms in Norwegian children with epilepsy aged 8-13 years: effects of age and gender? *Epilepsia* 2011; 52: 1231-8.
- American Academy of Child and Adolescent Psychiatry. Practice parameter for the assessment and treatment of children and adolescents with depressive disorders. *J Am Acad Child Adolesc Psychiatr* 2007; 46: 1503-25.
- Austin JK, Harezlak J, Dunn DW, *et al*. Behavior problems in children before first recognized seizures. *Pediatrics* 2001; 107: 115-22.
- Austin JK, Dunn DW, Johnson CS, Perkins SM. Behavioral issues involving children and adolescents with epilepsy and the impact of their families: recent research data. *Epilepsy Behav* 2004; 5 (Suppl 3): S33-41.
- Austin JK, Perkins SM, Johnson CS, *et al*. Self-esteem and symptoms of depression in children with seizures: relationships with neurological functioning and family variables over time. *Epilepsia* 2010; 51: 2074-83.
- Austin JK, Perkins SM, Johnson CS, *et al*. Behavior problems in children at time of first recognized seizure and changes over the following 3 years. *Epilepsy Behav* 2011; 21: 373-81.
- Barry JJ, Ettinger AB, Friel P, *et al*. Consensus statement: The evaluation and treatment of people with epilepsy and affective disorders. *Epilepsy Behav* 2008; 13 (Suppl 1): S1-29.
- Berg AT, Vickrey BG, Testa FM, *et al*. Behavior and social competency in idiopathic and cryptogenic childhood epilepsy. *Dev Med Child Neurol* 2007; 49: 487-92.
- Berg AT, Caplan R, Hesdorffer DC. Psychiatric and neurodevelopmental disorders in childhood-onset epilepsy. *Epilepsy Behav* 2011; 20: 550-5.
- Birmaher B, Brent DA, Kolko D, *et al*. Clinical outcome after short-term therapy for adolescents with major depressive disorder. *Arch Gen Psychiatry* 2000; 57: 29-36.
- Birmaher B, Brent DA. Depression and Dysthymia. In: Dulcan M (ed). *Dulcan's Textbook of Child and Adolescent Psychiatry*. Chicago: American Psychiatric Publishing, Inc, 2010, pp. 261-78.

- Bozkaya IO, Ahan E, Serdaroglu A, Soysal AS, Ozkan S, Gucuyener K. Knowledge of perception of, and attitudes toward epilepsy of schoolchildren in Ankara and the effect of an educational program. *Epilepsy Behav* 2010; 17: 56-63.
- Brent DA. Perper JA. Moritz G. Baugher M. Schweers J. Roth C. Firearms and adolescent suicide. A community case-control study. *Am J Dis Child* 1993; 147: 1066-71.
- Brent DA, Poling K, McKain B, Baugher M. A psychoeducational program for families of affectively ill children and adolescents. *J Am Acad Child Adolesc Psychiatr* 1993; 32: 770-4.
- Bridge JA, Iyengar S, Salary CB, *et al*. Clinical response and risk for reported suicidal ideation and suicide attempts in pediatric antidepressant treatment: a meta-analysis of randomized controlled trials. JAMA 2007; 297: 1683-96.
- Buelow JM, Austin JK, Perkins SM, *et al*. Behavior and mental health problems in children with epilepsy and low IQ. *Dev Med Child Neurol* 2003; 45: 683-92.
- Caplan R, Siddarth P, Gurbani S, Hanson R, Sankar R, Shields WD. Depression and anxiety disorders in pediatric epilepsy. *Epilepsia* 2005; 46: 720-30.
- Caplan R, Siddarth P, Stahl L, *et al*. Childhood absence epilepsy: behavioral, cognitive, and linguistic comorbidities. *Epilepsia* 2008; 49: 1838-46.
- Caplan R, Siddarth P, Levitt J, Gurbani S, Shields WD, Sankar R. Suicidality and brain volumes in pediatric epilepsy. *Epilepsy Behav* 2010; 18: 286-90.
- Carreno M, Gil-Nagel A, Sanchez JC. Strategies to detect adverse effects of antiepileptic drugs in clinical practice. *Epilepsy Behav* 2008; 13: 178-83.
- Chapieski L, Brewer V, Evanovich K, *et al*. Adaptive functioning in children with seizures: impact of maternal anxiety about epilepsy. *Epilepsy Behav* 2005; 7: 246-52.
- Cheung AH, Emslie GJ, Mayes TL. Review of the efficacy and safety of antidepressants in youth depression. *J Child Psychol Psychiatr* 2005; 46: 735-54.
- Costello EJ, Mustillo S, Erkanli A, Keeler G, Angold A. Prevalence and development of psychiatric disorders in childhood and adolescence. *Arch Gen Psychiatr* 2003; 60: 837-44.
- Cotterman-Hart S. Depression in epilepsy: why aren't we treaing? *Epilepsy Behav* 2010; 19: 419-21.
- Davies S, Heyman I, Goodman R. A population survey of mental health problems in children with epilepsy. *Dev Med Child Neurol* 2003; 45: 292-5.
- Dunn DW, Austin JK, Huster GA. Symptoms of depression in adolescents with epilepsy. *J Amer Acad Child Adolesc Psychiatr* 1999; 38: 1133-8.
- Dunn DW, Austin JK, Perkins SM. Prevalence of psychopathology in childhood epilepsy: categorical and dimensional measures. *Dev Med Child Neurol* 2009; 51: 364-72.
- Ekinci O, Titus JB, Rodopman AA, Berkem M, Trevathan E. Depression and anxiety in children and adolescents with epilepsy: prevalence, risk factors, and treatment. *Epilepsy Behav* 2009; 14: 8-18.
- Emslie GJ, Findling RL, Yeung PP, Kunz NR, Li Y. Venlafaxine ER for the treatment of pediatric subjects with depression: results of two placebo-controlled trials. *J Am Acad Child Adolesc Psychiatr* 2007; 46: 479-88.
- Ettinger AB, Weisbrot DM, Nolan EE, *et al*. Symptoms of depression and anxiety in pediatric epilepsy patients. *Epilepsia* 1999; 39: 595-9.
- Ferro MA, Avison WR, Campbell MK, Speechley K. The impact of maternal depressive symptoms on health-related quality of life in children with epilepsy: A prospective study of family environment as mediators and moderators. *Epilepsia* 2011; 52: 316-25.
- Goldsein TR and Brent DA. Youth Suicide. In: Dulcan M (ed). *Dulcan's Textbook of Child and Adolescent Psychiatry*. Chicago: American Psychiatric Publishing, Inc, 2010, pp. 531-41.
- Hanssen-Bauer K, Heyerdahl S, Ericksson AS. Mental health problems in children and adolescents referred to a national epilepsy center. *Epilepsy Behav* 2007; 10: 255-62.

- Hazell P, O'Connell D, Heathcote D, et al. Tricyclic drugs for depression in children and adolescents. *Cochrane Database Syst Rev* 2002; 2: CD002317.
- Hermann BP, Jones JE. Depression and anxiety disorders in children with epilepsy. In: Duchowny M, Cross JH, Arzimanoglou A (eds). *Pediatric Epilepsy*. New York, McGraw Hill Medical, 2013, pp. 330-6.
- Hesdorrfer DC, Hauser WA, Olafsson E, Ludvigsson P, Kjartansson O. Depression and suicide attempts as risk factors for incident unprovoked seizures. *Ann Neurol* 2006; 59: 39-41.
- Hesdorrfer DC, Caplan R, Berg AT. Familial clustering of epilepsy and behavioral disorders: evidence for a shared genetic basis. *Epilepsia* 2012; 53: 301-7.
- Hirfanoglu T, Serdaroglu A, Cansu A, Soysal AS, Derle E, Gucuyener K. Do knowledge of, perception of, and attitudes toward epilepsy affect the quality of life of Turkish children with epilepsy and their parents? *Epilepsy Behav* 2009; 14: 71-7.
- Kanner AM, Schachter SC, Barry JJ, Hersdorffer DC, Mula M, Trimble M, et al. Depression and epilepsy, pain and psychogenic non-epileptic seizures: clinical and therapeutic perspectives. *Epilepsy Behav* 2012; 24: 169-81.
- Kanner AM, Dunn DW. Diagnosis and management of depression and psychosis in children and adolescents with epilepsy. *J Child Neurol* 2004; 19 (Suppl. 1): S65-72.
- Lewinsohn PM, Pettit JW, Joiner TE Jr., Seeley JR. The symptomatic expression of major depressive disorder in adolescents and young adults. *J Abnormal Psychology* 2003; 112: 244-52.
- Li Y, Ji C, Qin J, Zhang Z. Parental anxiety and quality of life of epileptic children. *Biomed Environ Sci* 2008; 21: 228-32.
- Luby JL, Mrakotsky C, Heffelfinger A, Brown K, Spitznagel E. Characteristics of depressed preschoolers with and without anhedonia: evidence for a melancholic depressive subtype in young children. *Am J Psychiatry* 2004; 161: 1998-2004.
- March J, Silva S, Petrycki S, et al. Fluoxetine, cognitive behavioral therapy, and their combinations for adolescents with depression: Treatment for Adolescents with Depression Study (TADS) randomized control trial. *JAMA* 2004; 292: 807-20.
- Martinović Z, Simonović P, Djokić R. Preventing depression in adolescents with epilepsy. *Epilepsy Behav* 2006; 9: 619-24.
- McNelis A, Musick B, Austin J, Dunn D, Creasy. Psychosocial care needs of children with new-onset seizures. *J Neurosci Nurs* 1998; 30: 161-8.
- Mula M, Sander JW. Negative effects of antiepileptic drugs on mood in patients with epilepsy. *Drug Safety* 2007; 30: 555-67.
- Oğuz A, Kurul S, Dirik E. Relationship of epilepsy-related factors to anxiety and depression in children with epilepsy. *J Child Neurol* 2002; 17: 37-40.
- Peter T, Roberts LW, Buzdugan R. Suicidal ideation among Canadian youth: A multivariate analysis. *Arch Suicide Res* 2008; 12: 263-75.
- Pilowsky DJ, Wickramaratne P, Talati A, et al. Children of depressed mothers 1 year after the initiation of maternal treatment: findings from the STAR*D-Child study. *Am J Psychiatry* 2008; 165: 1136-11.
- Plioplys S. Depression in children and adolescents with epilepsy. *Epilepsy Behav* 2003; 4: S39-S45.
- Reilly C, Agnew R, Neville BGR. Depression and anxiety in childhood epilepsy: a review. *Seizure* 2011; 20: 589-97.
- Renaud J, Brent DA, Baugher M, Birmaher B, Kolko DJ, Bridge J. Rapid response to psychosocial treatment for adolescent depression: a two-year follow-up. *J Am Acad Child Adolesc Psychiatry* 1998; 37: 1184-90.
- Rodenburg R, Stams GJ, Meijer AM, Aldenkamp AP, Dekovi? M. Psychopathology in children with epilepsy: a meta-analysis. *J Ped Psychol* 2005a; 30: 453-68.

- Rodenburg R, Meijer AM, Dekovi? M, Aldenkamp AP. Family factors and psychopathology in children with epilepsy: a literature review. *Epilepsy Behav* 2005b; 6: 488-503.
- Rodenburg R, Marie Meijer A, Dekovi? M, Aldenkamp AP. Family predictors of psychopathology in children with epilepsy. *Epilepsia* 2006; 47: 601-14.
- Roeder R, Roeer K, Asano E, Chugani HT. Depression and mental health help-seeking behaviors in a predominantly African American population of children and adolescents with epilepsy. *Epilepsia* 2009; 50: 1943-52.
- Russ SA, Larson K, Halfon N. A national profile of childhood epilepsy and seizure disorder. *Pediatrics* 2012; 129: 256-64.
- Turky A, Beavis JM, Thapar AK, Kerr MP. Psychopathology in children and adolescents with epilepsy: an investigation of predictive variables. *Epilepsy Behav* 2008; 12: 136-144.
- Vega C, Guo J, Killory B, *et al*. Symptoms of anxiety and depression in childhood absence epilepsy. *Epilepsia* 2011; 52: e70-e74.
- Wagner KD. Pharmacotherapy for major depression in children and adolescents. *Prog Neuropsychopharmacol Biol Psychiatry* 2005; 29: 819-26 (10E).
- Weintraub D, Buchsbaum R, Resor SR, Hirsch LJ. Psychiatric and behavioral side effects of the newer antiepileptic drugs in adults with epilepsy. *Epilepsy Behav* 2007; 10: 105-10.
- Wood LJ, Sherman EM, Hamiwka LD, Blackman MA, Wirrell EC. Maternal depression: the cost of caring for a child with intractable epilepsy. *Pediatr Neurol* 2008; 39: 418-22.
- Yong L, Chengye J, Jiong Q. Factors affecting the quality of life in childhood epilepsy in China. *Acta Neurol Scand* 2006; 113: 167-73.

Health perception and socio-economic status of childhood onset epilepsy

Ada T. Geerts

Department of Neurology, Erasmus MC, Rotterdam, The Netherlands

---

After a diagnosis of epilepsy, the main focus lies on medical aspects such as etiology, seizure frequency, treatment, and prognosis. When seizures start during childhood, additional aspects become important, as epilepsy and its etiology may have consequences for cognitive, psychosocial and emotional development, education, and later employment. Moreover, epilepsy may negatively influence social functioning, self-esteem, and quality of life. On top of this, patients with epilepsy often have comorbidities which they have to deal with.

These topics were part of the Dutch study of epilepsy in childhood (DSEC). In this hospital based, prospective cohort study, consecutive children with epilepsy (age: 1 month-16 years) were followed since diagnosis for a mean duration of 15 years.

This chapter will discuss several of these aspects by a review of the results of both this study and other studies, with a special focus on patients with uncomplicated epilepsy.

■ Comorbidities

Patients with epilepsy are frequently burdened with comorbidities, which can have an additional effect on quality of life and psychosocial functioning. The mechanisms of association between these comorbidities and epilepsy sometimes are causal (like epilepsy following stroke) or resultant (like osteoporosis as a result of medication). However, some of these comorbidities beside epilepsy, such as migraine, cognitive impairment, behavioral or psychiatric disorders, might be a reflection of the same brain disorder (Jensen, 2011; Rogawski, 2012).

A recently published study shows the magnitude of comorbidities in adults. In this study, which was a large nationally representative household survey of 5,692 US adults, patients with epilepsy were significantly more likely to have at least one additional physical disorder than people without epilepsy (93.6% vs. 77.8%; $P < 0.001$; odds ratio 4.2), after controlling for age, sex and race (Kessler et al., 2012). These included any digestive disorder, migraine, headache and pain, respiratory disorder, or sensory disorder. In addition, the

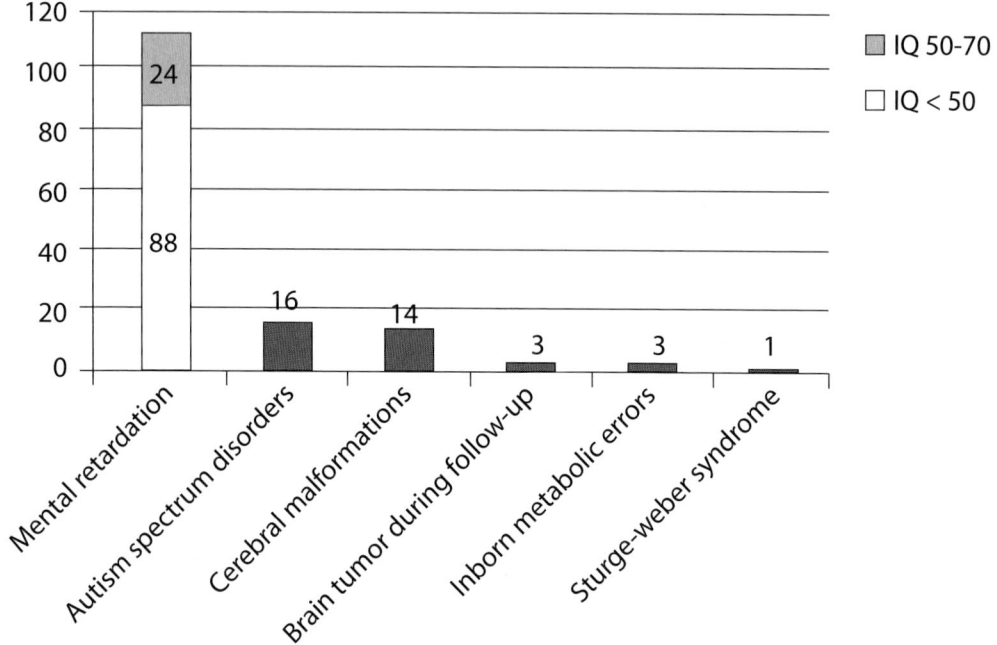

Figure 1. Brain-related comorbidities reported in the Dutch study of epilepsy in childhood.

lifetime DSM-IV/CIDI mental disorders were significantly more frequent in patients with epilepsy (67.9 vs. 47.0%, P = 0.011), particularly behavioral disorders, panic and post-traumatic stress disorders, and drug abuse.

Several other studies focused on comorbidities in childhood-onset epilepsy. One of these was the Finnish study of Jalava and Sillanpää (1996). After 35 years of follow-up a comparison was made between patients with epilepsy and two matched control groups. Somatic comorbidities were found in 89% of 220 patients versus 67% of 99 random controls (p < 0.05). Half of the patient group was mentally retarded. Somatic diseases with the exception of oral diseases were not significantly increased among patients with "epilepsy only" as compared with random or employee controls. No differences were found in migraine or headache frequencies. Psychiatric disorders, sleeplessness and a combination of psychiatric and either somatic or psychosomatic disorders were significantly more frequent in patients with "epilepsy only" than in both control groups. Patients still receiving AEDs had no more psychiatric or psychosomatic disorders than those whose medication had been discontinued.

In the well-known Connecticut study comprising 613 children with epilepsy, the effect of epilepsy and comorbidities on quality of life was assessed in a subset of children younger than 18 years old with a follow-up of 8-9 years (Baca et al., 2011). Of these children 39% had neurodevelopmental spectrum disorders (mainly developmental or language delay), 26% had psychiatric disorders (mainly ADHD), 15% suffered from migraine, and 24% reported chronic medical conditions (mainly asthma). They concluded that psychiatric comorbidities are strongly associated with quality of life in childhood-onset epilepsy, and suggest that comprehensive epilepsy care must include screening and treatment for these conditions, even if patients are in remission.

Another study on comorbidities was recently completed in Tanzania (Burton et al., 2012). They found that 85% of 112 children with epilepsy aged 6-14 years had comorbidities, with more than half of them reporting more than one, whereas only 27% of age-matched controls had these. Comorbidities consisted of cognitive impairment (64%), behavior disorder (61%), motor difficulties (26%), burns and other previous injuries (26%).

In contrast to the studies mentioned above, fewer patients in the Dutch study reported comorbidities, perhaps because a checklist was used, but despite this, half of the cohort reported one or more neurological brain-related morbidities or other impairments and disabilities (Geerts et al., 2011). In this study, 27% of the 413 subjects were mentally retarded. *Figures 1 and 2* show all reported comorbidities. With the exception of mental retardation, all mentioned problems are without doubt underreported.

Considering the above studies, it is clear that patients with childhood-onset epilepsy more often have comorbidities than subjects without epilepsy. The most frequently mentioned comorbidities are cognitive impairments, psychiatric and behavioral disorders.

■ Health perception

The health status of patients can be measured using objective criteria such as i.e. disease severity, amount of pain, disabilities as a result of a disease, but also by using subjective criteria. The best subjective measurement is probably quality of life, but also health status perception is an important health care outcome. In patients with epilepsy the health perception might be worse compared with patients having other chronic diseases, as epilepsy is probably more often associated with social stigma. The question is do patients with uncomplicated epilepsy or those in remission have a subjective health status that is comparable with that of healthy persons.

Figure 2. Other impairments and disabilities reported in the Dutch study of epilepsy in childhood.

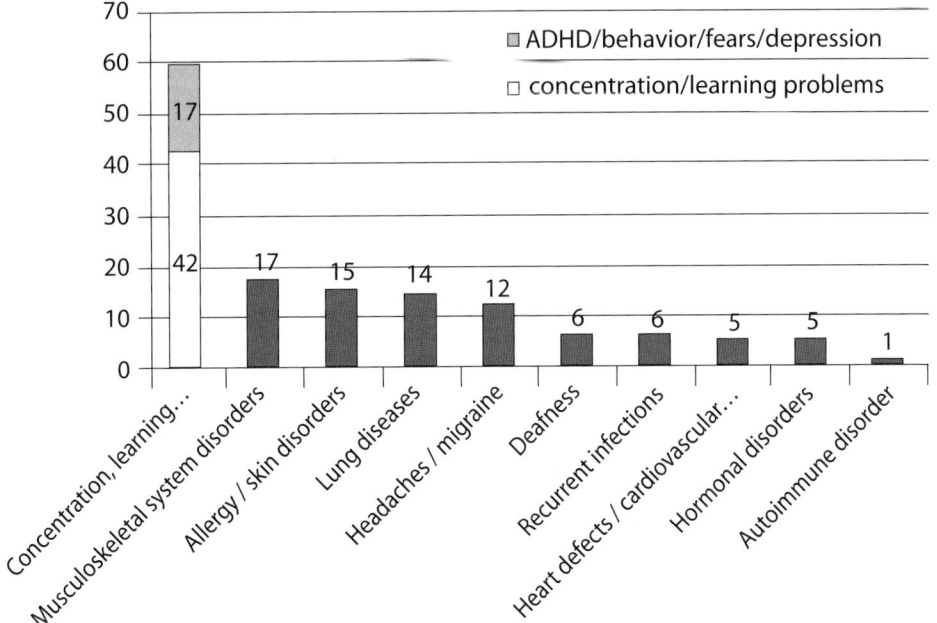

In the Dutch study of epilepsy in childhood, the health perception of normally intelligent patients with epilepsy was assessed and compared with that of age peers of the Dutch population. The age-adjusted standardized incidence rates (*Table I*) showed that subjects without remission had a worse health perception than respondents of the CBS Health Inquiry. Within this group, those without remission and still using antiepileptic drugs (AEDs) reported a worse health perception than those off AEDs [26.7% *vs.* 6.7%, 95% confidence interval (CI) of difference: 1.9-38.1, p < 0.05). Furthermore, fewer subjects with cryptogenic or symptomatic etiology reported a 'very good' health perception, whereas those with an idiopathic etiology or in remission showed no difference with their age peers (Geerts et al., 2011).

In a birth cohort population-based study, childhood epilepsy was associated with poor general health at 33 years on univariate analyses, but not after adjusting for childhood cognitive development or comorbidities and anxiety over acceptance by peers or adults at age 11 (Chin et al., 2011).

Koponen *et al.* showed that most of the patients with "epilepsy only" (79%) and almost all in the control group (87%) assessed their general health as good or very good. The difference was not significant (Koponen et al., 2007).

In a Finnish study, patients with childhood-onset epilepsy perceived their health status to be comparable with that of controls, irrespective of physical inactivity, continued seizures, or AED monotherapy. However, patients receiving AED polytherapy perceived their health as rather poor or very poor significantly more often than did controls (OR, 5.1; 95% CI, 1.2-21.3). In addition unmarried patients felt more often that their general health was "fairly poor" or "quite poor" (OR, 6.8; 95% CI, 1.3-36.5) compared with married patients with epilepsy (Jalava & Sillanpaa, 1997b; Jalava et al., 1997).

Beside the possible reasons of a poor health perception mentioned above, i.e. active epilepsy, ongoing use of medication (specifically polytherapy), and being unmarried, other factors may be detrimental for health perception. In 2007 a study in Portugal was performed in 200 patients with epilepsy with the aim to identify variables related to health status perception and quality of life (QOL) (Pais-Ribeiro et al., 2007). The mean age of the patients was 40 years, 99% were currently using AEDs and 95% had seizures in the last year. According to this study, optimism was the variable that best contributed to the mental health status perception and QOL, whereas seizure frequency did not.

Table I. Subjective health perception of 283 subjects (excluding those with an IQ < 70 and 18 subjects who gave no answer) compared with the respondents (excluding institutionalized subjects) of the Dutch Health Inquiry in the year 2005

Age-adjusted standardized incidence rates with 95% confidence interval (# p < 0.1, * p < 0.05)			
	Very good	Good	Less than good
Idiopathic (n = 184)	1.09 (0.83-1.41)	0.95 (0.78-1.15)	1.03 (0.63-1.59)
Cryptogenic/Symptomatic (n = 99)	0.66 (0.40-1.02)#	1.14 (0.89-1.45)	1.16 (0.60-2.02)
Remission (n = 223)	0.98 (0.76-1.25)	1.04 (0.88-1.23)	0.81 (0.49-1.27)
No remission (n = 60)	0.80 (0.44-1.34)	0.92 (0.63-1.29)	2.03 (1.08-3.46)*

Considering the results of these studies, most patients with epilepsy and normal intelligence and no additional neurological impairments have a good health perception. Having active epilepsy, ongoing use of medication or other epilepsy-related factors are probably strong predictors of a poor health perception.

■ Marriage or cohabitation

Children with epilepsy often grow into adults with significant social problems including decreased marriage rates, fewer social relationships, and living arrangements that differ from healthy persons. Learning disorders and mental handicap are the most consistent predictors of these social problems (Camfield & Camfield, 2007).

Several studies following patients with epilepsy focused on marriage rates, but not all of them presented these rates for each etiological group separately (Kokkonen et al., 1997; Shackleton et al., 2003; Novy et al., 2012). This is considered less informative as differences between these groups are to be expected. However, several cohort studies concentrated on uncomplicated epilepsy or epilepsy combined with normal intelligence.

In the Finnish study for example, 100 subjects with uncomplicated childhood-onset epilepsy were matched for sex, age, and place of birth with 99 random controls (Jalava & Sillanpaa, 1997a). At the mean age of 36 years, 60% of the patients were married *versus* 83% of the matched controls ($p < 0.0001$). This lower rate of marriage was not associated with age at onset, etiology, type of epilepsy, active epilepsy, ongoing treatment, educational level or present life satisfaction. However, patients aged 20-25 years were more often single in case they had persistent seizures compared with those in remission ($p = 0.0006$). In a later publication, the investigators showed that a lower marriage rate was also found for patients being in remission, even for those off medication (Sillanpaa et al., 2004).

Further, in the United Kingdom, a comparison was made between a subgroup of children with epilepsy (onset < age 16 years) from the 1958 National Child Development Study (birth cohort study of 17,414 children) with unaffected cohort members on outcomes at age 33 (Chin et al., 2011). Of the 101 patients with epilepsy, 69% had been married. Having had childhood epilepsy was an independent risk factor for not being married (OR 0.50, 95% CI 0.38-0.95). People with symptomatic epilepsy were 62% less likely (OR 0.38, 95% CI 0.13-0.86) to be married at age 33, whereas those with idiopathic epilepsy were 44% less likely to be married (OR 0.56, 95% CI 0.18-0.95) as compared with people who did not have childhood epilepsy. There was no statistical difference between the etiology groups in the likelihood of being married (21 of 32 symptomatic subjects *versus* 24 of 33 idiopathic subjects).

One other study on childhood-onset epilepsy found an overall lower rate of marriage for patients with epilepsy for 3 of the 4 age groups. But for 99 selected patients of normal intelligence only the younger age group had a significantly lower marriage rate, probably due to a relatively high rate of students in that age group (Wakamoto et al., 2000).

In the Dutch study of epilepsy in childhood, subjects with idiopathic or cryptogenic etiology did not differ regarding marriage or cohabitation from the Dutch population. The symptomatic group, however, had a significantly lower age-adjusted standardized incidence rate for living with a partner (0.39, 95% CI: 0.18-0.75, $p < 0.01$). On the other hand, patients with active epilepsy did not have a lower marriage rate than their healthy age peers (age-adjusted standardized incidence rate: 0.92; 95% CI: 0.69-1.21, ns). This was also demonstrated in a Japanese study that investigated the marital status of 278 adult patients (20-60 years) with epilepsy without mental retardation and who had been treated for > 5 years in one hospital. Only 30% of the men and 22% of the women had controlled seizures at the time of marriage (Wada et al., 2004).

In conclusion, most studies show a lower rate of marriage or cohabitation for subjects with childhood-onset epilepsy, even for those with idiopathic etiology or uncomplicated epilepsy. The most plausible reasons for lower marriage rates in subjects with a normal intelligence are social stigma, psychosocial functioning, and self-esteem. Possible reasons for the discrepancy of the Dutch study with the other mentioned studies might be the difference in study design (birth cohort *versus* hospital based studies, comparison with matched controls *versus* age peers of the general population). One other explanation might be that the majority of the Dutch cohort was still too young to get married or live together with a partner. In the Netherlands the average age to get married is more than 30 years (CBS, 2013). In that case, further follow-up might show a drop in marriage rates compared with the Dutch population once the majority of these patients reach the age of getting married or cohabiting. However, lower marriage rates for certain age groups do not always imply that these patients will remain unmarried, as they might get married at an older age.

■ Offspring

Several studies showed that patients with epilepsy less often have children (Dansky et al., 1980; Schupf & Ottman, 1996; Shackleton et al., 2003; Artama et al., 2004). This is partly due to lower marriage rates, comorbidities, AED-related reduced fertility, and more complications during pregnancy (*i.e.*, still births and spontaneous abortions) or socioeconomic factors (Artama et al., 2004; Tsuji, 2004). Beside this, some women voluntarily decide not to have children because of their epilepsy.

Most studies concentrate on all patients with epilepsy, irrespective of age of onset. In addition, these studies often do not focus on those patients with idiopathic etiology, uncomplicated epilepsy or those in remission. These groups are of special interest, as their lives are probably more or less comparable with those without illness. Only a few studies focused on the reproductive activity within childhood-onset epilepsy cohorts. In two cohorts, subjects with childhood-onset epilepsy had fewer children than expected (Sillanpaa et al., 2004; Chin et al., 2011). In the first cohort in which patients with uncomplicated epilepsy were compared with age, sex and place of birth matched controls, this was irrespective of being in remission or not (Sillanpaa et al., 2004). In the British childhood-onset epilepsy study (Chin et al., 2011), subjects with symptomatic etiology were less likely to be parents by age 33 years (OR 0.52, $p < 0.001$), but also those with idiopathic etiology (OR 0.75, $p < 0.004$). This was independent of cognition scores, attainment of A level/ higher education, and being employed by age 33 years. There was no statistical difference between etiology groups in the likelihood of being a parent (17/33 idiopathic, 17/32 symptomatic).

In contrast to these two studies, the Dutch study showed different results, as none of the group with symptomatic etiology had children, but the idiopathic and cryptogenic groups were similar to the general population. Although these results look interesting, again these divergent outcomes might result from the fact that the Dutch cohort was relatively young and that a comparison was made with the general population, which is probably less accurate.

While in the Dutch study none of the patients with symptomatic etiology had children, this group did have offspring in the study of Chin et al. A possible explanation might be that the severity of symptomatic epilepsy could be different between patients, leading to divergent rates in marriage and having offspring within the group of remote symptomatic etiology. In the Dutch study, 56% of the remote symptomatic group had a severe (IQ < 50) and 17% had a mild mental retardation (IQ = 50-70). However, these data were not available for the British study (Chin et al., 2011).

As only these three studies were available for studying the reproductive activity of patients with childhood-onset epilepsy, another study might be of interest. In 2011, respondents of the National Longitudinal Study of Adolescent Health from the US with or without childhood-onset cancer, heart disease, diabetes, or epilepsy were compared with young adults without these chronic illnesses in terms of marriage, having children and other outcomes (Maslow et al., 2011). Of the patients with onset before the age of 18 years (n = 295), 44% had epilepsy. Compared to those without chronic illness (n = 13.136), respondents with childhood-onset chronic illness had similar odds of marriage (OR = 0.89, 95% CI: 0.65-1.24), and having children (OR = 0.99, 95% CI: 0.70-1.42).

Considering the results of these studies on childhood-onset epilepsy, no firm conclusion can be drawn other than a lower birth rate in those having a remote symptomatic etiology. More long-term follow-up studies of cohorts with childhood-onset epilepsy are needed to investigate if patients with idiopathic etiology or uncomplicated epilepsy are reluctant or constrained in having children.

■ Education

Children with chronic illnesses are at risk of lower educational attainment, and central nervous system disease may put individuals at even greater risk (Lancashire et al., 2010; Maslow et al., 2011). Several studies focused on the cognitive and educational outcomes of children with epilepsy (Wakamoto et al., 2000; Zelnik et al., 2001; Vinayan et al., 2005; Sogawa et al., 2010).

In the Dutch study of epilepsy in childhood the educational achievement was studied in two ways. First, the present education of students was compared with that of age-matched peers of the Dutch population, including special education, excluding institutionalized subjects. More subjects with remote symptomatic etiology followed special education compared with Dutch students (42.5% vs. 1.3%, p < 0.01), and slightly fewer students with idiopathic etiology followed higher education (21% vs. 32%, p < 0.1). Lower educational levels were not a result of active epilepsy and/or ongoing treatment. This was demonstrated by the fait that significantly fewer subjects with idiopathic etiology having a 5-year terminal remission after a mean follow-up of 15 years at last contact studied at a university (Geerts, 2012).

In addition to the students' education, the highest educational attainment of employees and jobseekers was compared with age peers of the Dutch labor force. The age-adjusted standardized incidence rates for subjects with idiopathic etiology having attained higher education were significantly lower (0.44; 0.20-0.84, p < 0.01). This was also the case for all subjects in remission (0.42; 0.21-0.76, p < 0.01).

Many other studies on childhood-onset epilepsy reported a lower than average educational attainment for subjects with epilepsy (Kokkonen et al., 1997; Wakamoto et al., 2000; Sillanpaa et al., 2004; Koponen et al., 2007). Most of the latter studies also reported this trend for subjects with "epilepsy only", normal intelligence, and for those in remission and off AEDs.

In the study of Koponen et al. for example, 347 young adults with epilepsy with normal intelligence and no neurological disorders were compared with age- and gender-matched controls. More than 40% had their first seizure after 15 years of age. The highest level of education was significantly different between both groups (p = 0.027), with 40% of the epilepsy group having only a vocational school level *versus* 29% of the controls, and only 14.5% of the epilepsy group having a university level *versus* 21% of controls (Koponen et al., 2007).

In the birth cohort study of Chin et al., outcome at age 33 was investigated and patients with childhood-onset epilepsy were compared with those not having epilepsy. One third (31%) of the 65 patients with epilepsy attained the highest level of education. On univariate analysis, people with childhood epilepsy were less likely (OR 0.47, 95% CI 0.28-0.80) to have achieved A level/higher education qualification. However, on stratification, those with idiopathic epilepsy were just as likely to have attained A level/higher education (OR 0.6, 95% CI 0.3-1.2) but those with symptomatic epilepsy remained less likely (OR 0.35, 95% 0.2-0.8). On multivariate modeling, childhood epilepsy was not an independent risk factor for not attaining A level/higher education by age 33 years, whereas cognition scores (OR 1.06, 95% CI 1.06-1.07) and child anxiety about peer/adult acceptance at 11 years were risk factors (OR 0.60, 95% CI 0.49-0.71) (Chin et al., 2011).

With the exception of the latter study, the results of most studies strongly point to a lesser educational achievement for subjects with epilepsy having normal intelligence. There is increasing evidence that mild impairment of cognitive functions precedes the onset of epilepsy or is present at diagnosis, even in cases with "epilepsy only" (Schouten et al., 2001; Oostrom et al., 2003; Berg et al., 2005; Henkin et al., 2005; Vinayan et al., 2005; Beghi et al., 2006; Hermann et al., 2007; Taylor et al., 2010).

In the latter study (Taylor et al. 2010), a total of 155 untreated patients with newly diagnosed epilepsy, more than 15 years of age, and no known brain pathology, were assessed before the start of antiepileptic medication (min 0-max 13 days after of enrollment). Their scores across the neuropsychological measures were compared with 87 healthy age- and sex-matched controls from the general population. Patients with epilepsy performed significantly worse than did healthy volunteers on 6 of 14 cognitive measures, particularly in the domains of memory and psychomotor speed. Cognitive performance was not related to the number of seizures, type of epilepsy, or mood. When an impairment index was calculated, 53.5% patients had a least one abnormal score on the test battery compared with 20.7% of healthy controls This implies that childhood-onset epilepsy in neurologically intact children is not as innocent as it may seem and that there might be a shared cause for epilepsy and cognitive deficiencies. Special education services often preceded the onset of seizures (Berg et al., 2005), and progress at school may be worse before seizure onset, with more children repeating a school year (Schouten et al., 2001). This was also demonstrated in the study of Bailet & Turk, 2000, who found that children with idiopathic epilepsy and children with migraine more often received special education and repeated a grade compared with healthy siblings (special education: 19% of 74 children with epilepsy, 15% of the 13 children with migraine and 4% of the 23 controls; repeated a grade: 34%, 38%, and 13% respectively).

■ Employment status

Several studies reported on the employment rates of subjects with epilepsy, and some found that employment rates were not significantly lower for selected subjects with epilepsy (Kokkonen et al., 1997; Wakamoto et al., 2000; Geerts et al., 2011; Marinas et al., 2011).

In Finland, 81 non-institutionalized patients with epilepsy born between 1964 and 1967 at an average age of 22.3 years were compared to 211 controls drawn at random from a population cohort born in the same period (Kokkonen et al., 1997). No separation was made between subjects with normal intelligence and those who were retarded. Both in the patient group and in the control group more than 60% were part of the labor force. Within this group, 78% of the patients had a job *versus* 86% of the control group, but unemployment was almost twice as high in the patient group even though this difference was not significant *(Table II)*. The most remarkable finding was that significantly fewer patients had a permanent job.

In a Japanese population-based childhood-onset epilepsy study, employment rate for 99 subjects with normal intelligence was 95.2%. If the 49 subjects with mental retardation were included the rate was 67.4%. The employment status between the patients of normal intelligence and the general population did not differ (p = 0.47). Despite this positive finding and the fact that 76.4% of the employed patients were in remission, the authors emphasize the impact of epilepsy on employment. Thirteen employed patients (15.6%) had to change their jobs or had been denied employment due to their illness, even though eight of the 13 patients had no mental retardation. The latter issue demonstrates that comparing achievements – in this case employment status – of patients with epilepsy ± remission does not always show the factual situation and that the burden of epilepsy is not always immediately evident.

In the Dutch study of epilepsy in childhood, the employment status (defined as having a job for at least 12 hours per week) of subjects with idiopathic or cryptogenic etiology did not differ from that of the general population, but significantly fewer subjects with symptomatic etiology were employed *(Table III)*. In addition, patients without remission were less often employed, although this was not significant (Geerts et al., 2011).

Table II. Present employed status of young adults with epilepsy in childhood and in controls (Kokkonen *et al.*, 1997)

	Patients (n = 81)	Controls (n = 211)
On disability pension	10 (12%)	4 (2%)
Students	20 (25%)	70 (33%)
Labor force	51 (63%)	137 (65%)
Permanently	18 [35.3%]	71 [51.8%]
Temporarily	22 [43.1%]	47 [34.3%]
Unemployed	8 [15.7%]	11 [8.0%]
Other	3 [5.9%]	8 [5.8%]

$\chi^2 = 14.7$; P < 0.001.

Table III. Employment status of 352 subjects compared with the age peers of the Dutch population, excluding institutionalized subjects (Geerts et al., 2011)

Age-adjusted standardized incidence rates with 95% confidence interval (# $p < 0.1$, * $p < 0.05$, ** $p < 0.01$)			
	Employed	Unemployed	Dependent
Idiopathic (n = 183)	0.95 (0.76-1.18)	0.80 (0.35-1.58)	1.08 (0.87-1.33)
Cryptogenic (n = 68)	1.03 (0.71-1.44)	0.27 (0.01-1.50)	1.06 (0.73-1.48)
Symptomatic (n = 101)	0.46 (0.29-0.70)**	0.36 (0.04-1.30)	1.57 (1.24-1.96)**
Remission (n = 261)	0.88 (0.72-1.06)	0.56 (0.24-1.11)	1.18 (0.99-1.39)#
No remission (n = 91)	0.71 (0.48-1.01)#	0.60 (0.12-1.76)	1.34 (1.02-1.74)*

Dependent: This includes students, housewives, and persons who are ill or disabled

The study by Marinas et al. 2011 is of adults, but is mentioned here as it clearly demonstrates the importance of epilepsy severity variables and indicate that the severity of epilepsy is related to employment and unemployment status, even though the overall (un)employment rates did not differ between the study group and the population. In this cross-sectional multicenter epidemiological Spanish study, 872 consecutive adults with epilepsy were included. Mean age at onset of epilepsy was 18.9 years; patients were included if their diagnosis was made at least one year ago and if they were able to cooperate. A total of 58% were employed, 11% unemployed, 13% were incapable of working, and 18% were students or housewives. These data were similar to those recorded in the general population (employed = 59% and unemployed = 10%). However, among the patients in remission in the preceding year, 64.2% were employed compared with 55.7% of the patients without remission in the past year (p = 0.02). Patients with non-refractory epilepsy had higher employment and lower unemployment rates than those with refractory epilepsy (employment rate = 64.4% vs. 44.7%, unemployment rate = 8.6% vs. 16.8%). Among patients on monotherapy, 65.8% were employed *versus* 50.7% of those on polytherapy (p = 0.000,0).

In contrast to the studies above, some reported a lower employment rate for patients with uncomplicated childhood-onset epilepsy. According to Jalava et al. (1997), about two thirds of patients with epilepsy and 90% of random controls were employed full-time and Koponen et al.(2007) showed that the rate of employment was significantly lower only for those with comprehensive school but not for those with matriculation examination.

After having discussed the employment rates above, the unemployment rates need to be documented as well. In the Dutch study unemployment was defined as having no job or working 12 h/week, but willing to work for at least 12 h/week, being available and actively looking for work. As shown in *table III*, the unemployment rates were low in the Dutch study, even for those with symptomatic etiology (Geerts et al., 2011). In contrast, Sillanpää et al. (1998) showed that 20% of 66 patients with uncomplicated epilepsy who were in remission and without medication were not employed *versus* 8% of 99 matched controls (RR = 2.36, p < 0.03), but for those with idiopathic epilepsy in remission without medication (n = 42) no difference was found (7% vs. 8%, RR = 0.86, p = 0.81). However, six years later they found that the risk of being not employed in subjects in remission off medication was not significantly higher any more than that in controls (5% vs. 2%, RR = 2.2, p = 0.35), but in those still taking medication, the risk was high and was the same whether or not the subjects were in remission (Sillanpaa et al., 2004).

In addition, two other studies focused on unemployment rates for subjects with epilepsy. Kokkonen found an unemployment rate twice as high for the non-institutionalized patients, but this group also included patients with a remote symptomatic etiology (Kokkonen et al., 1997). Koponen et al. showed that the unemployment rate among young adults aged 22-25 years with "epilepsy only" was twice as high (23%) as in the control group (11%, $p < 0.001$). Importantly, those with seizures in the last year were significantly more likely to be unemployed than those having a 1-year remission (27% vs. 19%) ($p = 0.044$).

The contradictory results in employment and unemployment rates described above could be due to the small sample sizes, or to differences in control groups and definitions used. For example, in some studies no clear definition was given for "being unemployed". This could include students, housewives, jobseekers, and disabled persons, or it could include only the jobseekers, which would better illustrate the social stigma of colleagues and attitude of employers towards epilepsy.

■ Occupation

Most studies report only on the employment status, but almost none focused on the level of occupation, although this is an important issue too. Only one study investigated the distribution of occupations among patients with "epilepsy only" and two matched control groups (Jalava & Sillanpaa, 1996), but no relevant differences were found. The study of Wakamoto et al. reported the occupational levels but did not compare these with a control group (Wakamoto et al., 2000).

Table IV. Occupational level of 138 employees in the Dutch cohort compared with that of age peers of Dutch employees (Geerts et al., 2011)

Age-adjusted standardized incidence rates with 95% confidence interval (# $p < 0.1$, * $p < 0.05$)				
	Elementary	Lower	Intermediate	Higher/scientific
Idiopathic (n = 86)	0.52 (0.17-1.22)	1.26 (0.88-1.74)	1.16 (0.81-1.60)	0.56 (0.26-1.07)#
Cryptogenic (n = 32)	0.00	0.62 (0.25-1.28)	1.52 (0.90-2.41)	1.19 (0.48-2.45)
Symptomatic (n = 20)	3.00 (1.21-6.19)*	0.86 (0.31-1.86)	0.92 (0.37-1.90)	0.00
Remission (n = 108)	0.85 (0.41-1.56)	1.09 (0.78-1.49)	1.16 (0.85-1.55)	0.62 (0.33-1.06)#
No remission (n = 30)	0.52 (0.06-1.89)	0.89 (0.43-1.64)	1.39 (0.78-2.29)	0.62 (0.13-1.81)

Elementary: jobs with simple duties. *Lower*: jobs with duties at the level of preliminary vocational education. *Intermediate*: jobs with duties at the level of intermediate vocational education. *Higher/scientific*: jobs with duties at the level of higher vocational or scientific education.

In the Dutch study, the occupational level of all jobs of the patients with epilepsy was classified according to the International Standard Classification of Occupations (ISCO-88) (ISCO, 2010). A total of 138 patients had a job. The occupational level of all patients was compared with that of Dutch age peers (Table IV). Slightly fewer employees with idiopathic etiology had an occupation that was based on higher vocational or scientific education. This was also found for all subjects being in remission. None with symptomatic etiology had a job based on higher education: most of them had an elementary job with simple duties.

Another important issue is underemployment. In one study, subjects with "epilepsy only" were significantly more often underemployed compared with controls (Jalava et al., 1997). Underemployment was defined as having a level of education and training that was significantly higher than required for the present job. Of their patients, 23% were underemployed *versus* 9% of random controls, and 14% of employee controls.

In the Dutch cohort, 26% of employees had a job one or two levels beneath their educational level, which is comparable with the results of Javala *et al*. Comparison of the cohort with the Dutch age peers on this point was not possible as these data were not available for the Dutch population.

Concluding remarks

In this chapter aspects other than those related to seizures and medication were discussed. Not many cohort studies on childhood-onset epilepsy did focus on these points, and those that were available have limitations. The most important ones include: small sample sizes, not separating groups on the basis of etiology or intelligence, the choice of control groups, and differences in definitions being used. This makes comparison between studies difficult.

However, despite this, we can draw some firm conclusions. First of all it is clear that patients with childhood-onset epilepsy are frequently burdened with comorbidities, which can have an additional effect on quality of life and psychosocial functioning. Most of these comorbidities are related to cognition, and behavioral or psychiatric disorders. Some of them are reversible when they are the direct consequence of seizures, interictal epileptic discharges or medication. However, most of them seem to be permanent, many of them preceding the onset of seizures. The question is whether these comorbidities and epilepsy reflect the same underlying brain disorder (Jensen, 2011; Rogawski, 2012). If this is true, understanding the shared cause might create new opportunities for drug development.

Second, the subjective health perception of subjects with childhood-onset epilepsy and normal intelligence is not fundamentally worse than that of controls. Considering the results of the available studies on this topic, having either active epilepsy and requiring the ongoing use of medication or other epilepsy-related factors seem to be strong predictors of a poor health perception.

Further, most studies show a lower rate of marriage or cohabitation for subjects with childhood-onset epilepsy, even for those with idiopathic etiology or uncomplicated epilepsy. Even though not all studies agree on this point, it is possible that social stigma, lower self-esteem, vulnerability and other psychosocial aspects are contributors for patients with epilepsy and normal intelligence not to be able to find a partner. It is well possible that active epilepsy might not be a strong contributor.

Regarding reproductive activity and offspring, more research is needed as only three cohort studies reported on this topic. In two cohorts with childhood-onset epilepsy, subjects with uncomplicated or idiopathic epilepsy had fewer children than expected, whereas in the Dutch study subjects with idiopathic and cryptogenic etiology were comparable with their age peers.

The results of most studies strongly point to a lesser educational achievement for subjects with epilepsy having a normal intelligence. This might be the consequence of mild cognitive impairments, present before the onset of epilepsy or acquired due to seizure or AED usage. However, it is possible that for some patients "having epilepsy" was the reason for following education at a slower pace, or at a lower level, even though their cognitive abilities were not impaired. It is even possible that subjects with epilepsy may be less ambitious in life because of the associated stigma and are reserved to a certain extent by their fear of new seizures. More research is needed to confirm whether cognitive impairments or any of the above mentioned variables are possible explanations for lower educational achievement. As also previously mentioned, there is increasing evidence that mild impairment of cognitive functions likely precedes the onset of epilepsy or is present at diagnosis, even in cases with "epilepsy only".

Regarding employment rates, no clear cut conclusion can be drawn as studies do not show similar results. However, it seems that subjects with idiopathic etiology or those with uncomplicated epilepsy might do better than other subjects. As already said before, the employment status itself might not be a good measure, as some patients had to change jobs more often for various reasons and fewer subjects with epilepsy might have fulltime jobs, which is not reflected in the employment status. Nevertheless, more information is needed to clarify employment and unemployment status in patients with epilepsy having normal intelligence, preferably in large prospectively followed cohorts with matched controls. The definition of unemployment should be clear and clinical variables indicating the severity of epilepsy should be considered.

In the Dutch study, slightly fewer employees with idiopathic etiology and employees in remission had an occupation that was based on higher vocational or scientific education. This could be a result of a lower educational achievement or of underemployment. Unfortunately, hardly any other studies concentrated on occupational achievement or underemployment. The latter item would be a good measure to demonstrate the burden of epilepsy, as subjects with epilepsy sometimes choose to or have to work at a lower level as they were supposed to, based on their level of education. We recommend these concepts to be addressed in future cohort studies.

Overall, we conclude that childhood-onset epilepsy has a substantial impact on many aspects of life, especially for those with symptomatic etiology or with active epilepsy using AEDs. For those with idiopathic etiology, the impact is less severe, but still significant with regard to educational and occupational achievement. The disturbing finding that this group might have mild impairment of cognitive functions preceding the onset of epilepsy should be examined in more detail.

References

- Artama M, Isojarvi JI, Raitanen J, Auvinen A. Birth rate among patients with epilepsy: a nationwide population-based cohort study in Finland. *Am J Epidemiol* 2004; 159: 1057-63.
- Baca CB, Vickrey BG, Caplan R, Vassar SD, Berg AT. Psychiatric and medical comorbidity and quality of life outcomes in childhood-onset epilepsy. *Pediatrics* 2011; 128: e1532-43.
- Bailet LL, Turk WR. The impact of childhood epilepsy on neurocognitive and behavioral performance: a prospective longitudinal study. *Epilepsia* 2000; 41: 426-31.

- Beghi M, Beghi E, Cornaggia CM, Gobbi G. Idiopathic generalized epilepsies of adolescence. *Epilepsia* 2006; 47 (Suppl 2): 107-10.
- Berg AT, Smith SN, Frobish D, Levy SR, Testa FM, Beckerman B, Shinnar S. Special education needs of children with newly diagnosed epilepsy. *Dev Med Child Neurol* 2005; 47: 749-53.
- Burton K, Rogathe J, Whittaker RG, et al. Co-morbidity of epilepsy in Tanzanian children: a community-based case-control study. *Seizure* 2012: 21: 169-74.
- Camfield CS, Camfield PR. Long-term social outcomes for children with epilepsy. *Epilepsia* 2007; 48 (Suppl 9): 3-5.
- Cbs Statistics Netherlands. 2013. Available: http://statline.cbs.nl/StatWeb/publication/?DM=SLNL&PA=37772ned&D1=a&D2=54&HDR=G1&STB=T&VW=T.
- Chin RF, Cumberland PM, Pujar SS, Peckham C, Ross EM, Scott RC. Outcomes of childhood epilepsy at age 33 years: A population-based birth-cohort study. *Epilepsia* 2011; 52: 1513-21.
- Dansky LV, Andermann E, Andermann F. Marriage and fertility in epileptic patients. *Epilepsia* 1980; 21: 261-71.
- Geerts A, Brouwer O, Van Donselaar C, et al. Health perception and socioeconomic status following childhood-onset epilepsy: the Dutch study of epilepsy in childhood. *Epilepsia* 2011; 52: 2192-202.
- Geerts A. *Course and Long-Term Outcome of Childhood-Onset Epilepsy. Dutch study of epilepsy in childhood.* PhD, Erasmus MC, 2012.
- Henkin Y, Sadeh M, Kivity S, Shabtai E, Kishon-Rabin L, Gadoth N. Cognitive function in idiopathic generalized epilepsy of childhood. *Dev Med Child Neurol* 2005; 47: 126-32.
- Hermann B, Jones J, Dabbs K, et al. The frequency, complications and aetiology of ADHD in new onset paediatric epilepsy. *Brain* 2007; 130: 3135-48.
- Isco The International Standard Classification of Occupations. 2010. Available: http://www.ilo.org/public/english/bureau/stat/isco/index.htm.
- Jalava M, Sillanpaa M. Concurrent illnesses in adults with childhood-onset epilepsy: a population-based 35-year follow-up study. *Epilepsia* 1996; 37: 1155-63.
- Jalava M, Sillanpaa M. Reproductive activity and offspring health of young adults with childhood-onset epilepsy: a controlled study. *Epilepsia* 1997a; 38: 532-40.
- Jalava M, Sillanpaa M. Physical activity, health-related fitness, and health experience in adults with childhood-onset epilepsy: a controlled study. *Epilepsia* 1997b; 38: 424-9.
- Jalava M, Sillanpaa M, Camfield C, Camfield P. Social adjustment and competence 35 years after onset of childhood epilepsy: a prospective controlled study. *Epilepsia* 1997; 38: 708-15.
- Jensen FE. Epilepsy as a spectrum disorder: Implications from novel clinical and basic neuroscience. *Epilepsia* 2011; 52 (Suppl 1): 1-6.
- Kessler RC, Lane MC, Shahly V, Stang PE. Accounting for comorbidity in assessing the burden of epilepsy among US adults: results from the National Comorbidity Survey Replication (NCS-R). *Molecular psychiatry* 2012; 17: 748-58.
- Kokkonen J, Kokkonen ER, Saukkonen AL, Pennanen P. Psychosocial outcome of young adults with epilepsy in childhood. *J Neurol Neurosurg Psychiatry* 1997; 62: 265-8.
- Koponen A, Seppala U, Eriksson K, et al. Social functioning and psychological well-being of 347 young adults with epilepsy only-population-based, controlled study from Finland. *Epilepsia* 2007; 48: 907-12.
- Lancashire ER, Frobisher C, Reulen RC, Winter DL, Glaser A, Hawkins MM. Educational attainment among adult survivors of childhood cancer in Great Britain: a population-based cohort study. *Journal of the National Cancer Institute* 2010; 102: 254-70.
- Marinas A, Elices E, Gil-Nagel A, et al. Socio-occupational and employment profile of patients with epilepsy. *Epilepsy Behav* 2011; 21: 223-7.

- Maslow GR, Haydon A, Mcree AL, Ford CA, Halpern CT. Growing up with a chronic illness: social success, educational/vocational distress. *J Adolescent Health* 2011; 49: 206-12.
- Novy J, Castelao E, Preisig M, Vidal PM, Waeber G, Vollenweider P, Rossetti AO. Psychiatric co-morbidities and cardiovascular risk factors in people with lifetime history of epilepsy of an urban community. *Clin Neurol Neurosurg* 2012; 114: 26-30.
- Olafsson E, Hauser WA, Gudmundsson G. Fertility in patients with epilepsy: a population-based study. *Neurology* 1998; 51: 71-3.
- Oostrom KJ, Smeets-Schouten A, Kruitwagen CL, Peters AC, Jennekens-Schinkel A. Not only a matter of epilepsy: early problems of cognition and behavior in children with "epilepsy only" – a prospective, longitudinale, controlled study starting at diagnosis. *Pediatrics* 2003; 112: 1338-44.
- Pais-Ribeiro J, Da Silva AM, Meneses RF, Falco C. Relationship between optimism, disease variables, and health perception and quality of life in individuals with epilepsy. *Epilepsy Behav* 2007; 11: 33-8.
- Rogawski M. Migraine and Epilepsy†Shared Mechanisms within the Family of Episodic Disorders. In: Noebels Jl, AM, Rogawski Ma, Olsen Rw, Delgado-Escueta Av (eds). *Source Jasper's Basic Mechanisms of the Epilepsies [Internet].* Bethesda (MD): National Center for Biotechnology Information (US), 2012.
- Schouten A, Oostrom K, Jennekens-Schinkel A, Peters AC. School career of children is at risk before diagnosis of epilepsy only. *Dev Med Child Neurol* 2001; 43: 575-6.
- Schupf N, Ottman R. Reproduction among individuals with idiopathic/cryptogenic epilepsy: risk factors for reduced fertility in marriage. *Epilepsia* 1996; 37: 833-40.
- Shackleton DP, Kasteleijn-Nolst Trenite DG, De Craen AJ, Vandenbroucke JP, Westendorp RG. Living with epilepsy: long-term prognosis and psychosocial outcomes. *Neurology* 2003; 61: 64-70.
- Sillanpaa M, Jalava M, Kaleva O, Shinnar S. Long-term prognosis of seizures with onset in childhood. *N Engl J Med* 1998; 338: 1715-22.
- Sillanpaa M, Haataja L, Shinnar S. Perceived impact of childhood-onset epilepsy on quality of life as an adult. *Epilepsia* 2004; 45: 971-7.
- Sogawa Y, Masur D, O'dell C, Moshe SL, Shinnar S. Cognitive outcomes in children who present with a first unprovoked seizure. *Epilepsia* 2010; 51: 2432-9.
- Taylor J, Kolamunnage-Dona R, Marson AG, Smith PE, Aldenkamp AP, Baker GA. Patients with epilepsy: cognitively compromised before the start of antiepileptic drug treatment? *Epilepsia* 2010; 51: 48-56.
- Tsuji S. [Social aspects of epilepsy: marriage, pregnancy, driving, antiepileptic drug withdrawal and against social stigma]. *Rinsho Shinkeigaku* 2004; 44: 865-7.
- Vinayan KP, Biji V, Thomas SV. Educational problems with underlying neuropsychological impairment are common in children with Benign Epilepsy of Childhood with Centrotemporal Spikes (BECTS). *Seizure* 2005; 14: 207-12.
- Wada K, Iwasa H, Okada M, *et al.* Marital status of patients with epilepsy with special reference to the influence of epileptic seizures on the patient's married life. *Epilepsia* 2004; 45 (Suppl 8): 33-6.
- Wakamoto H, Nagao H, Hayashi M, Morimoto T. Long-term medical, educational, and social prognoses of childhood-onset epilepsy: a population-based study in a rural district of Japan. *Brain Dev* 2000; 22: 246-55.
- Zelnik N, Sa'adi L, Silman-Stolar Z, Goikhman I. Seizure control and educational outcome in childhood-onset epilepsy. *J Child Neurol* 2001; 16: 820-4.

What if quality of life better expressed outcomes for epilepsy?

Kathy Nixon Speechley

Departments of Paediatrics and Epidemiology & Biostatistics, Western University, London, Ontario, Canada

The International League Against Epilepsy (ILAE) Commission on Epidemiology contends that health-related quality of life can "be regarded as the broadest and most important outcome of any chronic health condition" (Thurman et al., 2011). For years, there has been widespread agreement that the overall goal for the management of childhood epilepsies is optimizing quality of life. Efforts have broadened from a focus on minimizing seizures to include efforts to also minimize associated sequelae, both medical and psychosocial (Jones, 1998; Schachter, 2000). Despite the relatively good long-term prognosis for seizure control (Shinnar & Pellock, 2002), many children with epilepsy still experience problems in multiple areas of functioning, including behavioural adjustment, social competence, academic achievement, and family life that extend into adolescence and adulthood (Camfield & Camfield, 2010; Sillanpaa et al.,1998). Acknowledging these potential psychosocial sequelae of epilepsy means that controlling seizures remains an essential, core component of the management of epilepsy but cannot be considered sufficient to declare successful management of epilepsy has been achieved. This chapter discusses the outcome of quality of life in childhood epilepsies and how consideration of quality of life adds to our knowledge about the prognosis for children with epilepsy (CWE).

■ Definitions

The World Health Organization (WHO) defines quality of life as "individuals' perception of their position in life in the context of the culture and value systems in which they live and in relation to their goals, expectations, standards and concerns. It is a broad ranging concept affected in a complex way by the person's physical health, psychological state, level of independence, social relationships, personal beliefs and their relationship to salient features of their environment" (WHOQOL, 1997).

Health-related quality of life (HRQL) is the aspect of quality of life that is particularly relevant to the delivery of health care. It refers to the impact, both subjective and objective, of dysfunction associated with illness or injury, medical treatment, and health care policy. Most descriptions of HRQL refer to four core domains of quality of life: disease state and physical symptoms, functional status, psychological functioning, and social functioning (Spieth & Harris, 1996). A key element of the definition of HRQL is that it incorporates *subjective* as well as objective components of the impact that a health condition and/or its management has on an individual. It is a patient's subjective assessment of the various aspects of current life that is more difficult to empirically quantify and likely more relevant within the context of delivering health care (Cummins, 2005).

The Patient-Centered Outcomes Research Institute's (PCORI) standards for patient-centered outcomes research articulates that patient outcomes selected for assessment must be those that resonate with patients and caregivers as being important, citing HRQL as one of the examples of such outcomes (PCORI, 2012). Within the context of health regulatory agency approval processes, HRQL is accepted as a specific type of patient-reported outcome (PRO) characterized by multidimensionality, such that claims of improvement in HRQL must be supported by evidence of significant change in the majority of relevant domains (U.S. Department of Health and Human Services, 2006; EMEA, 2005).

■ Research related to the outcome of HRQL

A large body of literature related to the outcome of HRQL in childhood epilepsies now exists. The studies can be characterized as falling into two categories: 1) those that focus on individual domains of HRQL such as psychological or social functioning; and 2) those that conduct multidimensional assessments of HRQL.

Studies in the first category collect patient – or parent – reported information to describe the prevalence of a particular aspect of HRQL (*e.g.*, behavior problems, social competence). They use validated, multi-item scales or a series of single questions designed to assess current status using dichotomous response options. The latter type of dichotomous classification is most often used in long-term follow-up of patients into adulthood to assess conventional indicators of success in adulthood, such as current employment status measured as employed *vs.* unemployed. These indicators are often used in conjunction with an assessment of the extent to which patients are satisfied with particular aspects of their lives (*e.g.*, employment, relationships, overall state of life) using Likert scales.

Studies in the second category aim for comprehensive assessments of HRQL using one of two main types of validated multidimensional measures: disease-specific, designed specifically for CWE to accurately capture aspects of HRQL that may be unique to epilepsy, or generic, to ensure all aspects of HRQL relevant to children are covered and to allow comparisons with children living with other conditions and those from the general population. There are now several validated scales available in both the categories of disease-specific and generic from which to choose. As part of the Common Data Elements Project developed by the National Institute of Neurological Disorders and Stroke (NINDS) (Loring *et al.*, 2011), a comprehensive review of these measures was conducted offering recommendations regarding measures to employ (NIH, NINDS, 2012).

The decision to include in this discussion, not only those studies where a validated measure of HRQL was employed, but also those that assessed a particular aspect of HRQL is based on the argument that the latter type of work has contributed considerably to developing our current level of understanding of HRQL and has a role to play in determining the next phase of clinical and research priorities. What follows is not intended to offer a comprehensive review of the literature reporting on HRQL in CWE. Instead, a few examples have been drawn from the two categories of investigation to illustrate the themes that have emerged out of the findings to date.

Assessments of specific domains of HRQL

The majority of empirical investigations in CWE have targeted individual aspects or domains of HRQL such as psychological well-being, behavior, and social competence. Among these studies, there are many examples of how epilepsy can negatively impact daily lives. For example, CWE have poorer social skills and are less assertive than their siblings (Tse et al., 2007). They have a higher prevalence of problems in the area of social competency (defined as impaired academic performance, peer relationships and participation in activities) compared to population norms (Connolly et al., 2006; Räty et al., 2003). Epilepsy can have a negative impact on academic achievement (Austin & Dunn, 2000). There is also substantial evidence that CWE have an elevated prevalence of behavioural and emotional problems (Freilinger et al., 2006; Plioplys et al., 2007). It is noteworthy that CWE are not only more likely to experience mild cognitive problems, problems in executive function and psychosocial problems than healthy controls but they also more likely to experience 2 or 3 of these problems simultaneously, as observed in a sample of CWE without severe non-verbal cognitive problems (Hoie et al., 2008). Children with epilepsy can feel stigmatized by their disorder, regardless of whether they have actually experienced discrimination (Jacoby & Austin, 2007).

Several studies have sought to identify significant correlates of individual domains of HRQL. Epilepsy-related factors such as intractability, number and types of AED therapy, medication neurotoxicity, seizure severity, etiology, age at onset, and having a learning disability have been found to be related to social outcomes (e.g., Tse et al., 2007; Freilinger et al., 2006; Devinsky, 1999). Others have found that some epilepsy factors such as seizure frequency were not related to psychosocial outcome in children (Wirrell et al., 1997). The few studies that considered family factors, offered preliminary indication that characteristics of the family environment warranted attention as significant correlates as well (Tse et al., 2007).

A few notable long-term follow-up studies have also reported on specific domains of HRQL in adulthood among those with childhood-onset epilepsy. The population-based incidence cohort of almost 700 children in Nova Scotia was followed for as long as 25-30 years. Subjects had experienced two or more unprovoked seizures with onset from one month to 16 years of age and between the years of 1977 and 1985 (Camfield et al., 1993). Subjects reported in semi-structured interviews on outcomes including school success, employment, family and romantic relationships, friendships, social activities, financial success, substance abuse, pregnancies, and interventions for mental illness. Subjects also rated their satisfaction with their current health, overall state of life, employment, friendships and social activities.

A common theme in the findings is the large proportion classified as having at least one marker of poor social outcome such as: failure to complete high school, unplanned pregnancy, depression, unemployment, living alone, or not having had a romantic relationship longer than three months. For example, 74% of those with juvenile myoclonic epilepsy had at least one major negative social outcome 25 years later (Camfield & Camfield, 2009), as did 76% of those with idiopathic generalized epilepsy with generalized tonic-clonic seizures (IGE-GTC) at 20 years (Camfield & Camfield, 2010). The results for the small group with IGE-GTC offer evidence that poor social outcomes in adulthood are also observed in some children diagnosed with relatively benign epilepsy, in that 77% had learning difficulties during high school, 40% did not complete high school, 33% were unemployed, and 27% had a psychiatric diagnosis (Camfield & Camfield, 2010). The 20-year social outcomes for patients who developed symptomatic generalized epilepsy indicated that 29% had a "moderate" outcome defined as unable to live independently but independent for most daily activities, and 58% experienced a "poor" outcome defined as dependent for nearly all activities (Camfield & Camfield, 2008).

In Finland, a population-based cohort of 245 subjects with two or more unprovoked seizures identified through hospital records and the National Health Service records registry in 1964, was enrolled in a longitudinal study of outcomes in 1972 (Sillanpaa et al., 1998). In 1992, age- and sex-matched control subjects were chosen and in 1997 measures of social function were administered using a mailed survey returned by 91 subjects with uncomplicated epilepsy and 90 controls. Among those with epilepsy, 67% were in remission off medication, 14% were in remission on medications, and 19% were not in remission. The key findings from this > 30-year follow-up were continued long-term repercussions on several outcomes conventionally viewed as societal indicators of success in adulthood (education, employment, marriage, driver's license) even among those who were seizure free and off medication. Those not in remission or in remission but still on treatment had the worst outcomes. Remaining on medication, regardless of whether one is in remission, had a major negative impact on long-term outcome (Sillanpaa et al., 2004).

Another long-term study assessed all patients with a diagnosis of epilepsy before age 16 years between 1961 and 1992 treated at a hospital in a rural region of Japan who were at least 20 years old. Patients were followed-up in 1998 using medical chart review and telephone interviews with parents (Wakamoto et al., 2000). Results for 155 patients indicated that medical prognosis was favourable for the majority in terms of seizure remission and few psychiatric complications, but similar to other long-term study results, the sample was disadvantaged compared to the general population on educational achievements, rates of employment, marriage, and driver's licenses. Contrary to other studies' results, patients of normal intelligence did not appear to differ from the general population on social and educational outcomes.

There has also been a recent report of health and social outcomes in adulthood based on the National Child Development Study (NCDS), a national birth cohort study of over 17,000 children, 98% of those born in one week in Britain in 1958 (Chin et al., 2011). Sixty-five of 101 persons identified as part of the NCDS as having onset of epilepsy before age 16 were surveyed at age 33 to compare their results with all other NCDS cohort members without epilepsy. Those with childhood epilepsy had poorer outcomes on general and mental health, were less likely to have "A level" or higher education or be employed, and less likely to be married or be parents, based on univariable analyses. However, using multivariable modeling, childhood epilepsy was not an independent risk factor for health, education or employment outcomes. It was poor cognitive development, having comorbidities and not feeling accepted by peers when assessed at age 11 that predicted poor outcomes at age 33. Those with normal to high cognitive scores had outcomes similar to the general population.

Summary

To date, the majority of studies of individual domains of HRQL in CWE have been cross-sectional studies based on prevalence samples. A few prospective investigations have reported long-term outcomes by following population-based cohorts for many years into adulthood. Taken together, this body of research has added substantially to our knowledge regarding the impact that living with epilepsy has on the daily lives of children and their families. We have learned that, as a group, CWE experience substantial deficits in multiple domains of HRQL. These deficits are not explained solely by the clinical characteristics of epilepsy – even those with "benign" epilepsy and those who obtain good seizure control in childhood can experience significant psychosocial, academic, and vocational disadvantage in adulthood. Family characteristics may play a role in social outcomes. There are inconsistencies across studies in the associations between epilepsy-related factors and social outcomes. Some negative impacts of epilepsy and its treatment persist into adulthood.

There are limitations associated with these studies. They do not capture the element of multidimensionality that is viewed as the hallmark of HRQL in that they focus on individual domains, which offer an important but incomplete picture of the impact of dysfunction associated with epilepsy and its treatment. Variability in the measurement of outcomes and the types of patient groups studied make it difficult at times to compare across studies. Finally, it cannot be assumed that the reported prevalence of the various so-called "poor social outcomes", or the "good social outcomes" for that matter, reflects patients' and families' subjective assessment of the impact epilepsy has on them. There are some notable discrepancies when one compares the evaluation of a patient population's quality of life based on conventional markers of positive social functioning to the same group's self-report on satisfaction with these aspects of their lives. Finally, these studies provide limited insights into the pathways that led patients to good *versus* poor outcomes.

■ Multidimensional assessments

Studies offering a comprehensive, multidimensional assessment of HRQL associated with childhood epilepsy have mostly described outcomes for particular sub-samples of children and youth with epilepsy studied cross-sectionally. One example is a study of children with intractable/refractory epilepsy that found compromised HRQL regardless of level of intellectual ability, but that those who were intellectually normal did score higher on several subscales of HRQL (Sabaz, 2001). Other studies have focused on those at a particular stage of development such as adolescence. For example, Stevanovic (2007) found HRQL among adolescents who had active, uncomplicated epilepsy for more than five years, which was well-controlled, was generally good to satisfactory but that there was great variation among subjects.

There have also been cross-sectional investigations comparing HRQL in CWE to healthy children and those with other chronic health conditions. HRQL in CWE is compromised compared to aged-matched healthy children (Miller *et al.*, 2003). One longitudinal study that compared HRQL in CWE to normative data from a general population sample found that CWE had worse HRQL both after diagnosis and two years later, and that the difference was smaller at the two-year follow-up (Speechley *et al.*, 2012). CWE also have worse HRQL than children with asthma on the psychological, social domains with only the physical domain not being significantly different (Austin *et al.*, 1994). Children's HRQL also appears to be more impacted by epilepsy than by diabetes (Hoare *et al.*, 2000).

Recently, two prospective studies have reported on HRQL in children with newly-diagnosed epilepsy employing validated multidimensional measures. One assessed HRQL in 124 children 2-12 years of age recruited from a new-onset seizure clinic in the United States over a 7 month period (Modi et al., 2011). HRQL was assessed using the Pediatric Quality of Life Inventory (PedsQL), a generic parent-report measure. HRQL was constant over time, except that emotional functioning showed a positive trend. Type and side-effects of AEDs and seizure frequency predicted HRQL over time. The authors suggest that the results speak to the value of proactively communicating to families about the possible effects of AEDs to present the opportunity for parents to anticipate and participate in shared decision making around treatment. On a related note, the authors advocate for the investigation of family environment in future work.

The other study, the Health-Related Quality of Life in Children with Epilepsy Study (HERQULES) followed 374 children in Canada aged 4-12 years newly diagnosed with epilepsy for 24 months (Speechley et al., 2012). HRQL was measured post-diagnosis and 6, 12, and 24 months later using parent reports on an epilepsy-specific measure, Quality of Life in Children with Epilepsy Questionnaire (QOLCE) and a generic measure, Child Health Questionnaire-Parent Form, (CHQ-PF50). On average, HRQL was relatively good but individual trajectories showed considerable variability. Scores on subscales were generally lowest at post-diagnosis and highest at 24 months. Improvement in HRQL was most rapid during the first 6 months after diagnosis and then stabilized. About half the children experienced either no clinically important improvement or a clinically important decline over the 2 years following diagnosis. Significant predictors at diagnosis for good HRQL two years later, controlling for baseline HRQL, were: absence of cognitive problems in children, better family functioning and fewer family demands. There was a qualitative interaction between baseline HRQL and cognitive problems, offering some indication that cognitive problems may be the driving force in the cases where HRQL declines over the 2 years.

Summary

These studies employing validated measures of HRQL offer the advantage of being able to capture a comprehensive overview of this outcome by simultaneously collecting information on all core domains of HRQL. The overall conclusion that emerges, similar to that from the studies that focused on individual domains, is that CWE experience diminished HRQL relative to their peers from the general population and to children with other chronic conditions.

The majority of these studies are based on relatively small samples, including few covariates, often focusing entirely on epilepsy-related factors and not incorporating the potential effects of other child and family characteristics. The variability in the clinical characteristics of epilepsy included as potential risk factors for HRQL is confusing to interpret. With only a few exceptions, studies have been cross-sectional, thus providing only a "snap-shot" of outcomes at one point in time. The two recent reports of incidence cohorts being followed prospectively present the opportunity to assess the course of HRQL across time and evaluate true risk factors for HRQL, rather than just correlates. It will be important to maintain cohorts such as these to continue to lengthen the follow-up period beyond two years past diagnosis. The fact that the longest follow-up to date from diagnosis found changes in levels of HRQL over the two-year period, as well as considerable variability in individual trajectories, points to the importance of extending the observation period.

The identification of risk factors other than epilepsy-related factors, such as family factors, has potential implications for epilepsy management strategies, if these initial findings are replicated.

■ Where we are and the road ahead

It is clear that despite relatively good prognosis for seizure control, many children with epilepsy still experience compromised HRQL. It is also the case that some children achieve good HRQL, at times in the face of rather poor clinical prognosis. It has become evident that level of HRQL cannot be fully explained by epilepsy-related factors alone. Often there is considerable variability in HRQL across patients, and over time that may not be captured by reporting "average" levels. There are initial indications that there may be several different individual trajectories of HRQL determined by a complex interplay of epilepsy factors, child characteristics, family environment and health care system factors. In addition, HRQL is likely dynamic over time.

Research on HRQL for CWE has been dominated by reports of "average", "static" outcomes, however, with a predominant focus on epilepsy-related predictors. Our focus needs to shift to more effectively describing variation across the population of CWE in terms of who does better, who stays the same, and who gets worse over time. As well, we need to broaden our search beyond epilepsy-related factors to identify the relative importance of several risk and protective factors, some of which will likely be child characteristics in addition to epilepsy-related factors, family environment and health care system factors, and to investigate potential significant interactions among these factors to produce their effect on HRQL.

Another key issue requiring attention relates to the methods used to practically interpret HRQL scores obtained by CWE. Specifically, we need to know how large the changes observed in HRQL scores must be to be viewed as meaningful. Minimal clinically important difference (MCID) refers to "the smallest difference in a score of a domain of interest that patients perceive as beneficial and that would mandate, in the absence of troublesome side effects and excessive costs, a change in the patient's management" (Jaeschke et al., 1989). MCID is important not only to patients and their families, but also to clinicians for use as a threshold by which to recommend a therapy to their patients, and to regulatory agencies to evaluate the effectiveness of treatments.

The research methods required to meet the challenges on the road ahead should utilize prospective investigation of large population-based incidence samples and multivariate, multilevel models of analysis. Such models should be built on a conceptual framework that incorporates the role of factors on three levels: child (including characteristics beyond those directly epilepsy-related), family, and interactions with the health care system, each supported by empirical evidence. An integrative approach is essential in the investigation of HRQL to ensure that both the *patient's subjective assessment* as well as the *multidimensionality of the model*, the mainstay of this key patient-reported outcome, is evaluated.

References

- Austin J, Dunn D. Children with epilepsy: quality of life and psychosocial needs. *Ann Rev Nurs Res* 2000; 18: 26-47.
- Austin J, Smith M, Risinger M, McNelis A. Childhood epilepsy and asthma: comparison of quality of life. *Epilepsia* 1994; 35: 608-15.
- Camfield C, Camfield P. Juvenile myoclonic epilepsy 25 years after seizure onset: A population-based study. *Neurology* 2009; 73: 1041-5.
- Camfield C, Camfield P, Gordon K, Smith B, Dooley J. Outcome of childhood epilepsy: a population-based study with a simple predictive scoring system for those treated with medication. *J Pediatr* 1993; 122: 861-8.
- Camfield P, Camfield C. Idiopathic generalized epilepsy with generalized tonic-clonic seizures (IGE-GTC): a population-based cohort with >20 year follow up for medical and social outcome. *Epilepsy Behav* 2010; 18: 61-3.
- Camfield P, Camfield C. Twenty years after childhood-onset symptomatic generalized epilepsy the social outcome is usually dependency or death: a population-based study. *Dev Med Child Neurol* 2008; 50: 859-63.
- Chin R, Cumberland P, Pujar S, Peckham C, Ross E, Scott R. Outcomes of childhood epilepsy at age 33 years: a population-based birth-cohort study. *Epilepsia* 2011; 52: 1513-21.
- Connolly A, Northcott E, Cairns D, et al. Quality of life of children with benign rolandic epilepsy. *Pediatr Neurol* 2006; 35: 240-5.
- Cummins RA. Moving from the quality of life concept to a theory. *J Intellect Disabil Res* 2005; 49: 699-706.
- Devinsky O, Westbrook L, Cramer J, Glassman M, Perrine K, Camfield, C. Risk factors for poor health-related quality of life in adolescents with epilepsy. *Epilepsia* 1999; 40: 1715-20.
- European Medicines Agency (EMEA), Committee for Medicinal Products for Human Use (CHMP). Reflection paper on the regulatory guidance for the use of health-related quality of life (HRQL) measures in the evaluation of medicinal products [online] 2005. Available from: http: //www.emea.europa.eu/pdfs/human/ewp/13939104en.pdf.
- Freilinger M, Reisel B, Reiter E, Zelenko M, Hauser E, Seidl R. Behavioral and emotional problems in children with epilepsy. *J Child Neurol* 2006; 21: 939-45.
- Hoare P, Mann H, Dunn S. Parental perception of the quality of life among children with epilepsy or diabetes with a new assessment questionnaire. *Qual Life Res* 2000; 9: 637-44.
- Hoie B, Sommerfelt K, Waaler P, Alsaker F, Skeidsvoll H, Mykletun A. The combined burden of cognitive, executive function, and psychosocial problems in children with epilepsy: a population-based study. *Dev Med Child Neurol* 2008; 50: 530-6.
- Jaeschke R, Singer J, Guyatt G. Measurement of health status: ascertaining the minimal clinically important difference. *Con Clin Trial* 1989; 10: 400-15.
- Jacoby A, Austin J. Social stigma for adults and children with epilepsy. *Epilepsia* 2007; 48 (Suppl 9): 6-9.
- Jones M. Consequences of epilepsy: why do we treat seizures? *Can J Neurol Sci* 1998; 25: S24-26.
- Loring DW, Lowenstein DH, Barbaro NM, et al. Common data elements in epilepsy research: Development and implementation of the NINDS epilepsy CDE project. *Epilepsia* 2011; 52: 1186-91.
- Miller V, Palermo T, Grewe S. Quality of life in pediatric epilepsy: demographic and disease-related predictors and comparison with healthy controls. *Epilepsy Behav* 2003; 4: 36-42.
- Modi A, Ingerski L, Rausch J, Glauser T. Treatment factors affecting longitudinal quality of life in new onset pediatric epilepsy. *J Pediatr Psychol* 2011; 36: 466-75.

- National Institute of Health, National Institute of Neurological Disorders and Stroke (NINDS). Common Data Elements: Quality of Life Scales Pediataric Measures, April 2012: http://www.commondataelements.ninds.nih.gov/epilepsy.aspx#tab=Data_Standards
- Patient-Centered Outcomes Research Institute (PCORI) Methodology Standards. Published December 14, 2012: http://www.pcori.org/research-we-support/methodology
- Plioplys S, Dunn D, Caplan R. 10-year research update review: psychiatric problems in children with epilepsy. J Am Acad Child Adolesc Psychiatry 2007; 46: 1389-402.
- Raty L, Wilde Larsson B, Soderfeldt B. Health-related quality of life in youth: a comparison between adolescents and young adults with uncomplicated epilepsy and healthy controls. J Adolesc Health 2003; 33(4): 252-8.
- Sabaz M, Cairns D, Lawson J, Bleasel A, Bye A. The health-related quality of life of children with refractory epilepsy: a comparison of those with and without intellectual disability. Epilepsia 2001; 42: 621-8.
- Sabaz M, Lawson JA, Cairns DR, et al. The impact of epilepsy surgery on quality of life in children. Neurology 2006; 66: 557-61.
- Schachter S. Epilepsy: quality of life and cost of care. Epilepsy Behav 2000; 1: 120-7.
- Shinnar S, Pellock J. Update on the epidemiology and prognosis of pediatric epilepsy. J Child Neurol 2002; 17 (Suppl 1): S4-17.
- Sillanpaa M, Haataja L, Shinnar S. Perceived impact of childhood-onset epilepsy on quality of life as an adult. Epilepsia 2004; 45: 971-7.
- Sillanpaa M, Jalava M, Kaleva O, Shinnar S. Long-term prognosis of seizures with onset in childhood. N Engl J Med 1998; 338: 1715-22.
- Speechley K, Ferro M, Camfield C, et al. Quality of life in children with new-onset epilepsy: a 2-year prospective cohort study. Neurology 2012; 79: 1548-55.
- Spieth L, Harris C. Assessment of health-related quality of life in children and adolescents: an integrative review. J Pediatr Psychol 1996; 21: 175-93.
- Stevanovic D. Health-related quality of life in adolescents with well-controlled epilepsy. Epilepsy Behav 2007; 10: 571-5.
- Thurman DJ, Beghi E, Begley CE, et al., for the ILAE Commission on Epidemiology standards for epidemiologic studies and surveillance of epilepsy. Epilepsia 2011: 52 (Suppl.7): 2-26.
- Tse E, Hamiwka L, Sherman E, Wirrell E. Social skills problems in children with epilepsy: prevalence, nature and predictors. Epilepsy Behav 2007; 11: 499-505.
- US Department of Health and Human Services FDA Center for Drug Evaluation and Research. Guidance for industry: patient-reported outcome measures: use in medical product development to support labeling claims: draft guidance. Health Qual Life Outcomes 2006; 4: 79.
- Wakamoto H, Nagaob H, Hayashia M, Morimotoc T. Long-term medical, educational, and social prognoses of childhood-onset epilepsy: a population-based study in a rural district of Japan. Brain Dev 2000 22: 246-55.
- WHOQOL – Measuring Quality Of Life, 1997. Available from: http://www.who.int/mental_health/media/68.pdf.
- Wirrell E, Camfield C, Camfield P, Dooley J, Gordon K, Smith B. Long-term psychological outcome in typical absence epilepsy. Arch Pediatr Adolesc Med 1997; 151: 152-8.

IMPRIM'VERT®

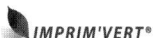

Achevé d'imprimer par Corlet, Imprimeur, S.A.
14110 Condé-sur-Noireau
N° d'Imprimeur : 154111 - Dépôt légal : mai 2013
Imprimé en France